PHLEBOTOMY

H A N D B O O K

PHLEBOTOMY
H A N D B O O K

Blood Collection Essentials

sixth edition

Diana Garza, EdD, MT(ASCP), CLS
Adjunct Associate Professor
Department of Laboratory Medicine
The University of Texas M.D. Anderson Cancer Center
Houston, Texas

Kathleen Becan-McBride, EdD, MT(ASCP)
Director, Community Outreach and Education
Coordinator, Texas-Mexico Border Health Services
Professor, UT-H Medical School, Dept. of Family Practice & Community Medicine
School of Public Health, School of Nursing
The University of Texas-Houston Health Science Center
Texas Medical Center, Houston, Texas
Assistant Director for Academic Partnerships, Greater Houston AHEC

Prentice
Hall

Upper Saddle River, New Jersey 07458

Library of Congress Cataloging-in-Publication Data

Garza, Diana.
    Phlebotomy handbook : blood collection essentials / Diana Garza, Kathleen
Becan-McBride.—6th ed.
      p. cm.
    Includes bibliographical references and index.
    ISBN 0-13-092887-9
    1. Phlebotomy—Handbooks, manuals, etc. I. Becan-McBride, Kathleen II. Title.
    [DNLM: 1. Phlebotomy—Handbooks. QY 39 G245p 2002]
RB45.15 .G37 2002
616.07'561—dc21   2001036276

Publisher: *Julie Levin Alexander*
Acquisitions Editor: *Mark Cohen*
Director of Production and Manufacturing: *Bruce Johnson*
Managing Production Editor: *Patrick Walsh*
Manufacturing Buyer: *Patrick Brown*
Production Liaison: *Julie Li*
Production Editor: *Amy Gehl, Carlisle Publishers Services*
Creative Director: *Cheryl Asherman*
Cover Design Coordinator: *Maria Guglielmo*
Cover Designer: *Joseph DePinho*
Editorial Assistant: *Melissa Kerian*
Composition: *Carlisle Production Services*
Printing and Binding: *R. R. Donnelley & Sons*

Notice: The authors and the publisher of this volume have taken care that the information and
technical recommendations contained herein are based on research and expert consultation,
and are accurate and compatible with the standards generally accepted at the time of
publication. Nevertheless, as new information becomes available, changes in clinical and
technical practices become necessary. The reader is advised to carefully consult
manufacturers' instructions and information material for all supplies and equipment before use,
and to consult with a healthcare professional as necessary. This advice is especially important
when using new supplies or equipment for clinical purposes. The authors and publisher
disclaim all responsibility for any liability, loss, injury, or damage incurred as a consequence,
directly or indirectly, of the use and application of any of the contents of this volume.

Pearson Education LTD.
Pearson Education Australia PTY, Limited
Pearson Education Singapore, Pte. Ltd
Pearson Education North Asia Ltd
Pearson Education Canada, Ltd.
Pearson Educación de Mexico, S.A. de C.V.
Pearson Education—Japan
Pearson Education Malaysia, Pte. Ltd
Pearson Education, Upper Saddle River, New Jersey

10 9 8 7 6 5 4 3 2 1
ISBN 0-13-092887-9

To my husband, Peter McLaughlin; my children, Lauren, Kaitlin, and Kevin; and my parents for their affection, patience, and constant support.

Diana Garza

To my husband, Mark; my sons, Patrick and Jonathan; my parents; my sister; and my parents-in-law for their support and devotion.

Kathleen Becan-McBride

Contents

IV. SPECIAL PROCEDURES AND POINT-OF-CARE TESTING / 303

V. QUALITY MANAGEMENT AND LEGAL ISSUES / 441

Preface

This book, *Phlebotomy Handbook: Blood Collection Essentials, Sixth Edition,* is designed for health care students and practitioners who are responsible for blood and specimen collections (i.e., nurses, phlebotomists, clinical laboratory technicians and technologists, respiratory therapists, and others). The primary goal of the book is to link the phlebotomist (blood collector) to the latest information, techniques, skills, and equipment for the provision of safe and effective collection procedures, for the improvement of diagnostic and therapeutic laboratory testing, for enhancement of customer satisfaction, and ultimately, for the promotion of better health outcomes. It provides a wide range of competencies, including communication, clinical, technical, and safety skills that any health care worker will use in the practice of phlebotomy and other specimen collection procedures. In addition, the book provides a background of general knowledge and insights to support the technical skills.

The book highlights trends in the health care industry that have forced greater efficiency, higher quality standards, safer devices and practices, and increased cost effectiveness. Also, methods of delivering health care services have continued shifting toward ambulatory care, client-based approaches to empowering patients and families with more information and education, decreasing stress and pain, improving customer service and communication skills, streamlining processes, cross-training clinical tasks, such as phlebotomy, and using shared decisions to meet an individual's needs. The role of the blood collector has expanded to encompass additional patient care duties and clinical responsibilities, a more patient-sensitive role, and improved interpersonal skills to deal effectively with patients, their families, and health care teams. Even the traditional title *phlebotomist* has changed in many facilities to *patient associate, patient care technician,* or *clinical assistant.* The practice of phlebotomy is presented in this industry context.

The order in which the material is presented generally follows the way in which a phlebotomist approaches the patient (i.e., beginning with important communication skills, a basic understanding of physiologic aspects, moving to safety considerations in preparation for the phlebotomy procedure, preparation of supplies and equipment, actual venipuncture or skin puncture, and potential complications). Specialty tests and, finally, a review of quality management and legal issues is presented toward the end. In addition, appendices are included that detail important terms, phrases, and symbols.

The content is divided into five major parts:

I. *Overview* provides a knowledge base of the roles and functions of a phlebotomist in the health care industry and the basics of anatomy and physiology with an emphasis on the circulatory system.

II. *Safety Procedures* provides information about safety and infection control in the workplace and the documentation and transportation procedures needed for safe handling of biohazardous specimens.

III. *Equipment and Procedures* provides the most updated information about blood collection equipment, provides a comprehensive description of the actual techniques used in phlebotomy, and reviews clinical and technical complications that may occur during the procedure.
IV. *Special Procedures and Point-of-Care Testing* provides information about pediatric phlebotomy procedures, arterial and IV collections, and special considerations for the elderly, homebound, and long-term care patients.
V. *Quality Management and Legal Issues* covers quality management issues for blood and specimen collection services and legal issues important to phlebotomy practice.

Key features of the *Phlebotomy Handbook: Blood Collection Essentials, Sixth Edition,* include the following:

- Latest information about the standards related to the Needlestick Prevention Act.
- Updated industry product information for blood collection safety devices.
- New color plates have been added including the veins, arteries, and heart.
- Expanded discussion of age-related competencies and transcultural communication.
- Expanded sections related to ethical issues.
- Performance Checklists have been added to specific chapters.
- Glossary of Terms.
- Clinical alert symbols indicate procedures or concepts that have vitally important clinical consequences for the patient. The clinical alert indicates that "extra caution" should be taken by the health care worker to comply with the procedure, thereby avoiding adverse outcomes for the patient.
- Procedural information is presented in comprehensive descriptions, using an "on the job" perspective.
- Exercises for improving communication skills are included to "get the feel" of being a patient and being an effective part of a health care team.
- Case studies are presented after each major section.
- Key terms, objectives, and study questions are provided for each chapter.
- A color chart indicating blood collection tubes, appropriate color codings, and additives.
- Appendices containing Spanish phrases, units of measurement and symbols, and formulas and calculations used in laboratories.
- Contrasting color tables and figures.
- Larger text format that makes it easy-to-read.

In summary, the authors have created a book that health care professionals and students will use as a central authority of information about blood collection practices. Instructors can also use this as the central body of information to teach specimen collection skills.

Phlebotomy Handbook, Sixth Edition, has companion resources that are cross-referenced to the text. Prentice Hall's *Q&A Review for Phlebotomy, Sixth Edition,* is an aid to students and health care workers preparing for a certification examination. It has an accompanying CD-ROM, a simulated board examination consisting of 100 multiple choice questions with referenced explanatory answers. Students can practice taking the simulated examination in print or via computer. A diagnostic report identifies those topics that need further review and study and provides the score for each content area. An *Instructor's Guide* is also available.

Acknowledgments

We are indebted to many individuals, product suppliers, manufacturing companies, and health care organizations for their assistance in preparing the previous editions of this textbook. The first edition was conceptualized in the early 1980s as the field of phlebotomy became more complex and teaching materials were scarce. As products, procedures, competencies, and safety measures expanded, so did our textbook. Each version has used the previous edition as a framework for redesigning, updating, and improving the next. We thank many phlebotomists, medical technicians, nurses, photographers, artists, and medical technologists who have given us countless editorial tips and practical approaches to the blood collection process over many years. We are grateful to all the health care workers, researchers, and safety advocates who took the time to seek new and better ways of providing services.

We are particularly grateful to BD VACUTAINER Systems *Preanalytical Solutions,* the College of American Pathologists, the American Society of Clinical Pathologists, The University of Texas M.D. Anderson Cancer Center, Texas Woman's University, and The University of Texas-Houston Health Science Center for their support. We thank Estella Woodard, MT(ASCP), and Peter McLaughlin, MD, for their assistance with the venipuncture photography through many editions of this textbook.

We also greatly appreciate our editors and copy editors, past and present, who have encouraged us and improved our writing through six editions. Special thanks go to Jane Licht, Cheryl Mehalik, Lin Marshall, and Mark Cohen.

We also would like to thank the following reviewers:

Timothy Guirl, MT(ASCP)
North Seattle Community College
Seattle, Washington

Roger W. Lamphere, MT(ASCP)
Rock Valley College
Rockford, Illinois

Rita Highland, MS, MT(ASCP)
Rock Valley College
Rockford, Illinois

Dr. C. Thomas Somma, MT(ASCP) SC
Chair and Associate Professor
School of Medical Laboratory Sciences
Old Dominion University
Norfolk, Virginia

And, last but not least, we are thankful for our families who have quietly and supportively tolerated the thousands of hours we have spent writing the previous and current editions of this textbook.

PHLEBOTOMY

HANDBOOK

OVERVIEW

THE PRACTICE OF PHLEBOTOMY, LIKE ANY other health professional skill, has certain characteristics that balance knowledge and theory with practical expertise. These characteristics include a recognizable definition or identity, a means of assigning tasks and responsibilities, and an established network for communication with other members of the health care team. These skills and responsibilities are now performed in a variety of health care settings, ranging from hospital intensive care units to an individual's home. Furthermore, phlebotomy practice is more widely performed by all types of health professionals, including nurses, respiratory therapists, clinical laboratory professionals, and others. Essential basic functions of the human body must also be well understood before technical skill and expertise can be acquired. Over the years, the practice of phlebotomy has developed these characteristics in sophisticated and elaborate ways. Part I, comprising the first three chapters of this book, defines phlebotomy practice in the current environment and creates a foundation of essential knowledge of the human body. In addition, the color atlas in Part I includes color illustrations pertaining to the anatomy and physiology that is particularly important during blood collection procedures.

Chapter 1, Phlebotomy Practice and Health Care Settings, describes a working framework for the phlebotomist (e.g., nurse, respiratory therapist, patient care technician, clinical assistant) in a health care environment that is rapidly changing. Emphasis is on roles and responsibilities, communication, and the vital link that the phlebotomist plays in providing quality health care services.

Chapter 2, Basic Anatomy and Physiology of Organ Systems, provides an overview of the structure and function of each body system. Particular emphasis is on identifying the anatomic regions of the body, the structural levels of the body, the role of homeostasis, and the relation of body functions to testing for diagnostic, therapeutic, and monitoring purposes.

Chapter 3, The Circulatory System, highlights the structures and functions of the circulatory system, and describes the specific role of the heart, vessels, and blood. Emphasis is on the arterial and venous system, blood flow and oxygen transport, identification of veins that are used for venipuncture, the cellular and noncellular components of blood, the phases of hemostasis, and blood pressure.

ONE

■

Phlebotomy Practice and Health Care Settings

CHAPTER OBJECTIVES

Upon completion of Chapter 1, the learner is responsible for the following:

1. Define phlebotomy practice and list the essential competencies for individuals performing phlebotomy/blood collection procedures.
2. Identify health care providers who generally perform phlebotomy procedures.
3. Identify the importance of phlebotomy procedures to the overall care of the patient.
4. List skills for active listening and effective verbal communication.
5. List examples of positive and negative body language.
6. Describe various health care settings, both inpatient and ambulatory, where phlebotomy services are routinely performed.
7. Describe the role of the clinical laboratory in blood collection and testing services.

■ THE GENERAL PRACTICE OF PHLEBOTOMY

The development of modern diagnostic techniques, clinical laboratory automation, computer technology, and changes in the delivery of health care services have increased the variety and number of laboratory testing options available for clinical decisions. As a result, various health care workers (e.g., phlebotomists, laboratorians, nurses, respiratory therapists, medical assistants, and others) are taking greater roles in phlebotomy and other specimen collection processes. Regardless of specific job backgrounds, however, there are common elements about the practice of phlebotomy that should be known by all who perform or are responsible for blood collections.

DEFINITION

The term *phlebotomy* is derived from the Greek words, *phlebo,* which relates to veins, and *tomy,* which relates to cutting. Therefore the definition can be summarized as the incision of a vein for blood letting (e.g., blood collection). Other synonomous, but less used, words are venesection or venisection.

The **phlebotomist** is the individual who practices phlebotomy or the "blood collector." The term *phlebotomist* will be used throughout this book even though it is interchangeable with *blood collector.* It is also important to keep in mind that phlebotomists often assist in the collection and transportation of specimens other than venous blood (e.g., arterial blood, urine, tissues, sputum). In addition, they may perform numerous other clinical, technical, or clerical functions in a health care facility.

According to the **American Society of Clinical Pathologists (ASCP),** "phlebotomy is more than just a skill, it is also an art." Furthermore, the ASCP suggests that phlebotomists have common characteristics. "They like challenge and responsibility. They are accurate, work well under pressure and communicate effectively. They set high standards for themselves and expect quality in the work they do. But, above all, they are deeply committed to quality health care delivery." A phlebotomy technician "collects blood specimens in a skillful, safe reliable manner."[1]

FUNCTION

Since the role of the phlebotomist has evolved according to specific work assignments and differing environments, individuals who practice phlebotomy may have many responsibilities in addition to blood collection. Regardless of what background the health care professional has, however, the primary function of the phlebotomist is to assist the health care team in the accurate, safe, and reliable collection and transportation of specimens for clinical laboratory analyses.

PURPOSE

Blood and other specimen collections are vitally important to the entire health assessment of patients. Laboratory analyses of a variety of specimens are used for three important purposes:

Diagnostic testing is used to figure out what is wrong with the patient.

Therapeutic assessments are used to develop the appropriate therapy or treatment of the medical condition.

Monitoring of a patient's health status is used to make sure the therapy or treatment is working to alleviate the medical condition.

If specimens are incorrectly acquired, labeled, or transported, laboratory tests are not useful and can even be harmful to patients.

■ PROFESSIONAL COMPETENCIES

Usually, the phlebotomist or blood collector must have a high school diploma or its equivalent to enter a phlebotomy training program. Training sessions may be conducted in a variety of settings, such as hospitals, community colleges, continuing education courses, and technical schools. Typically, the length of training varies from a few weeks to months, depending on the location and size of the facility, the complexity of patients being served, or both. Some employers require or recommend phlebotomy certification, which is accomplished by passing a national certification examination. Certification can provide advantages through job opportunities and increased chances for advancement.

There are professional organizations that recognize phlebotomists independently. All are sponsors of certification examinations for health care workers. (Refer to Box 1–1). Many of these organizations have developed **competency statements** to describe the entry-level skills, tasks, and roles performed by designated health care workers. Box 1–2 describes one organization's list of competencies for entry-level phlebotomy technicians.

In a work setting, at minimum, the phlebotomists' performance will be evaluated using these types of competencies. Additional measures of ability and performance might include the following:

- Compliance with all types of organizational policies
  - Dress Code
  - Infection Control
  - Fire and Safety

BOX 1–1. PROFESSIONAL ORGANIZATIONS FOR PHLEBOTOMISTS

Each of at least five organizations has board certification tests in phlebotomy. A reader intending to apply for one or more of the board examinations should determine which particular phlebotomy examinations are better known or accepted in the local community or state.

The American Society of Clinical Pathologists (ASCP)

ASCP
Board of Registry
P.O. Box 12277
Chicago, IL 60612-0277
(312) 738-1336 or 800-621-4142
www.ascp.org

ASCP allows nonphysician members to gain associate membership status. Through the ASCP Board of Registry, a Phlebotomy Technician Examination, PBT (ASCP), is offered quarterly. This is a criterion-referenced examination model. It covers the entry-level skills of a phlebotomist and uses taxonomy levels that assess recall (recognize facts), interpretive skills (use knowledge to interpret numeric data), and problem-solving skills (use applications of specific information to solve problems). Over 13,000 phlebotomists have been certified by ASCP since 1989, when the first phlebotomy examination was administered.

The National Phlebotomy Association (NPA)

NPA
1901 Brightseat Road
Landover, MD 20785
(301) 386-4200
www.scpt.com

NPA was established in 1978 to recognize the phlebotomist as a distinctive and identifiable part of the health care team. NPA offers annual certification examinations and results in a CPT (NPA).

The American Society for Clinical Laboratory Science (ASCLS) and The National Credentialing Agency for Laboratory, Inc. (NCA)

NCA	ASCLS
P.O. Box 15945-289	7910 Woodmont Ave., Suite 530
Lenexa, KS 66285	Bethesda, MD 20814
(913) 438-5110	(301) 657-2768
www.nca-info.org	www.ascls.org

ASCLS has recognized clinical laboratory personnel for more than 50 years. Several types of memberships are available, depending on the education and experience of the individual. Currently, phlebotomists join ASCLS as associate members as part of the Phlebotomy Section and take a certification examination through the NCA. The certification is a CLP16 (NCA).

American Medical Technologists (AMT)

AMT
710 Higgins Rd.
Park Ridge, IL 60068
(847) 823-5169
(800) 275-1268
www.amt1.com

BOX 1–1.   *(continued)*

American Society of Phlebotomy Technicians (ASPT)

ASPT
P.O. Box 1831
Hickory, NC 28603
(828) 294-0078
www.aspt.org

ASPT offers a certification examination that results in a CPT (ASPT) certification. One year of experience is required or, 6 months' experience with a letter from a supervisor documenting completion of a specified number of venipunctures.

National Healthcareer Association (NHA)

194 Route 46E
Fairfield, NJ 07004
(800) 499-9092
www.nha2000.com

The NHA offers a certification examination that requires a high school diploma and graduation from an approved training program or equivalent experience documented by an employer. The certification is a CPT(NHA).

- Communication skills
  - Verbal and nonverbal
  - Listening skills
  - Tone of voice
  - Dealing with angry patients
  - Interactions with peers and coworkers
  - Telephone etiquette
- Satisfaction of the patients
  - Waiting time
  - Complications during the procedure
  - Courtesy
  - Degree of discomfort or pain
- Clerical responsibilities
- Unexcused absences or tardiness
- Knowledge of medical and/or laboratory terminology
- Measures of efficiency and quality
  - Number of uncomplicated blood draws in a specified time period
  - Number of unacceptable laboratory specimens
  - Blood culture contamination rate

There are many ways for supervisors to assess competency, e.g., direct observation, videotaping, reviewing worksheets or log books, reviewing quality control records, providing simulations similar to real life situations, and/or providing written examinations. The benefits of competency assessment have been described for the employee, the patient, and the supervisor as follows:[2]

- Provides performance feedback
- Identifies performance problems early

> ## BOX 1–2.   AMERICAN SOCIETY OF CLINICAL PATHOLOGISTS–BOARD OF REGISTRY COMPETENCY STATEMENTS FOR THE PHLEBOTOMY TECHNICIAN, REVISED JUNE, 1999.
>
> In regard to Anatomy and Physiology, Specimen Collection, Specimen Processing and Handling and Laboratory Operations related to Phlebotomy, and in accordance with established procedures, the Phlebotomy Technician, PBT(ASCP), at career entry:
>
> ### Applies Knowledge of
>
> - Principles of basic and special procedures
> - Medical terminology
> - Potential sources of error
> - Safety measures/infection control
> - Standard operating procedures
> - Fundamental biological characteristics
>
> ### Selects Appropriate
>
> - Course of action
> - Quality control procedures
> - Equipment/methods/reagents
> - Site for blood collection
>
> ### Prepares Patient and Equipment
>
> ### Evaluates
>
> - Specimen and patient situation
> - Possible sources of error or inconsistencies
> - Quality control procedures
> - Common procedural/technical problems
> - Appropriate actions and methods
> - Corrective actions
>
> (From the American Society of Clinical Pathologists Board of Registry, 1999, with permission.)

- Promotes consistency among all workers
- Encourages employees to stay abreast of policies and procedures
- Pinpoints opportunities for improvement in procedures
- Reminds staff of important facts that might have been forgotten over time
- Demonstrates that personnel are competent to perform tasks
- Ensures high quality standards

PROFESSIONAL ETHICS

The principles of right and wrong conduct, as they apply to professional problems, are the ethics for that profession. Professions set standards of conduct for members, and members are expected to adhere to those standards of performance in their work. Standards of behavior are implied in the codes of ethics for each member of the health care team. The three major points common to most ethical standards are:

1. Do no harm to anyone intentionally.
2. Perform according to sound technical ability and good judgment.
3. Respect the patients' rights (which include confidentiality, privacy, the right to know about their treatment, and the right to refuse treatment).

As examples, the ASCP and the **National Phlebotomy Association (NPA)** developed codes of ethics for laboratory professionals and health care workers involved in specimen collection. The major themes of the codes involve responsibilities for accuracy and reliability of laboratory test results and patient confidentiality. Also, the concepts of honesty, integrity, and regard for the dignity of other human beings continue to be the personal foundations for the ethical behavior of health care workers.

Many hospitals and health service organizations across the country have also established specific codes of ethics for their employees, statements of organizational values, or both. Often these codes deal with professional expectations for employees as they relate to the functions or mission of the organization. For further discussion of ethical issues in phlebotomy, refer to Chapter 18.

PROFESSIONAL BEHAVIOR

Professional behavior cannot be prescribed or calculated in a mathematical equation. Each health care worker has a personal responsibility for providing the best possible care. Important character attributes for health care workers who practice phlebotomy follow.

- *Sincere interest in health care.* Health care workers should be compassionate and possess an intense desire to serve people and become knowledgeable in blood and specimen collection practices. They should also have the emotional stability and maturity to deal successfully with seeing others in pain, handling blood and body fluids, facing injury and trauma, seeing disease sites, and the possibility of observing death. Responses of health care workers to harsh situations must be prompt, professional, and reassuring to the patient, their families, and the health care team.
- *Accountability for doing things right.* Personal integrity, veracity (telling the truth), or "doing what's right when no one is looking" (e.g., washing hands between patient collections, observing precautions to gown and scrub in isolation, reporting one's own mistakes, and collecting timed tests at the proper time), reflects a health care worker's personal accountability or individual responsibility for actions.
- *Dedication to high standards of performance.* Health care workers involved in specimen collections must continually upgrade and maintain the quality of their skills. They must know about new techniques and safety procedures, new supplies and equipment, changing time constraints on tests, computer technology, and changes in scientific knowledge. They should be willing to ask for assistance when dealing with a difficult patient or procedure. They should only collect the specimens ordered and only those that they have been trained to collect. They must respect patients' rights to privacy and confidentiality.
- *Propensity for cleanliness.* Health care workers must protect themselves and patients by accepting that sterile techniques, good personal hygiene, and cleanliness affect

safety and quality health care. This is more important than saving time or cutting corners to save money.

- *Pride, satisfaction, and self-fulfillment in the job.* Health care workers involved in specimen collection should attain professional satisfaction from continually improving their professional skills and knowledge, from knowing that others are dependent on their work, and from knowing that their skills contribute to the betterment of patients. The most successful, highly regarded phlebotomists are those who are most gratified with their work.

Only the individual dealing with patients on a one-to-one basis knows for sure whether the work that he or she performs each day is based on tenets for optimum professional behavior.

WORKING WITH HEALTH CARE TEAM MEMBERS

In recent years, most health care organizations have reorganized and downsized to provide increasingly efficient services in a more patient-oriented manner. In addition, advanced laboratory technology has enabled laboratory testing to be performed closer to the point of care (e.g., at the patient's bedside, at ancillary or mobile sites, or even in the home). These special testing procedures are more fully covered in Part IV, Special Procedures and Point-of-Care Testing.

As a result of these trends, shifts in job roles and responsibilities for phlebotomists have been tremendously affected. More than ever in the past, the role of the phlebotomist has become more involved and coordinated with other health care processes. In some cases, health professionals, such as nurses, respiratory therapists, patient care technicians, and others, have been cross-trained to assume phlebotomy duties. In other cases, traditional laboratory-based phlebotomists have been cross-trained to assume other clerical or patient care duties. Whatever the case, the role of the health care worker as a team player will continue to evolve and change. Change begins from within, and phlebotomists must be flexible enough to work with a variety of health care professionals in a wide range of settings.

Teams can improve skills (more talent, expertise, and technical competence), communication (more ideas, mutual respect, crossing departmental lines), participation (increased job satisfaction, combined efforts are greater than individual efforts), effectiveness (solutions are more likely to be implemented, the team has ownership of the shared decisions).[3–6] There are several common sense traits and interpersonal skills that are needed in order for teams to be effective. These are listed in Box 1–3.

■ COMMUNICATION SKILLS IN THE PATIENT CARE ENVIRONMENT

As a vital member of the health care team, the phlebotomist provides the link between the patient and laboratory analytical area. The quality of the blood specimen determines the quality of the diagnostic test result. The ease of collection of these specimens, however, depends on the skills and abilities of the health care worker to perform the collection techniques and interact successfully with the patient.

BOX 1–3.   SKILLS NEEDED FOR EFFECTIVE TEAMS

Each team member should:

1. Understand the mission of the organization
2. Know the basic skills for group process and team dynamics (e.g., active listening, setting norms)
3. Understand relevance and commitment to team goals
4. Be reliable and dependable in work assignments
5. Be able to communicate ideas and feelings
6. Actively participate in decision making
7. Learn how to be flexible in decision making
8. Constructively manage conflicts
9. Contribute to the cohesion of the team
10. Contribute to problem-solving strategies
11. Support and encourage other team members

BEDSIDE MANNER

The climate established by the health care worker upon entering a patient's room will affect the entire patient encounter. The feeling of confidence that comes from the knowledge that the collection tray is clean and completely stocked is the first step in a good bedside manner. A pleasant facial expression, neat appearance, and professional manner set the stage for a positive interaction with the patient. The first 30 seconds after the phlebotomist enters the patient's room determines how that patient perceives the quality of patient care offered by that hospital. Most patients admit that the procedure they dread most is being "stuck" for blood collection, so phlebotomists should make every effort to minimize the negative effects of the situation.

Upon entering the patient's room, the blood collector should introduce him- or herself and state that he or she is part of the hospital unit or laboratory staff, whichever is the case. The patient should be informed that the specimen is being collected for a test ordered by the physician. A statement indicating that this is routine hospital protocol often reassures the patient. A lengthy discussion of why a certain test was ordered or what tests were ordered is inappropriate. These questions should be referred to the patient's physician.

During all the steps of the venipuncture, the health care worker should remain calm, compassionate, and professional with conversations limited to essential information. Sometimes patients are comforted by letting them know about how the procedure is going (e.g., "this is going well," or "it is almost over"). Care should be taken not to be distracted from the phlebotomy procedure by excessive talk of unrelated issues. Before leaving the room, the patient should be thanked for cooperating.

COMMUNICATION ISSUES IN THE HOME AND AMBULATORY SETTINGS

As previously mentioned, blood collection and testing at the point-of-care is in great demand because of the convenience, reliability, and rapid turnaround time for test results. Various terms are used for laboratory testing in settings outside the inpatient hospital unit. These include on-site testing, alternate-site testing, near-patient testing, patient-focused testing, point-of-care testing, and bedside testing. Because this can take place in different environments, ranging from clinics to physicians' offices to mobile vans to an individual's home, the setting may be more casual than in a hospital room. Nevertheless, professional behavior should remain particularly important.

Methods for communication in ambulatory settings or the home usually require more time for the following reasons:

- The phlebotomist must introduce him- or herself and clearly explain the purpose of the interaction.
- The patient should be directed to an appropriate place to sit or recline during the procedure. This may involve walking to a private area, blood collection booth, or special recliner.
- If the phlebotomy procedure is taking place in an unfamiliar setting, such as the patient's home, the phlebotomist must take extra time to find the nearest bathroom (for hand washing, blood spillage) and the nearest bed in case there are complications to the phlebotomy procedure (fainting).
- In a patient's home, the phlebotomist may need to find a phone or bring a mobile phone to clarify laboratory orders or inquire about patient information.
- Information about the procedure should be fully explained (especially if it is a first-time blood collection for the patient or if it has been a long time since the last blood collection).
- Identifying the patient should be done meticulously and cautiously, using various methods to identify the patient positively (e.g., driver's license or identification card, confirmation of birthday and home address, or social security number, if available).
- The phlebotomist must assure that the puncture site has been appropriately cared for and that the patient is physically fit to leave the area after the phlebotomy procedure. If the patient is homebound, the phlebotomist must assure that the patient is no longer bleeding, the puncture site has been appropriately bandaged, and that the patient is able to stay by him- or herself.

PATIENT INTERVIEW

Health care organizations differ slightly in their guidelines for patient interviews. All agree that proper patient identification is essential. If the patient is hospitalized, this should be accomplished by a match between the test requisition or labels and the armband, and by verbal confirmation from the patient. If a hospitalized patient does *not* have an armband, a positive confirmation must be made by a unit nurse who knows the patient. This process should be well documented by the phlebotomist.

Special identification procedures should also be well documented for ambulatory patients, especially in cases of homebound patients, mobile vans, and other off-site locations. Armbands are not commonly used in ambulatory settings; however, an identification card usually is. It may include some demographic data and other identifying information, such as the patient's identification number, date of birth (DOB), address, or a combination of these. This information should be confirmed by the patient prior to blood collection. The patient should always be asked, "What is your name?" *not* "Are you Ms. Smith?" The first question is a more reliable and direct way of confirming identity. The second question is inappropriate and less reliable because a patient who is heavily medicated will often agree with anything that he or she is asked.

Some health care facilities insist that the health care worker ask for the patient's complete address, whereas others require the mention of the patient's hometown, birthdate, or street name to reinforce and confirm identity. Some prefer that patients spell an unusual last name. This portion of the specimen collection procedure ensures that the remainder of the diagnostic testing protocol provides information on the correct person.

It is important for the health care worker to remember that verbal and nonverbal cues (body language) play an important part in the communication of what the patient perceives and how he or she responds. In addition, listening skills are a valuable part of patient communication. Both of these skills are discussed further later in this chapter.

TEACHING PATIENTS

For most phlebotomy procedures to be successful the patient must participate and cooperate. The phlebotomist must be willing and able to provide sufficient, understandable instruction to the patient for the protocols to be accomplished. For example, in some clinical situations, patients with diabetes need to be instructed on the use of mechanical aids to perform finger sticks on themselves at home to check blood glucose levels.

Nursing staff or unit personnel may have instructed the inpatient that he or she will be fasting or will have "nothing by mouth" until after the early morning blood collections. The health care worker should listen to patients' comments, such as, "I didn't have breakfast yet," and "they won't feed me." Even a question or comment about food may inspire a response to confirm that the patient was truly fasting. When in doubt, simply asking the patient if they have eaten or had anything to drink other than water will confirm that the patient has been fasting.

Even more critical are the timed tests, such as the glucose tolerance test. In this test, patient understanding is essential. For the procedure to yield valid and reliable results, the patient must stay fasting, be in his or her room at the specified time, and drink enough water to provide the timed urine specimens. If the patient is a child, the parents or guardian must receive and understand the instructions. If the patient begins to feel ill or faint, the phlebotomist should know how to cope with the situation, depending on the setting. If the patient is experiencing excessive pain during the procedure, the phlebotomist must know how and when to discontinue the venipuncture. Usually the appropriate nursing staff should be notified to aid in the patient's care; however, in ambulatory situations, nursing staff may not always be available, and the phlebotomist should be trained on how to monitor the patient and cope with the circumstances. A bed and bathroom should be convenient to the collection area to provide for the patient's comfort and safety. Complications in blood collection, such as fainting (syncope), are discussed further in Chapter 10, and other first aid topics are reviewed in Chapter 5.

Other times at which the health care worker is involved with teaching patients about specimen collection involve 24-hour urine specimens, urine specimens for microbiologic culture, and sputum and stool specimens. These are more thoroughly discussed in Chapter 15.

COMMUNICATION STRATEGIES

Communication is essential not only for teaching and interacting with patients but also for everyday effectiveness in all areas of the workplace. Effective verbal interactions can be depicted as a communication loop. The message must leave the sender and reach the receiver (Box 1–4). The receiver usually provides feedback to the sender. Without feedback, the sender has no way of knowing whether the message was accurately received or if the message was somehow blocked by extraneous factors. The factors can "filter out" meaning from a message. Filters can be damaging to effective communication. When there are cultural, behavioral, or language differences among health care workers and patients, there is an increased risk that patients will not understand care instructions. Health care workers need to be sure that the message they send is the same message received by the patient. In the following sections, communication is broken down into its three more-detailed components:

1. Verbal communication
2. Nonverbal communication
3. Active listening

BOX 1–4.   PATIENT–PHLEBOTOMIST COMMUNICATION LOOP

Sender/Phlebotomist

"Hello, please excuse the interruption, my name is Brenda and I work on this unit as a blood collector. I am here to collect a blood sample."

Filters

(Television is on, patient is about to eat breakfast, two family members are in the room talking about the football game last night, and a volunteer walks in to deliver mail.)

Receiver/Patient

"This is not going to hurt, is it? By the way, why are you doing this?"

Sender/Phlebotomist Feedback

(The phlebotomist should read verbal and nonverbal cues from the patient and family members to discern the patient's comfort level with the request to draw blood. Based on these impressions, his or her questions should be answered and additional issues should be clarified prior to proceeding with patient identification and specimen collection.)
"Would you mind if I turn down the volume on the television while we discuss this? It is important that a blood sample be taken prior to your breakfast so that the laboratory can run the tests your doctor has ordered. The procedure hurts a little, but it should be over quickly. Do you have any other questions about this procedure? Your family members may stay in your room if you are more comfortable with them here."

Feedback Loop Is Completed by Confirmation From the Receiver/Patient

"I don't have any other questions, and you can go ahead with the stick. I would like my family members to stay for moral support."

Verbal Communication

Keep in mind that talking with strangers about personal things such as your body is never easy and can be particularly difficult for young teenage patients or patients from different cultural backgrounds than the health care worker. Encouraging patients to talk about themselves or to accept a health care worker usually involves the following:[6]

1. Show empathy (for waking them up, disturbing them, or interrupting their meal)
2. Show respect (for their privacy, for their condition, for their family members)
3. Build trust (maintain confidentiality, explain procedures clearly, tell the truth)
4. Establish rapport (common courtesy, show interest)
5. Listen actively (face the patient, maintain nonauthoritative posture, lean toward the patient, establish eye contact, relax and listen intently)
6. Provide specific feedback (about their behavior, about a procedure)

A basic understanding of the language is needed for any health care worker to communicate with all patients, young and old. There are filters or barriers to simple verbal communication, however, that can interfere greatly with the patient-phlebotomist relationship.

Language.   Many members of the health care team use jargon or medical terminology to explain procedures to the patient. This can be confusing to lay people. In addition, the meaning of words varies with the context and age of the speaker. To promote understanding, a vocabulary that is easily understood should be used with patients whenever possible. This is particularly true with children.

Patients must *not* be told, "This won't hurt." Most blood collection procedures are slightly painful; therefore, it is important that the patient be forewarned and prepared. This is even more important when dealing with children. To help ease anxiety, the child can be asked to hold something (e.g., a bandage) while the procedure is taking place. This allows the child to feel helpful and provides a distraction from the procedure.

Hearing Impairments.   The more complex the directions, the greater the need to communicate. Thus, the health care worker should be more sensitive to patients who have impaired hearing. A question such as, "Is there a step you would like me to repeat before we begin?" yields better clues that the patient has heard and understood than saying, "Do you understand?" If it is obvious that the patient did not hear, all efforts should be made to write down instructions for the patient. It is strongly recommended that writing tools be kept at the bedside of these patients and also be accessible in ambulatory settings.

Other distracting noises can also interfere with hearing. A busy hallway, visitors, a television or radio in the room, or headphones can prevent the patient from hearing accurately. In these cases, the phlebotomist should take steps in a polite and professional manner, to reduce the sound level so the patient can hear necessary instructions. Examples might include phrases such as the following:

- *To visitors:* "Excuse me please, it is important for me to explain this procedure to Mr. Jones. Would you mind if we have a quiet moment together for a few minutes? Thank you for your cooperation."
- *For the television:* "Mr. Jones, I am sorry to disrupt your television show, but would you mind if we lower the volume for a few minutes so we can go over the procedure for collecting your blood sample? Thank you, this should only take a few minutes."

- *For headphones:* "Mr. Jones, it is important that we discuss this procedure before beginning. Would you mind taking off your headphones for a few minutes? I will be brief. Thank you for your cooperation."

Languages Other than English.   The diversity of languages spoken in this country is extensive. In many parts of the United States, one sees signs in multiple languages. Patients who do not speak English can understand some basics from nonverbal cues, such as sign language, but the phlebotomist must know how to locate an interpreter, if possible. Often there may be volunteers to perform language interpretations. If a large segment of the patient population speaks another language, the health care facility should provide interpreters who know the basic use of that language. In the absence of an interpreter, written instructions in other languages may facilitate the process. Printed cards in different languages can be used to transmit information.

In many regions of the United States, it is important to develop some skill in Spanish. It is recommended that the health care worker practice the phrases with someone who can speak the language before attempting to communicate with a patient because mispronounced words may lead to more confusion. (Basic requests in Spanish are listed in the Appendices.)

Keep in mind that English language skills and understanding may vary greatly in the United States. The cultural diversity in this country lends itself to language differences. The health care worker should always speak respectfully, in a highly professional manner, and with phrases that are clearly articulated. The dignity of the patient, whether he or she is English-speaking or not, is of utmost importance. If a health care worker feels frustrated by an inability to communicate with a patient, he or she should seek assistance from a supervisor, translator, family member, or physician. Each patient should be treated compassionately, fairly, and with the utmost of dignity, regardless of language abilities.

Age.   The vocabulary of a teenager is different from that of someone 70 to 80 years old. Phlebotomists should be sensitive to word usage for each age. Communication issues for various age groups are discussed further in later chapters.

Tone of Voice.   The tone of one's voice and the inflection used can change a positive sentence into a negative-sounding statement. The pitch, or tone, of voice should match the words that are spoken. Sarcasm is usually communicated just by tone of voice. Health care workers can avoid sending mixed messages to patients by practicing a calm, soothing, and confident tone of voice. Box 1–5 is a practice exercise for health care professionals to use in observing their own facial expressions and voice tones.

Emergency Situations.   Emergency, or "STAT," blood collections are common in emergency rooms and in some complicated surgical or medical cases. These phlebotomy procedures require extra speed and accuracy without jeopardizing the "personal touch." Patients in emergency rooms may not have identification information with them and may be unconscious. All facilities, however, should have documented procedures for the identification process with which phlebotomists should be familiar. Individual patients should be considered in terms of their dignity and individual needs, not by nicknames, such as, "Mr. L down the hall," or "the broken leg in 3C." Each is entitled to professional, respectful care in all circumstances.

BOX 1–5. EXERCISE TO IMPROVE TONE OF VOICE AND FACIAL EXPRESSIONS

The following exercise is useful for improving verbal and nonverbal communication skills. Practice it in front of a mirror or with a co-worker.

Step 1. Using a *nice tone of voice* (i.e., calm, compassionate, clear, professional tone), with a smile on your face, practice saying the following phrases:

- "Please . . ."
- "Good morning."
- "How was your breakfast?"
- "Have you had lunch?"
- "May I check your identification bracelet?"
- "Thank you."

Step 2. Now, using a *degrading tone of voice* (i.e., sarcastic, whiny, angry tone), with a frustrated, disdainful look on your face, repeat the phrases listed in step 1.

Step 3. List the specific features you liked about the first method with those features you disliked about the second method. Try to contrast details of facial features (wrinkled eyebrows or smiling face), how the voice lowers or raises at the end of the statements, and how you feel when speaking in the two manners.

Step 4. Keep a mental impression (or actually take a picture) of the way you look and sound during the first step. *Remember:* A simple smile can often force a positive change in voice tone.

Nonverbal Communication

Some educators believe that communication is comprised of 10 to 20 percent words and 80 to 90 percent nonverbal cues. These nonverbal cues, or body language, can be positive and helpful to understanding, or it can be negative and hinder effective communication. These cues are summarized in Box 1–6.

BOX 1–6. NONVERBAL COMMUNICATION, OR BODY LANGUAGE

Positive Body Language

Maintaining erect posture	Communicating at eye level when possible
Having relaxed hands, arms, shoulders	Displaying good grooming habits
Communicating face to face	Maintaining zone of comfort
Maintaining eye contact	Smiling

Negative Body Language and Distracting Behaviors

Slouching, shrugging shoulders	Wrinkling forehead
Rolling eyes, wandering eyes	Thumbing through books or papers
Looking at ceiling or window, staring blankly	Chewing gum
Rubbing eyes, blinking excessively	Repeatedly looking at clock or watch
Squirming	Lining up objects on a desk
Tapping foot, fingers, pencil	Stretching, yawning
Sighing deeply, moaning, groaning	Sitting backward on a chair (i.e., straddling it)
Crossing arms, clenching fists	Peering over eyeglasses
	Pointing a finger at someone

Positive Body Language

Smiling.   A simple, compassionate smile can set the stage for open lines of communication. It can make each patient feel that he or she is the most important person at that moment. In addition, most people look better with smiles on their faces than they do with frowns. It takes fewer muscle movements to smile than it does to frown.

Eye Contact and Eye Level.   The most expressive parts of the human face are the eyes. Therefore eye contact is important in effective communication. Eye contact promotes a sense of trust and honesty between the patient and phlebotomist. It can make the entire procedure less traumatic for the patient if he or she sees a compassionate expression in the phlebotomist's eyes. There is an expression that says "the eyes are the windows of the soul."

Eye level is also a consideration. Bedridden patients must always look up to those in the room, including the health care team members. This can create a feeling of intimidation, of being "looked down on," or of weakness. Most of the time, phlebotomists do not have the extra time to spend finding a chair to sit in so that they are at eye level; however, if a health care worker must explain a lengthy procedure or if it is noted that the patient is particularly nervous about the procedure, the explanation should be done while seated at eye level with the patient. Box 1–7 is an exercise for understanding what it feels like to be bedridden.

A word of caution about eye contact is necessary when dealing with patients of certain cultures. Generally speaking, Americans view eye contact as a positive aspect of human nature; avoidance of eye contact might mean that someone is not being truthful. However, some Asians and Native Americans believe that prolonged eye contact is rude and an invasion of privacy. Muslim women may avoid eye contact due to modesty.[6] Patients may not appreciate direct eye contact with a health care provider because it may make them feel self-conscious; it may be unacceptable in their culture, or may not be acceptable with the opposite gender. The health care worker should take cues from the patient. If the patient does not look at the health care worker when she is speaking, perhaps she or he would feel more comfortable with more space between them or less direct eye contact. The health care worker can take the interaction at a slower pace to monitor the patient's comfort level.

Face-to-Face Communication.   Phlebotomists should face patients directly. Otherwise, the patient may feel neglected, that they are being avoided, or that information is

---

BOX 1–7.   PRACTICE EXERCISE FOR DEVELOPING SENSITIVITY TO BEDRIDDEN PATIENTS

Health care workers should strive to be as compassionate as possible. Bedridden patients often feel intimidated because health care workers must repeatedly "look down" on them to provide care. Sometimes these patients are depressed because of their condition or prognosis. This exercise will help you imagine yourself in the patient's condition and can make you a more compassionate member of the health care team. Practice the exercise with a co-worker.

1. Lie on a bed while your co-worker stands directly over you, looking down.
2. Have the co-worker go through the motions of a venipuncture procedure, including the greeting and identification process. Try to imagine the anticipation of the needle stick. Have the co-worker maintain eye contact with you while conversing.
3. Repeat step 2, without eye contact.
4. Mentally note the positive and negative aspects of this procedure.

being withheld. If a patient turns away from a phlebotomist, however, it should be taken as a cue that the patient is uncomfortable for some reason. The phlebotomist should do everything possible to make the patient feel more comfortable during the phlebotomy procedure.

Zone of Comfort.   Most individuals begin to feel uncomfortable when strangers get too close to them physically. A **zone of comfort** is the area of space around a patient that is private territory, so to speak. For Western cultures, there are four zones of interpersonal space[6]:

- Intimate space (direct contact up to 18 inches)—for close relationships and health care workers who bathe, feed, dress, and perform venipunctures
- Personal space (18 inches to 4 feet)—for interactions among friends and many patient encounters
- Social space (4 feet to 12 feet)—for most interactions of everyday life
- Public space (more than 12 feet)—for lectures, speeches, etc.

When a stranger gets too close, it can cause the patient to feel nervous, fearful, or anxious. Health care workers must be understanding and approach nervous patients slowly and gently to avoid causing feelings of being threatened. This is particularly true with children, many of whom have a wide zone of comfort; that is, they do not like anyone to approach them except close relatives or friends. A skilled health care worker must be aware of his or her threat to a patient and use a calm, professional, and confident manner.

Cultural Sensitivity

Culture is a system of values (individualism, importance of education and financial security, competition vs. cooperation, etc.), beliefs (spiritual orientation, family bonding), and practices (food, music, traditions) that stems from one's concept of reality. Culture influences decisions and behaviors in many aspects of life. Learning about various ethnic groups and cultures is important for health care professionals so as to understand the reasons for patients' behaviors during times of health and illness. Specific traits that vary among cultures have been addressed previously, (e.g., eye contact and zone of comfort). However, with the changing demographics of the U.S. population, it is vital for all health care workers to become more sensitive and compassionate about accepting cultural practices that vary from our own. When a health care worker is unsure or unaware of acceptable patterns of behavior for a patient, the recommended action is to "follow the patient's lead."[6] For example, if a patient speaks softly and slowly, speak the same way. If the patient turns to a family member when speaking to you, include the family member in the conversation. If a patient moves closer to you during the conversation, try not to back away from the patient's zone of comfort. The best way to become more culturally competent is to allow patients to teach us, to become active observers of how culturally diverse patients interact with each other and with health professionals. Becoming keen observers of mannerisms, gestures, and facial expressions of group members, reading about cultural groups, watching films and videos, reading novels that depict groups, and reading newspapers published by cultural groups will make health care workers better and more informed at what they do.[6]

   In some cultures, the zone of comfort may be wide, and in others, people naturally speak more closely to each other. How much at ease a person feels with physical closeness can also vary with gender. Some women feel very uncomfortable having a male health care worker standing over them preparing to draw a blood specimen, and vice versa. It is particularly considerate if a phlebotomist recognizes this and responds accordingly. Again, respect for the patient's needs and dignity must be considered. Phlebotomists can practice having the sensation that someone is "too close for comfort" by using role reversal. Box 1–8 provides a brief exercise.

Negative Body Language and Distracting Behaviors

Wandering Eyes.   When people roll their eyes upward, they convey the sense of being bored, inattentive, or unwilling to perform a duty. Because this behavior is distracting, it should be avoided when a phlebotomist is communicating with, listening to, or observing patients, co-workers, or supervisors.

The same can be said about gazing out the window or looking up at the ceiling. If a phlebotomist enters a patient's room and begins addressing the patient while looking out the window, the patient will feel neglected and the phlebotomist will appear unconcerned. If the window is too tempting to avoid a glance, the phlebotomist can include the patient in his or her observations. A friendly comment about the weather might be appropriate; then the phlebotomy procedure can be continued when full attention can be given to the patient. The objective is to make the patient feel at ease through good communication techniques so that the procedure can be successful.

Nervous Behaviors.   Behaviors, such as squirming or tapping a pencil or a foot, can be very distracting. They can make a patient feel nervous, hurried, or anxious about the venipuncture. A calm and confident image maximizes the patient's comfort and trust. It is also helpful to recognize these behaviors in patients, especially children, so that efforts can be made to reduce fear. Allowing a few extra moments of conversation or preparation may help.

Breathing Pattern.   A deep sigh can convey a feeling of being bored or a reluctance to do the job. Phlebotomists should avoid sighing, especially when communicating with an

---

BOX 1–8.   ROLE REVERSAL EXERCISE

Having respect for an individual's personal space, or zone of comfort, is part of being a compassionate health care worker. The comfort zone of each person varies with sex, culture, and situation. However, most people feel uneasy when strangers are touching them or are "too close for comfort." An example of this uncomfortable sensation is in a crowded elevator. People take great measures to move so that they are not touching strangers, and as people exit the elevator, the remaining people move and shift to provide more space around themselves. This same sense of uneasiness is felt by patients who are approached by unfamiliar health care workers.

To simulate a real patient–health care worker interaction, practice the following exercise with a co-worker who is not a close friend. Eye contact should be made during this exercise.

1. Lie on a bed as if you are a patient.
2. Have the co-worker slowly approach you. He or she should begin 10 feet away and pause between steps.
3. Note at what distance you begin to feel awkward or uncomfortable. (Usually, this distance is about 2 to 4 feet from the bed.) This distance is the boundary of your zone of comfort.
4. Repeat the exercise with the same co-worker. You will probably require a smaller zone of comfort because a person becomes a little more at ease after initial contact with an unfamiliar person.

angry, uncooperative patient. Likewise, if a patient sighs deeply or moans at the mere sight of the phlebotomist, this should be a cue that a little extra attention, conversation, or a smile might ease the patient's reluctance for the procedure.

Other Distracting Behaviors.   Many other actions can convey negative or defensive emotions. Among these are crossed arms, a wrinkled forehead, frequent glances at a clock or watch, rapid thumbing through papers, chewing gum, yawning, or stretching. Health care workers should realize that these behaviors can detract from their professional image when they are communicating with patients, families, visitors, co-workers, and supervisors. It is also important to realize what these cues mean if a patient exhibits them. The most effective communicators can detect these signs immediately and deal with them in an honest, compassionate, and professional manner. Regular in-services or continuing education programs can be directed at reminding phlebotomists to be aware of positive and negative body language, both in their own behavior and that of patients.

Active Listening

Another component of effective communication is the art of listening. **Active listening** helps close the communication loop by ensuring that the message sent can indeed be repeated and understood. Listening skills do not depend on intellect or educational background; they can be learned and practiced. Box 1–9 provides tips for becoming an active listener.

BOX 1–9.   STEPS FOR ACTIVE LISTENING

The following steps are presented as a starting point for the development of listening skills by health care workers. Because individuals can mentally process words faster than they can speak them, a good listener must concentrate and focus on the speaker to keep his or her mind from wandering. Development of these skills can help an individual in professional life as well as in personal life.

1. Concentrate on the speaker by "getting ready" to listen. Take a moment to clear your mind of distracting thoughts. Begin the interaction with an open, objective mind. Sometimes taking a deep breath can help clear your mind and prepare it to receive more information.
2. Use silent pauses in the conversation wisely by mentally summarizing what has been said.
3. Let the speaker know that someone is listening. Use simple phrases, such as "I see," "Oh," "Very interesting," and "How about that," to reassure the speaker and communicate understanding and acceptance.
4. Keep personal judgments to yourself until the speaker finishes relaying his or her idea.
5. Verify the conversation with feedback. Make sure that everything was clarified. Ask for more explanation if necessary.
6. Mentally review the key words to summarize the overall idea being communicated.
7. Pay attention to body language and ask for clarification. Simple prompts, such as "You look sad," and "You seem upset or nervous," can add more meaning to the conversation and encourage the speaker to verbalize feelings.
8. Listen for true meaning in the message, not just the literal words.
9. Maintain eye contact to communicate interest or concern.
10. Encourage the listener to expand his or her thoughts by using simple phrases, such as "Let's discuss it further," "Tell me more about it," and "Really?"
11. Paraphrase the idea or conversation to ensure complete understanding.
12. Practice active listening at work and at home.

■ APPEARANCE, GROOMING, AND PHYSICAL FITNESS

POSTURE

Phlebotomists usually perform their work while standing. There are occasions, however, particularly with ambulatory patients, when it is more effective to sit adjacent to the patient for the blood collection procedure. Erect posture conveys a sense of confidence and pride in job performance. Slouching conveys a sense of laziness and apathy.

Good posture is helpful for both the phlebotomist and the patient. It minimizes the health care worker's back and neck strain and eases the patient's mind about the confidence of the phlebotomist. Relaxed hands, arms, and shoulders enable the health care worker to work more freely and to show the patient how to relax their arms and shoulders as well.

GROOMING

Physical appearance communicates a strong impression about an individual. Neatly combed hair, clean fingernails, a clean, pressed uniform, protective garb, and an overall tidy appearance communicate a commitment to cleanliness and infection control, and they instill confidence in a person. This is particularly important in today's health care environment, where patients and employees are deeply concerned about the spread of infectious diseases, such as hepatitis, tuberculosis, and human immunodeficiency virus (HIV).

PERSONAL HYGIENE

A professional appearance is completed by careful attention to personal hygiene. A daily bath or shower followed by the use of deodorant is recommended. Perfume or aftershave lotions should be used sparingly because patients may be allergic or may find some scents overpowering and distasteful when they are sick.

NUTRITION, REST, AND EXERCISE

The role of a health care worker requires physical stamina. Good health improves the health care worker's appearance, attitude, job performance, and ability to cope with stress. Appropriate eating habits, rest during lunch and break periods, and off-duty exercising are essential to an individual's well-being. Practicing a healthy lifestyle while on and off duty will facilitate a return to work with a refreshed and more productive attitude.

In most health care environments, the pace is hectic, and overtime work is common. Therefore, it is helpful to know how to deal with stress. Box 1–10 gives some tips for dealing with stress.

PROTECTIVE EQUIPMENT AND CLOTHING

Employers of health care workers are legally required to provide **personal protective equipment (PPE)** or barrier protection for workers handling biohazardous, infectious substances. This type of garb includes gowns, gloves, masks, laboratory coats or aprons, and face shields. Due to latex sensitivities and allergies, employers must provide an array of sizes and styles of gloves and gowns in order to protect their employees. Careful compliance with safety standards minimizes the risk of occupational exposures to blood-borne pathogens. Safety considerations are covered in more detail in Chapter 5.

BOX 1–10.   TIPS FOR DEALING WITH STRESS

Take time to manage time effectively.

Plan time to rest, even at work during breaks.

Associate with gentle people and share your feelings with them.

Learn and practice relaxation skills and alternate with physical exercise.

Eat nutritious foods and exercise to improve health.

Engage in satisfying, meaningful work and hobbies.

Find time for privacy.

Keep a journal.

Read interesting books and articles to get new ideas.

■ PATIENTS' RIGHTS

All members of the health care team must recognize that their first responsibility is to the patient's health, safety, and personal dignity. Many organizations, such as the **American Hospital Association (AHA),** have recognized rights for patients in health care organizations. The AHA originally adopted a **Patient's Bill of Rights** in 1973, and it has revised and/or reaffirmed it as needed. The key elements involve a patient's rights to the following[7]:

- Respectful and considerate care.
- Accurate information about diagnosis, treatment, and prognosis.
- Informed consent.
- Refusal of treatment.
- Privacy.
- Confidentiality.
- Advance directives.
- Review records about his/her own treatment.
- Provision of health care services during a transfer.
- Information about the identity and role of personnel involved in his or her care.
- Information about research procedures involved in his or her care.
- Billing information and explanation of business relationships of those providing services.

ISSUES IN SPECIMEN COLLECTION

There are occasions during specimen collections when a patient's rights are particularly important. The patient may be rude, ill tempered, demanding, uncooperative, or a combination of these. It is important, however, for members of the health care team to always deliver the best quality of care that they can give, while being careful to show consideration, fairness, compassion, and respect for each patient.

Requests for certain laboratory tests and the results of clinical laboratory tests are part of the patient's medical record and are *strictly confidential*. This rule of confidentiality applies in all areas inside and outside of the work site. A health care worker should never discuss patient information with individuals who are not directly responsible for some aspect of patient care. Nor should patient information be discussed in public places, such as an elevator, hallway, or cafeteria. Family members or friends may overhear and would not have the benefit of a full explanation. Joking in the work area about a patient's condition, physical feature, or character trait is completely inappropriate and unprofessional. These situations could be interpreted as a violation of confidentiality and are subject to legal action.

Clinical laboratory requisitions and reports also contain demographic data that should not be exposed to the public, even if the analytic results are not yet recorded. The health care facility is responsible for the security of data in electronic information storage and retrieval systems and for making the information available only to those who specifically need it. Health care workers are, however, also responsible for doing their part in maintaining confidentiality.

In general, the patient's primary care giver, usually a physician, is responsible for discussing information about why laboratory tests were ordered, the results, the testing methodologies, or the medical decisions that will be made based on the results. Health care workers involved in specimen collection should refrain from giving information of this nature to patients, their families, or their friends. This can be correctly handled by saying to the patient or family member, "Your physician ordered blood to be drawn for testing; it would be best to discuss the tests with him or her."

Sometimes, a talkative patient may want to share information of a personal and sensitive nature with the health care worker. It is appropriate to stop the patient politely from disclosure and continue the collection procedure.

As part of the principle of informed consent, the health care worker should briefly explain to the patient the procedures used to collect the blood sample. The patient also has the right to know that the blood-drawing team member is part of the organization's staff and who he or she is. It is important for the phlebotomist to stress that the physician has ordered the tests. The patient also has the right to know if someone involved in his or her care is a student. It is helpful if the student's supervisor can reassure the patient of the student's competency to perform the procedure. Every effort should be made to have student–patient interactions be positive.

If a patient refuses to have a blood specimen drawn, the health care worker is responsible for reminding the patient that the physician ordered the clinical laboratory tests as part of the patient's medical care. If the patient still refuses, the health care worker should inform his or her supervisor and, if possible, the physician. Emotional confrontations or conflicts with the patient should be avoided. All actions and discussions should be documented.

FAMILY, VISITORS, AND SIGNIFICANT OTHERS

Family members and friends of patients are often present when phlebotomists need to acquire specimens. It is important to realize that they can make the patient more secure and comfortable. Sometimes, however, families and visitors are much more difficult to deal with than the patients. They may make requests that are beyond the scope of acceptable or authorized responsibilities for the health care worker. For example, unless specifically authorized to do so, a health care worker should not give food to hospitalized patients. It is better to inform the appropriate health care team member of the family member's request.

If several visitors are in the room with the patient, they may be asked to step into the hall while the blood specimen is being drawn. If the health care worker believes that assistance is required, a family member may be asked to assist. This can make the family members feel helpful, as well as provide reassurance to patients, particularly children.

Physicians, priests, and chaplains have the right to visit privately with patients. Unless the blood specimen is timed, the health care worker should respect that privacy and return to the patient after completing the other draws in the unit or area. If the procedure is timed or stat, the health care worker can apologize for the interruption, explain the nature of the request, and ask permission to collect the specimen.

Families and visitors of patients should not be permitted in the clinical laboratory or provided with patient information, except by prior arrangement and permission. Their safety and the confidentiality of patient records must be considered. Frequently, patients do not want their family members to know test results.

■ HEALTH CARE ORGANIZATIONS

Health care organizations have evolved into different levels of care. **Primary care** is given to maintain and monitor normal health and to prevent diseases by means of laboratory screening tests and immunizations. Blood cholesterol screening and blood glucose screening for diabetes are examples. Other examples of primary care include treatment of minor injuries, diagnosis and treatment of colds or sore throats, well-baby checkups for infants, immunizations, prenatal care during a normal pregnancy, and treatment of chronic illnesses and diseases, such as diabetes mellitus.

Primary care physicians are usually trained in family practice or internal medicine. Other primary health care workers include nurse practitioners, nurse midwives, nurse specialists, and physician assistants (PAs). When patients need a higher level of care, the primary care professionals are responsible for referring patients to the appropriate specialist.

Secondary care refers to specialized care involving a physician who is an expert on a particular group of diseases, a group of organ systems, or an organ. For example, an ophthalmologist is a specialist who diagnoses and treats eye disorders.

Tertiary care is highly specialized and oriented toward unusual and complex diagnoses and therapies. Sophisticated instrumentation and technology or invasive procedures, such as open-heart surgery, are used in an acute care hospital environment. **Acute care** hospitals are characterized by hospital stays of less than 30 days. **Long-term care** refers to care needed longer than 30 days. Hospitalized patients are often referred to as **inpatients.**

HOSPITAL INPATIENT SERVICES

There are approximately 6,000 hospitals in the United States. They vary according to the following:

- Mission (patient care, education, research).
- Bed size.
- Ownership (public or nonprofit, governmental, for profit or proprietary).
- Length of stay (short term [e.g., less than 30 days]; long term [e.g., greater than 30 days]).
- Type of care provided (general acute care hospitals; and specialty care hospitals, such as birthing centers, cancer centers, psychiatric hospitals, pediatric hospitals, and rehabilitation hospitals).
- Location (urban or rural).
- Relationship to other health facilities (integrated hospital systems, religious multihospital systems, independent hospitals).

Traditional hospitals have been organizationally structured around departments according to medical or surgical specialties. The typical hospital departments of the 1980s and early 1990s are shown in Table 1–1 and sometimes are still used. Subspecialized departments are usually organized around organs or organ systems as shown in Table 1–2. Sometimes, departments or ancillary services are organized around therapy services or procedures offered to the patient. Phlebotomists should become knowledgeable about these areas of the hospital because patients spend time in them prior to, during, and after their phlebotomy procedures. There are factors that may affect the outcome of the laboratory test that relate to these departments. Typical hospital services are listed in Box 1–11.

Hospitals are in a state of flux due to reengineering and restructuring, and new organizational structures have surfaced. Many traditional hospital departments have been merged

Table 1–1. Departments Found in Most Large Health Care Facilities

DEPARTMENT	BRIEF DESCRIPTION
Internal medicine	General diagnosis and treatment of patients for problems of one or more internal organs
Pediatrics	General diagnosis and therapy for children
Surgery	Diagnosis and treatment in which the physician physically alters a part of the patient's body
Anesthesiology	Preparing the patient for specialized treatment and/or surgery
Pathology and laboratory medicine	Diagnosis, both before and after treatment, using anatomic and/or clinical laboratory test results
Obstetrics/gynecology	Diagnosis and treatment relating to the sexual reproductive system of females, using both surgical and nonsurgical procedures
Psychiatry/neurology	Diagnosis and treatment for people of all ages with mental, emotional, and nervous system problems, using primarily nonsurgical procedures
Radiology/medical imaging	Diagnosis and treatment, primarily through the use of x-ray, ultrasonography, and other internal imaging procedures
Allergy	Diagnosis and treatment of persons who have allergies or "reactions" to irritating agents
Geriatrics	Diagnosis and treatment of the elderly population
Oncology	Diagnosis and treatment of malignant (life-threatening) tumors
Proctology	Diagnosis and treatment of diseases of the anus and rectum
Rheumatology	Diagnosis and treatment of joint and tissue diseases, including arthritis
Family medicine/general practice	Care of medical problems of all family members so that a different physician is not necessary for each family member by age level or sex
Neonatal–perinatal	Study, support, and treatment of newborn and prematurely born babies and their mothers
Physical medicine	Diagnosis and treatment of disorders and disabilities of the neuromuscular system
Plastic surgery	Correction of the deformity of tissues, including skin

Table 1-2. Medical Departments Listed by Organs and Organ Systems

DEPARTMENT	BRIEF DESCRIPTION
Orthopedics	Bones and joints
Ophthalmology	Eyes
Otolaryngology	Ears, nose, and throat
Urology	Sexual and reproductive system for males and renal system for females and males
Cardiology	Heart
Dermatology	Skin
Neurology	Nervous system
Hematology	Blood system
Immunology	Immune system
Gastroenterology	Esophagus, stomach, and intestines
Nephrology	Kidneys
Endocrinology	Organs and tissues that produce hormones (e.g., estrogens, testosterone, cortisol)
Cardiovascular	Heart and blood circulation
Pulmonary	Lungs

or eliminated. Hospitals, in some cases, have taken on nontraditional services, such as hotel management, music therapy, etc. Another trend for hospitals has been to expand their services to provide more of a continuous system from birth through death. Community outreach efforts have been expanded to reach new managed care markets. This often includes patients enrolled in **Medicare** (federal program covering health services for the elderly) and **Medicaid** (joint federal and state program covering health services for the poor and other special populations).

In summary, for the next few years, the hospital industry will continue to experiment with models of health care delivery that will affect all health care workers.

AMBULATORY AND HOME HEALTH CARE SERVICES

Ambulatory care is personal health care provided to an individual who is not bedridden. Trends in the health care industry have led to a wide range of ambulatory services delivered in a variety of settings. The shift from inpatient hospital services to ambulatory or "outpatient" services has been facilitated by technologic advances, computer applications that allow for portability, and more efficient models of delivering quality care outside the hospital. In addition, with the "aging of America" the fastest growing segment of the population is the elderly. Many health care services have been established to make it more accessible and comfortable for elderly individuals with chronic conditions to seek treatment outside the hospital setting. Long-term care services may involve inpatient and/or ambulatory services.

Home health care services are expanding in response to the aging population. Home health care involves the provision of services in a patient's home under the direction of a physician. Phlebotomists, nurses, home health assistants and aides, and others are

BOX 1–11.   TRADITIONAL HOSPITAL ANCILLARY SERVICES OR DEPARTMENTS

- *Laboratory medicine/pathology:* uses sophisticated instrumentation to analyze blood, body fluids, and tissues for pathological conditions. Laboratory results are used in diagnosis, treatment, and monitoring of patients' health status.
- *Occupational therapy:* assists the patient in becoming functionally independent within the limitations of the patient's disability or condition. Occupational therapists (OTs) collaborate with the health care team to design therapeutic programs of rehabilitative activities for the patient. The therapy is designed to improve functional abilities or activities of daily living (ADLs).
- *Physical therapy:* assists the patient in restoring physical abilities that have been impaired by illness or injury. Rehabilitation programs often use heat/cold, water therapy, ultrasound or electricity, and physical exercises designed to restore useful activity.
- *Pharmacy:* dispenses medications ordered by physicians. Pharmacists also collaborate with the health care team on drug therapies. Phlebotomists may collect blood specimens at timed intervals to monitor the level of the drug in the patient's bloodstream.
- *Nutrition and dietetics:* perform nutritional assessments, patient education, and design special diets for patients who have eating-related disorders (i.e., diabetes, obesity).
- *Diagnostic imaging/radiology:* uses ionizing radiation for treating disease, fluoroscopic and radiographic x-ray instrumentation and imaging methods for diagnosis, and radioisotopes for both diagnosing and treating disease. Fluoroscopic, tomographic, and radiographic analyses of the human body are performed. In this department, patients and employees are protected from exposure to unnecessary radiation. Sometimes patients are injected with dye that might interfere with some laboratory tests. The phlebotomist should document the circumstances as appropriate. In addition, the phlebotomist should be aware of applicable safety requirements.
- *Nuclear medicine:* uses radioactive isotopes or tracers in the diagnosis and treatment of patients and in the study of the disease process. The radioactive substance is injected into the patient and emits rays that can be detected by sophisticated instrumentation. Phlebotomists should be knowledgeable of special safety requirements for entering this area. Also, the radioisotopes may interfere with laboratory testing so this should be documented.
- *Electroencephalography:* uses the electroencephalograph (EEG) to record brain wave patterns.
- *Electrocardiography:* uses the electrocardiograph (ECG or EKG) to record the electric currents produced by contractions of the heart. This assists in the diagnosis of heart disease.
- *Radiotherapy:* uses high-energy x-rays, such as from cobalt treatment, in the treatment of disease, particularly cancer. Safety precautions are again important to avoid unnecessary irradiation.
- *Other support services:* housekeeping, physical plant, maintenance, security, information system management, purchasing, personnel, and laundry.

employed by companies and hospitals offering these services. These health care workers usually perform multiple tasks at homes throughout the community. They then transport the blood to the clinical laboratory for testing. Box 1–12 describes a range of ambulatory care settings.

Many of these settings provide on-site laboratory services. In some cases, however, blood and other patient specimens are sent by courier to a larger independent laboratory or back to a hospital-based laboratory for testing. In other cases, blood tests may be done at the site of the collection, e.g., **point-of-care** testing.

> ## BOX 1–12.   AMBULATORY CARE SETTINGS
>
> Hospital-based clinics
> Hospital-based emergency centers
> Physician group practices
> Individual or solo medical practices
> Specialty practices
> Rehabilitation centers
> Mobile vans for blood donations
> Mobile vans for primary care delivery
> Mobile mammography units
> Free-standing surgical centers
> Health department clinics
> Community health centers (CHCs)
> Rural health clinics
> Community-based mental health centers
> School-based clinics
> Prison health clinics
> Dialysis centers
> Multiphasic screening centers
> Home health agencies
> Home hospice agencies
> Durable medical equipment suppliers
> Health maintenance organizations (HMOs)

THE CLINICAL LABORATORY'S ROLE IN SPECIMEN COLLECTION SERVICES

A typical hospital-based clinical laboratory can have two components: **clinical pathology** and **anatomic pathology.** In the clinical pathology area, blood and other types of body fluids and tissues are analyzed (e.g., urine, cerebrospinal fluid [CSF], sputum, gastric secretions, synovial fluid). In the anatomic pathology area, autopsies are performed and cytologic procedures and surgical biopsy tissues are analyzed. Laboratories can also be independently owned and operated outside the hospital setting. Regardless of the type of laboratory, it is important to understand that the phlebotomist plays a vital role in the process of analysis. Reliability and accuracy of test results depend on the *preanalytic* process of specimen collection.

Personnel who work on the *analytic* phase of laboratory testing may have different educational backgrounds:

- *Pathologists:* physicians who have extensive training in pathology, which is the study and diagnosis of disease through the use of laboratory test results.
- *Administrative staff:* individuals who usually have a graduate degree in health care administration or business. Often these individuals have extensive clinical experience as well.

- *Technical supervisors:* clinical laboratory scientists (also known as medical technologists) with additional experience and education in a laboratory specialty area, such as hematology, microbiology, or clinical chemistry.
- *Clinical Laboratory Scientists (CLS) or Medical Technologists (MT):* individuals with a bachelor's degree in a biological science. Educational requirements include 1 or more years of study in a CLS program. Licensing is required in some states. Roles and responsibilities include performing chemical, microscopic, microbiologic, or immunologic tests pertaining to patient care; recording and reporting test results; participating in research and development of new test methods; performing preventive maintenance, troubleshooting, and quality control of instruments and reagents; maintaining safety in the clinical laboratory; and teaching residents and fellows in pathology and laboratory sciences.
- *Medical Laboratory Technicians (MLT) or Clinical Laboratory Technicians (CLT):* these individuals have a 2-year certificate or associate degree. The MLT may perform designated tests and procedures, prepare specimens for testing and transport, prepare reagents, perform quality control measures, and assist the CLS in numerous preanalytic and postanalytic processes.
- *Other laboratory personnel:* laboratory information systems (LIS) operators and programmers, clerical staff, quality management staff, infection control officers, and biomedical equipment specialists.

Large clinical laboratories may cluster testing processes according to the following subsections:

- Clinical chemistry.
- Hematology and coagulation.
- Microbiology and parasitology.
- Immunohematology (blood banking) or transfusion medicine.
- Immunology and serology.
- Cytology.
- Histology.
- Cytogenetics.
- Urinalysis.

Examples of the types of commonly performed tests in each of these sections are listed in Table 1–3. The importance of specific test procedures will be discussed further in Chapters 2 and 3.

Smaller laboratories can be located in remote locations or clinics, physician offices, and in mobile vans. Health care workers who perform the testing must maintain the same high standards of quality as are found in larger, high-volume laboratories.

The federal government also regulates all clinical laboratories through the **Clinical Laboratory Improvement Amendments of 1988 (CLIA 1988).** Regulations apply to *any* site that tests human specimens, including small **physician's office laboratories (POLs)** or screening tests done at a hospital bedside. The regulations include establishing qualifications for health care personnel who perform the tests, periodic inspections, proficiency assessments, and the investigation of complaints. Laboratory tests are grouped into three categories according to the level of complexity of the testing procedure and the risk involved for the patient if errors are made in performing or interpreting the test. The tests

Table 1–3. Summary of Major Tests Performed in the Clinical Laboratory Sections

CLINICAL CHEMISTRY PROCEDURES

Total proteins

Glucose and glucose tolerance

Glycated hemoglobin

Triglycerides

Total cholesterol

HDL cholesterol

Iron

Total iron-binding capacity (IBC or TIBC)

Electrolytes (sodium [Na^+], potassium [K^+], chloride [Cl^-], bicarbonate [HCO_3^-])

Magnesium

Blood gases (pH, partial pressure of carbon dioxide [Pco_2], partial pressure of oxygen [Po_2])

Creatinine

Uric acid

Blood urea nitrogen (BUN)

Enzymes (e.g., lactate dehydrogenase [LD], alanine aminotransferase [ALT], creatine phosphokinase [CPK])

Drug analysis (e.g., gentamicin, tobramycin, primidone, phenytoin, digoxin, quinidine, salicylates, blood alcohol, barbiturates)

Bilirubin

Hormones (e.g., thyroxine [T_4], insulin, testosterone, luteinizing hormone, parathyroid hormones, prolactin, cortisol)

CLINICAL MICROBIOLOGY PROCEDURES

Acid-fast bacilli (AFB) smear	Fungus direct smear	Pinworm preparation
Anaerobic cultures	GC cultures	Stool cultures
Culture and sensitivity (C&S)	Gram staining	Strep screening
AFB culture	Occult blood	Urine cultures
Fungus cultures	Nose/throat cultures	
Blood cultures	Ova and parasites	

HEMATOLOGY AND COAGULATION PROCEDURES

CSF cell count	Hemoglobin	Reticulocyte count
Differential	Hemoprofile	Sedimentation rate
Eosinophil count	LE cell preparation	Sickle-cell preparation
Fecal leukocyte count	Nasal eosinophil count	WBC count
Hematocrit	Platelet count	Thrombin time
CBC	Partial thromboplastin time (PTT)	
Fibrin split product	Prothrombin time (PT)	
Fibrinogen	RBC count	

(continued)

Table 1–3. *(continued)*

CLINICAL MICROSCOPY AND URINALYSIS PROCEDURES

Routine UA		Miscellaneous UA
pH	Nitrites	Hemosiderin
Specific gravity	Urobilinogen	Pregnancy test
Protein	Ascorbic acid	Synovial fluid analysis
Sugar	Occult blood	Seminal fluid analysis
Ketones	Leukocytes	
Bilirubin		

IMMUNOHEMATOLOGY PROCEDURES (TRANSFUSION MEDICINE)

ABO and Rh$_o$ (D) typing	Hepatitis B surface antigen	Antibody titer
ABO grouping	(HB$_s$Ag) and antibody	Direct Coombs' test
Antibody identification	HIV testing	Rh phenotyping and
Hepatitis B core antigen and	Antibody screen indirect	genotyping
antibody	Coombs' test	Rh$_o$ (D) typing

CLINICAL IMMUNOLOGY/SEROLOGY PROCEDURES

Amebiasis screening	*Francisella tularensis* antibody	Rubella HIA
Antinuclear antibody (ANA)	Legionnaires' disease antibody	Rheumatoid factor
ASO screening	Cold agglutinins	RPR
ASO titer	CSF/VDRL	RPR quantitative
Brucella antibody	Syphilis antibody (FTA-ABS)	*Salmonella* agglutinins
C-reactive protein	Infectious mononucleosis	Q fever
Borrelia burgodorferi	MHA-TP	
(Lyme disease) antibody	*Proteus* OX antibodies	

Abbreviations: ASO, anti-streptolysin O; CBC, complete blood count; CSF, cerebrospinal fluid; FTA-ABS, fluorescent treponemal antibody absorption; GC, gonococcus; HDL, high-density lipoprotein; HIA, hemagglutination-inhibition antibody; HIV, human immunodeficiency virus; LE, lupus erythematosus; MHA-TP, microhemagglutination—*Treponema pallidum;* RBC, red blood cell; RPR, rapid plasma reagin; UA, urinalysis; VDRL, Venereal Disease Research Laboratory; WBC, white blood cell.

may also be reclassified from one category to another as technology advances. The categories are listed next.

Waivered tests are those tests that are the easiest to perform, the least susceptible to error, and the least risky to patients. Examples include urinalysis, urine pregnancy tests, blood glucose screening tests, rheumatoid factor tests or mononucleosis tests using blood agglutination, occult blood detection from stool samples, spun microhematocrits, and erythrocyte sedimentation rates. These are tests that are commonly done in ambulatory settings, on hospital units near the bedside, and in other remote locations.

Moderate complexity tests are those tests that are simple to perform but may involve more risk to the patient if results are inaccurate. Examples include white and red blood cell counts, hemoglobin, hematocrit, blood chemistries, and urine cultures.

High complexity tests are those tests that are complex to perform and may allow for reasonable risk of harm to the patient if results are inaccurate. These include tests that require sophisticated instrumentation and oversight by a pathologist or Ph.D.-level scientist. Examples include molecular probe analyses, bone marrow evaluations, immunoassays, flow cytometry, cytogenetics analysis, and electrophoresis.

Other regulatory agencies also have oversight of clinical laboratories, depending on the type of testing they do and the reimbursement they receive for the procedures. Among these are the Health Care Financing Administration (HCFA), the Food and Drug Administration, the American Association of Blood Banks, the American Society for Clinical Pathologists, and the Joint Commission for the Accreditation of Healthcare Organizations.

SELF STUDY

KEY TERMS

Active Listening
Acute Care
Ambulatory Care
American Hospital Association
(AHA)
American Nurses Association
(ANA)
American Society for Clinical
Laboratory Science
(ASCLS)
American Society of Clinical
Pathologists (ASCP)
Anatomic Pathology
Clinical Laboratory
Improvement Amendments
of 1988 (CLIA 1988)
Clinical Pathology
Competency Statement
Culture

Home Health Care Services
Inpatients
Long-term Care
Medicaid
Medicare
National Phlebotomy
Association (NPA)
Patient's Bill of Rights
Personal Protective Equipment
(PPE)
Phlebotomist
Physician's Office Laboratories
(POLs)
Point-of-Care
Primary Care
Secondary Care
Tertiary Care
Zone of Comfort

STUDY QUESTIONS

The following questions may have *one* or *more* answers.

1. Which of the following are important trends in health care?

   a. cost containment
   b. the "aging of America"

   c. shift from in- to outpatient settings
   d. restructuring the health care team

2. Examples of nonverbal, distracting behaviors include which of the following:

   a. chewing gum
   b. gazing outside the window

   c. direct eye contact
   d. glancing at the clock

3. Which of the following statements is inappropriate during a phlebotomy procedure?

   a. "This won't hurt a bit!"
   b. "Your name is Mrs. Jones,
      isn't it?"

   c. "You are required to cooperate with this
      procedure."
   d. "Could you please spell
      your last name for me?"

4. Which of the following are key elements in effective communication?

   a. active listening

   b. nonverbal cues

   c. verbal skills

   d. "point-of-care" procedures

5. The AHA adopted the Patient's Bill of Rights. These include which of the following?

   a. informed consent

   b. refusal of treatment

   c. privacy

   d. confidentiality

6. Which of the following is/are considered primary health care providers?

   a. nurse

   b. nurse midwife

   c. cardiologist

   d. internal medicine doctor

7. Which of the following procedures would be considered primary care?

   a. immunizations

   b. prenatal checkups

   c. blood glucose screening

   d. CAT scan

8. Hospitals differ according to which of the following?

   a. bed size

   b. length of stay

   c. mission

   d. ownership

9. PPE might include which of the following items?

   a. clipboard for requisitions

   b. gloves

   c. gowns or aprons

   d. face shields

References

1. American Society of Clinical Pathologists: *Careers in the Laboratory Series-Phlebotomist,* ASCP Board of Registry, Box 12277, Chicago, IL 60612-0277, 1997.

2. Gerbasi, S: Competency Assessment in a Team-Based Laboratory, *Medical Laboratory Observer* 2000 (Sept.); 46–54.

3. Johnson, DW, Johnson, RT: *Joining Together, Group Theory and Group Skills,* 6th ed. Boston; Allyn & Bacon: 2000.

4. Mears, P: *Healthcare Teams, Building Continuous Quality Improvement.* Delray Beach, FL; St. Lucie Press: 1994.

5. Parsons, ML, Murdaugh, CL: *Patient-Centered Care: A Model for Restructuring.* Gaithersburg, MD; Aspen Publishers: 1994.

6. Luckman, J: *Transcultural Communication in Health Care.* Albany NY; Delmar: 2000.

7. American Hospital Association: *A Patient's Bill of Rights,* Revision approved by AHA Board of Trustees, Oct . 21, 1992; www.aha.org/resources/pbillofrights.asp.

TWO

∎

Basic Anatomy and Physiology of Organ Systems

CHAPTER OUTLINE

CHAPTER OBJECTIVES

Upon completion of Chapter 2, the learner is responsible for the following:

1. Define the terms *anatomy, physiology,* and *pathology.*
2. Describe the directional terms, anatomic surface regions, and cavities of the body.
3. Describe the eight structural levels of the human body ranging from atoms to cells to the entire organism.
4. Describe the role of homeostasis in normal body functioning.
5. Define the terms *metabolism, catabolism,* and *anabolism.*
6. Describe the purpose, function, and structural components of the 11 body systems.
7. Recognize examples of disorders associated with each organ system.
8. List common diagnostic tests associated with each organ system.

■ ANATOMIC REGIONS

The human body has distinctive characteristics; that is, a backbone, bisymmetry, body cavities, and 11 major organ systems: integumentary, skeletal, muscular, nervous, respiratory, digestive, urinary, reproductive, endocrine, lymphatic, and cardiovascular. This chapter highlights the basic **anatomy** (structural components of the body) and **physiology** (functional components) of each system except the circulatory or cardiovascular system, which is covered in Chapter 3. This chapter also covers common diseases or disorders of the major organ systems. **Pathology** is the study of all aspects of disease and abnormal conditions in the body.

Body regions can be categorized in various ways. One way is to begin at the top and work down. In this manner, the body can be described as having the following regions:[1]

- Head and neck.
- Upper torso.
- Lower torso (female and male).
- Back.
- Arms.
- Legs.
- Hands and feet.

The body can also be described by surface regions, body planes, and body cavities. The front, **anterior,** or **ventral** surface of the body is separated into thoracic, abdominal, and pelvic cavities. The back, **posterior,** or **dorsal** surface is divided into cranial and spinal cavities. Each of these cavities houses one or more organs. Areas and directions of the body can be described by their distance from or proximity to one of the **body planes** (Fig. 2–1 and Table 2–1). The **sagittal plane** runs lengthwise from front to back, dividing the body into right and left halves. The **frontal plane** runs lengthwise from side to side, dividing the body into anterior and posterior sections. The **transverse plane** runs crosswise, or horizontally, dividing the body into upper and lower sections. **Medial** means toward the midline, and **lateral** means toward the sides of the body. *Normal anatomic position* refers to an erect standing position with arms at rest and palms forward.

■ STRUCTURAL ORGANIZATION

The design of the human body is elaborate and sophisticated. A human body can be divided into eight structural levels (Fig. 2–2): atoms, molecules (chemical constituents), small structures within cells or organelles, cells (the basic living units of all plants and animals), tissues (groups of similar cells), organs (two or more tissues), organ systems (groups of organs), and the organism (the human body) itself. Trillions of cells make up each individual. Similar groups of cells are combined into tissues, such as muscles or nerves, and tissues are combined into systems, such as the circulatory or reproductive system. These organ systems work simultaneously to serve the needs of the body. No one system works independently of the others.

Before the major organ systems and their functions are discussed, a basic understanding of the human cell is necessary. Figures 2–3 and 2–4 illustrate a basic cell and its structures and some examples of specific cell morphologies. The size and shape of a cell depend on its function. Some cells fight disease-causing viruses and bacteria; some transport gases, such

Figure 2–1. Body planes.

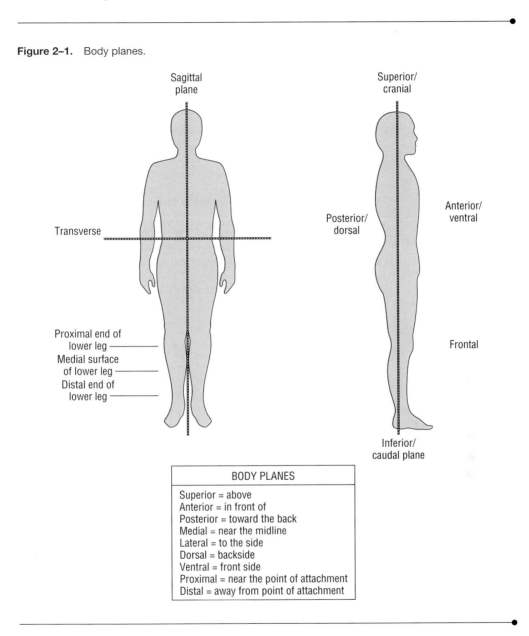

Sagittal plane

Transverse

Proximal end of lower leg
Medial surface of lower leg
Distal end of lower leg

Superior/ cranial

Posterior/ dorsal

Anterior/ ventral

Frontal

Inferior/ caudal plane

BODY PLANES
Superior = above
Anterior = in front of
Posterior = toward the back
Medial = near the midline
Lateral = to the side
Dorsal = backside
Ventral = front side
Proximal = near the point of attachment
Distal = away from point of attachment

as oxygen (O_2) and carbon dioxide (CO_2); some produce movement, store nutrients, or manufacture proteins, chemicals, or liquids; and others, such as the egg and the sperm, can create a new life. At the same time, other cells contribute to thoughts and emotions. Despite such diverse functions, several cells have basic structural elements in common. The cell membrane encloses the contents of the cell. This membrane serves as a protective barrier that selectively allows certain substances to move in or out. Nutrients and O_2 are taken in through the membrane only when needed, and wastes are eliminated as they build up. Most

Table 2–1.   Directional Terms for Body Position

TERM	DESCRIPTION AND EXAMPLE
Right/left	Toward the right/left side of the body. (Example: The patient has scar tissue on the right arm.)
Inferior/superior	A structure or organ below/above another. (Example: The forehead is superior to the nose. The nose is inferior to the eyes.)
Anterior (ventral)	Front of the body. (Example: Toes are anterior, or ventral, to the heel.)
Posterior (dorsal)	Back of the body. (Example: The spinal cord is posterior, or dorsal, to the heart.)
Proximal	Closer to the point of attachment to the body trunk. (Example: The knee is proximal to the ankle.)
Distal	Farther from the point of attachment to the body trunk. (Example: The toes are distal to the ankle.)
Lateral	Away from the midline of the body. (Example: The hip is lateral to the navel.)
Medial	Toward the midline of the body. (Example: The heart is medial to the arms.)
Superficial	Closer to the outer surface of the body. (Example: Skin is superficial to muscles or bone.)
Deep	Internal or farther from the outer surface of the body. (Example: The heart and lungs are deep organs.)

cells also have a **nucleus,** which is enclosed inside a nuclear membrane. The nucleus (*nuclei* for two or more) is commonly thought of as the control mechanism of the cell that governs the functions of the individual cell (i.e., growth, repair, reproduction, and metabolism). Inside the nucleus is a **nucleolus** and threadlike chromatin, which also aid in cell metabolism and reproduction. The nucleus contains a blueprint of itself in the genetic material so that it can reproduce itself when necessary. If the nucleus of a cell is damaged or destroyed, in most cases the cell will die; however, even though red blood cells (RBCs) lose their nuclei when they mature, the cells continue to live and carry O_2 for several months. Another component of the cell, the **cytoplasm,** contains mostly water with dissolved nutrients and fills up the rest of the cell membrane. Within the cytoplasm are smaller structures called *organelles.* The names and functions of these organelles are as follows:

- **Mitochondria.** Produce energy for the cell.
- **Ribosomes.** Assemble amino acids into proteins.
- **Endoplasmic reticulum.** Acts as transport channel between the cell membrane and the nuclear membrane.
- **Lysosomes.** Release digestive enzymes into vacuoles, or small pouches, for digestion of food particles.
- **Golgi apparatus.** Stores proteins.
- **Centriole.** Plays a role in cell division.

Cells communicate with each other in sophisticated reactions using electrical impulses (such as from one nerve cell to another) or in chemical reactions that result in the release of hormones or other enzymes and proteins to stimulate a particular function. The study of cellular structures and processes has captivated clinical laboratory scientists for years. With

Figure 2–2.   Levels of structural organization.

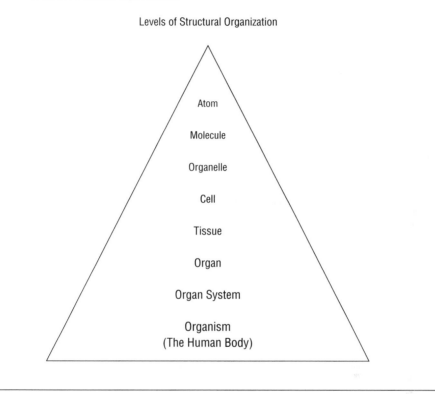

Levels of Structural Organization

Atom

Molecule

Organelle

Cell

Tissue

Organ

Organ System

Organism
(The Human Body)

technologies, such as flow cytometry, amplification of genetic material, and specific probing, the ways of seeking information about cellular functions continue to expand.

Deoxyribonucleic acid (DNA) is a long molecule commonly described as a *double helix*
or *twisted ladder.* The molecule contains thousands of **genes,** which carry the code for an individual's genetic makeup, such as eye color, sex, and height. An individual's DNA contains
the *DNA-coded blueprint* that was inherited from that person's parents. Genes also instruct
the body to make the proteins needed to sustain life. Although each nucleus has a complete
set of genes (except the egg and the sperm, each of which contains half a set), only certain
genes are used in each cell to perform the cell's specific functions. DNA also duplicates exact
copies of itself. An individual's DNA directs the development, growth, and functioning of all
body systems and makes each individual's body unique, except in the case of identical twins.

Survival is the primary function of the human body, and many complex processes work
independently and together to achieve this function. In human physiology, the body strives
for a **steady state,** or **homeostasis.** Literally, *homeostasis* means "remaining the same." It
is a condition in which a healthy body, although constantly changing and functioning, remains in a normal, healthy condition. Homeostasis, or a steady-state condition, allows the
normal body to stay in balance by compensating with changes. For example, if the body is
taking in too much water, it responds to this imbalance by excreting water from the kidneys
(urine), skin (perspiration), intestines (feces), and lungs (water in expiration) (Fig. 2–5).

Figure 2–3. Basic cellular structure and components.

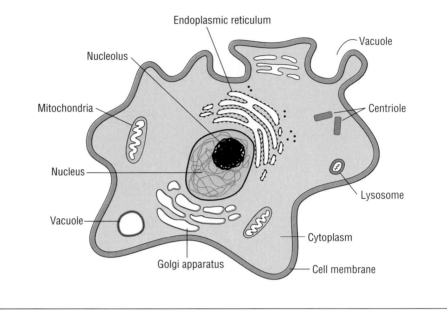

Figure 2–4. Various cell structures.

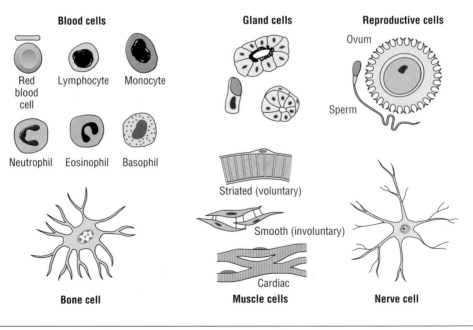

Figure 2–5. Homeostasis. The human body stays in balance by compensating with changes. When the body needs fluid, a person becomes thirsty and drinks water, which is then absorbed in the intestines. Conversely, if the body retains too much fluid, it reacts by excreting water from the kidneys (urine), skin (perspiration), intestines (feces), and lungs (water droplets as we exhale).

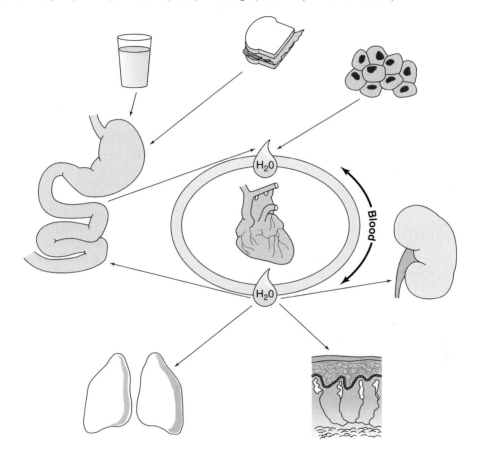

A healthy body maintains constancy of its chemical components and processes in order to survive. Each organ system and body structure plays a part in maintaining homeostasis.

Another important function of the human body is **metabolism.** This process involves making necessary substances or breaking down chemical substances in order to use energy. **Catabolism** is a series of chemical reactions produced in cells to change complex substances into simpler ones while simultaneously releasing energy. This process provides energy for all body functions, whether for moving a chair or for allowing a heart to beat. Conversely, **anabolism** is a process by which cells use energy to make complex compounds from simpler ones. It allows synthesis of body fluids, such as sweat, tears, saliva, and chemical constituents (enzymes, hormones, and antibodies). Both phases are required to maintain metabolic functions in a healthy individual.

As mentioned previously, in a normal, healthy body, structural and functional aspects work together. Organization of all the body structures, such as cells, tissues, organs, and systems, together with proper functioning, such as digestion, respiration, circulation, nerve sensitivity, movement, and secretion, provide for a healthy individual. Systems working together can keep a body metabolizing properly and in homeostasis, which is the basis of survival.

Laboratory testing can provide a wealth of information about the individual organ systems and the integrated processes. Specimens, such as blood, bone marrow, urine, cerebrospinal fluid (CSF), pleural fluid, biopsy tissue, seminal fluid, and others, can be microscopically analyzed, assayed, and cultured to determine pathogenesis.[1,2]

■ MAJOR ORGAN SYSTEMS

This section summarizes the functions of the 11 major organ systems (Table 2–2). For each body system, a corresponding box provides a brief summary of the structure, function, disorders, and common diagnostic tests for that system.

INTEGUMENTARY SYSTEM

The **integumentary system** consists of the skin, hair, sweat and oil glands, teeth, and fingernails (Box 2–1). It is primarily involved in protective and regulatory functions. Intact skin protects the deeper tissues by providing a barrier to entering microorganisms and foreign bodies and by protecting such tissues from heat, cold, and other hazardous exposures. The skin also prevents water loss or allows for perspiration as needed by the body during exercise, fever, or weather conditions. Sebaceous glands in the skin produce oils for hair and skin protection, and sweat glands produce perspiration, which helps cool the body as needed and eliminates some waste. **Melanin** in the skin provides skin color and protects underlying tissues from absorbing ultraviolet rays. Ultraviolet light stimulates production of inactive vitamin D in the skin. The liver and kidneys then activate vitamin D so that it is beneficial to the body. Other functions of the skin are to store fat in the layers next to the underlying tissues and to allow an individual to experience sensations, such as touch, temperature, pain, and

Table 2–2. Normal Body Functions Controlled by Organ Systems

NORMAL BODY FUNCTIONS	ORGAN SYSTEMS
Protection	Integumentary
Support	Skeletal
Movement	Muscular
Control	Nervous
Regulation	Endocrine
Fluid Regulation	Cardiovascular
Transport	Lymphatic
Environmental Control and Exchange	Respiratory
	Digestive
	Urinary
Birth	Reproductive

> **BOX 2–1.** INTEGUMENTARY SYSTEM
>
> **Components:**
>
> - Skin, sweat and oil glands
> - Hair
> - Fingernails
> - Teeth
>
> **Functions:**
>
> - Protects underlying tissues
> - Regulates body temperature
> - Eliminates some wastes
> - Receives sensory stimuli, such as touch, pressure, temperature, pain
> - Prevents water loss
>
> **Disorders:**
>
> - Acne
> - Burns
> - Carcinoma and other skin cancers
> - Fungal infections
> - Herpes
> - Impetigo
> - Keloid
> - Pediculosis
> - Pruritus
> - Psoriasis
>
> **Diagnostic Tests:**
>
> - Biopsies
> - KOH preparations for skin scrapings
> - Microbiological cultures
> - Tissue cultures

pressure. Hair on the head provides protection by acting as a heat insulator, eyebrows keep perspiration out of the eyes, eyelashes protect eyes from foreign objects, and hairs in the nasal passages filter out dust and harmful microorganisms. Likewise, fingernails protect the tips of the hands. Teeth aid in breaking up food to begin the digestive process.

Integumentary system disorders include bacterial infections, such as acne, impetigo (caused by *Staphylococcus aureus*), and decubitis ulcers; viral infections, such as fever blisters or cold sores, rubeola, rubella, chickenpox, and herpes zoster (shingles); fungal infections, such as ringworm and athlete's foot; allergic reactions, such as dermatitis and eczema; psoriasis; and skin cancers, such as malignant melanoma. Diagnostic tests for many of these conditions involve skin scrapings; bacteriologic, viral, or fungal tissue cultures; potassium hydroxide (KOH) preparations; or biopsy staining procedures.

SKELETAL SYSTEM

The **skeletal system** refers to all bones and joints of the body. This system comprises primarily two types of tissue: bone and cartilage. Bone is composed of cells surrounded by calcified intercellular substances that allow for a rigid structure. **Cartilage** is composed of similar cells, but these cells are surrounded by a gelatinous material, instead of calcified substances, that allows for more flexibility. Likewise, tendons and ligaments provide flexibility and leverage. The skeletal system serves the body in five major ways: support, protection for softer tissues (brain and lungs), movement and leverage, **hematopoiesis** (blood cell formation) in the bone marrow, and mineral storage (Box 2–2).

More than 200 bones are contained in the human body, and they are classified into four groups on the basis of their shapes. Long bones include leg bones (e.g., femur, tibia, fibula) and arm and hand bones (e.g., humerus, radius, ulna, phalanges). Short bones include carpals and tarsals, or wrist and ankle bones, respectively. Among flat bones are several cranial bones, the

BOX 2–2. SKELETAL SYSTEM

Components:

- Bones
- Cartilage
- Tendons
- Ligaments
- Joints

Functions:

- Provides support
- Protects organs
- Allows leverage and movement
- Produces blood cells
- Stores minerals

Disorders:

- Arthritis
- Bursitis
- Gout
- Osteomyelitis
- Osteoporosis
- Rickets
- Tumors

Diagnostic Tests:

- Alkaline phosphatase (ALP)
- Calcium
- Complete blood cell (CBC) count
- Erythrocyte sedimentation rate (ESR)
- Phosphorus
- Synovial fluid analysis
- Uric acid
- Vitamin D

ribs, and the scapulae (or shoulder blades). Finally, irregular bones include cranial bones (e.g., sphenoid, ethmoid) and bones of the vertebral column (e.g., vertebrae, sacrum, coccyx).

Bones are connected to each other by a variety of joints that permit flexion, extension, abduction (away from median), adduction (toward median), rotation, and combinations of these movements (Fig. 2–6). Bone structure differs between male and female skeletons. Besides being somewhat larger and heavier, the male has a pelvis that is deeper with a narrow pubic arch. In contrast, the female pelvis is shallow and broad and has a wider pubic arch to facilitate childbirth.

In general, bones consist of several layers covered by a membrane, the periosteum. The periosteum contains blood vessels that bring blood from inside the bone to the outer layer. The outer layer, or compact bone, is more rigid and heavier than the inner layer, which is like a honeycomb. This inner layer is called *spongy bone* but is just as strong as compact bone. In the center of a bone is the marrow, which produces most blood cells. Approximately 5 billion RBCs are produced daily by about 1/2 lb (227 g) of bone marrow. Marrow is located in all the bones of an infant, but in adults it is in the skull, sternum (or breastbone), vertebrae, hipbones, and ends of the long bones.[1]

Minerals stored in bones include calcium and phosphorus. When these minerals are needed in other parts of the body, they are released from the bone through the bloodstream.

Skeletal system disorders include inflammatory conditions such as arthritis and bursitis; gout; bacterial infections such as osteomyelitis; porous bone conditions such as osteoporosis; developmental conditions such as gigantism, dwarfism, and rickets; and bone tumors. Laboratory assessment of skeletal system disorders can include serum calcium and phosphate levels, serum alkaline phosphatase (ALP) levels, uric acid, vitamin D, erythrocyte sedimentation rate (ESR), complete blood cell (CBC) counts, microscopic analysis, and microbial cultures of the bone marrow and synovial fluid (fluid between joints and bones).

Figure 2–6. Skeleton.

MUSCULAR SYSTEM

The **muscular system** refers to all muscles of the body, including those attached to bones and those along walls of internal structures, such as the heart. On the basis of location, microscopic structure, and neural control, muscles are classified as follows: (1) **skeletal (striated voluntary) muscles**—attached to bones; (2) **visceral (nonstriated [smooth] involuntary) muscles**—line the walls of internal structures, such as veins and arteries; and (3) **cardiac (striated involuntary) muscles**—make up the wall of the heart (Box 2–3). Muscles provide movement, maintain posture, and produce heat. Movement takes place not only during locomotion, but also during body movements, changes in the size of openings, and propulsion of substances (e.g., propulsion of blood through veins or passage of food through intestines). Posture is maintained during sitting and standing by continued

---

BOX 2–3. MUSCULAR SYSTEM

Components:

- Skeletal muscle
- Cardiac muscle (heart)
- Smooth muscle (walls of hollow organs)

Functions:

- Permits movement
- Produces heat
- Maintains posture

Disorders:

- Atrophy
- Muscular dystrophy (MD)

- Myalgia
- Tendinitis

Diagnostic Tests:

- Autoimmune antibodies
- CK isoenzymes
- Creatine phosphokinase (CPK)
- Lactate dehydrogenase (LDH or LD)
- Lactic acid
- Myoglobin

---

partial contraction of specific muscles. Muscle cells that provide mechanical energy for movement also release energy in the form of heat. All three muscle types work by extending, contracting, conducting, and being easily stimulated.

Skeletal muscles (more than 400 in humans) compose approximately 40 percent of a man's body. In contrast, women have less muscle and more fat than that in men. Muscles are strongest at about age 25, but with proper nutrition and exercise, they can remain strong throughout life. Without sufficient exercise, muscles become smaller and weaker. Glycogen is the form of stored glucose in muscles. Without stores of glycogen, muscles must wait for glucose, which is transported through the bloodstream. Exercise increases the amount of glycogen available for muscles, which in turn allows them to function more easily.

Muscular system disorders include muscular dystrophy (MD), conditions that disrupt nerve stimulation (as in severe accidents or myasthenia gravis), muscle cramps and tendinitis, and viral infections, such as multiple sclerosis (MS) and polio.

Laboratory testing of muscular system disorders often involves clinical assays of specific muscle enzymes, such as creatine phosphokinase (CK) and lactate dehydrogenase (LDH), analysis of autoimmune antibodies, microscopic examination, or culturing of biopsy tissue.

NERVOUS SYSTEM

The **nervous system** provides communication in the body, sensations, thoughts, emotions, and memories. Nerve impulses and chemical substances regulate, control, integrate, and organize body functions. The nervous system is composed of specialized nerve cells **(neurons)**, the brain, the spinal cord, brain and cord coverings, fluid, and the nerve impulse itself. An estimated 10 billion neurons or more reside in the human body, most of which are in the brain. Sensory neurons transmit nerve impulses to the spinal cord or the brain from muscle tissues. Motor neurons transmit impulses to muscles from the spinal

Plate 1. Superficial anatomy of the heart. (Top) Anterior (sternocostal) view of the heart showing major anatomic features. (Bottom) Posterior (diaphragmatic) surface of the heart. (Coronary arteries are shown in red, coronary veins in blue.)

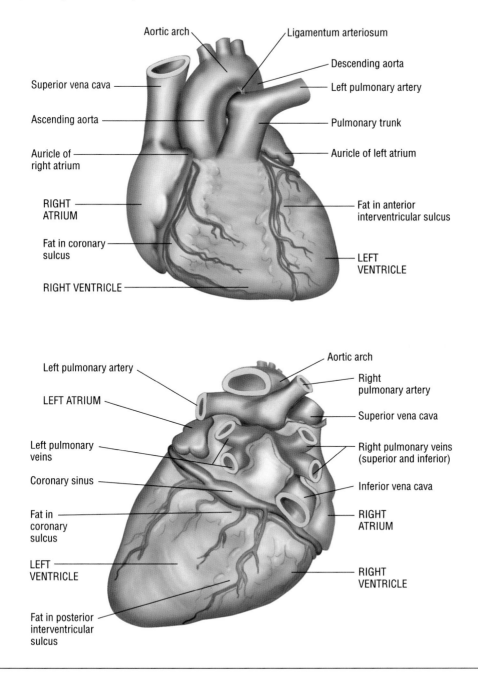

Plate 2. Sectional anatomy of the heart. A diagrammatic frontal section through the heart showing major landmarks and the path of blood flow through the atria and ventricles.

Aortic arch

Ligamentum arteriosum

Pulmonary trunk

Pulmonary semilunar valve

Superior vena cava

Right pulmonary arteries

Left pulmonary artery

LEFT ATRIUM

Right pulmonary veins

Left pulmonary veins

Interatrial septum

Aortic semi-lunar valve

Pectinate muscles

Cusp of left AV (bicuspid) valve

RIGHT ATRIUM

Chordae tendineae

Fossa ovalis

Papillary muscles

Cusp of right AV (tricuspid) valve

LEFT VENTRICLE

Inferior vena cava

Trabeculae carneae

RIGHT VENTRICLE

Descending (thoracic) aorta

Interventricular septum

Plate 3. The pulmonary circuit. The right ventricle of the heart pumps blood into the pulmonary artery (pulmonary trunk), which divides into the right and left pulmonary arteries that go to each lung. In the lungs the arteries branch extensively into small arteries and arterioles, then to capillaries. The capillaries surround the alveoli so that exchange of oxygen and carbon dioxide can take place. The capillaries flow into veins and finally into the two pulmonary veins that return blood to the heart through the left atrium. This oxygenated blood will then travel to the rest of the body. (Note that the pulmonary veins contain oxygenated blood. They are the only veins that carry blood with a high oxygen content. All other veins of the body carry blood with a low oxygen content.)

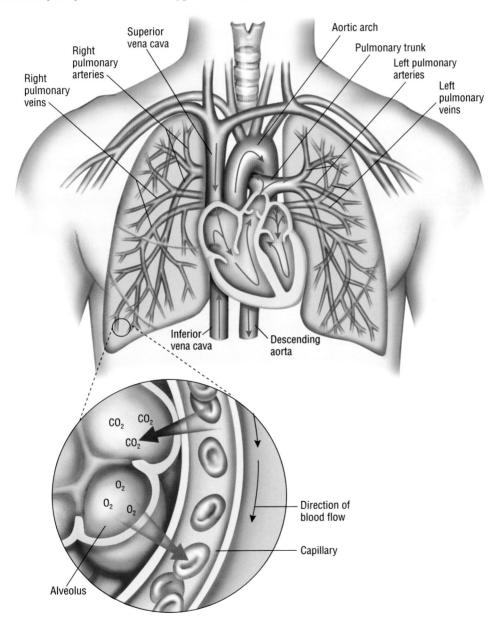

Plate 4. Exchange of gases in systemic and pulmonary capillaries. Oxygen (O_2) and carbon dioxide (CO_2) molecules are carried in red blood cells by hemoglobin (Hb) molecules. In the systemic or tissue capillaries, O_2 is released and CO_2 is picked up. When the red cell returns to the pulmonary capillaries in the lungs, CO_2 is released and O_2 is picked up.

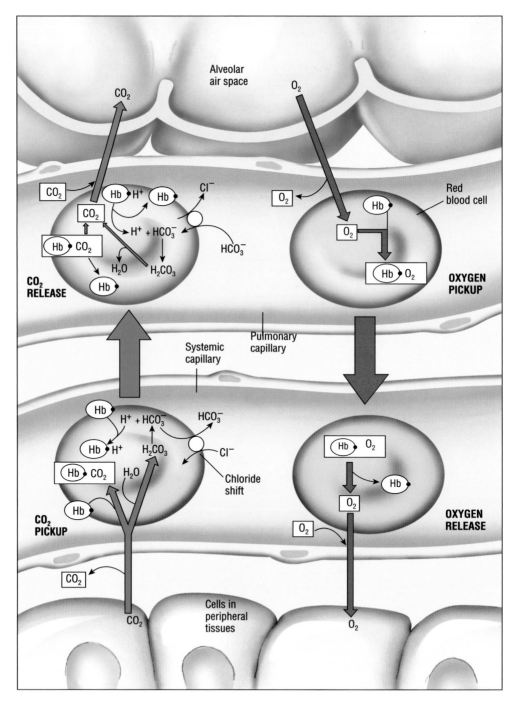

Plate 5. The arterial system.

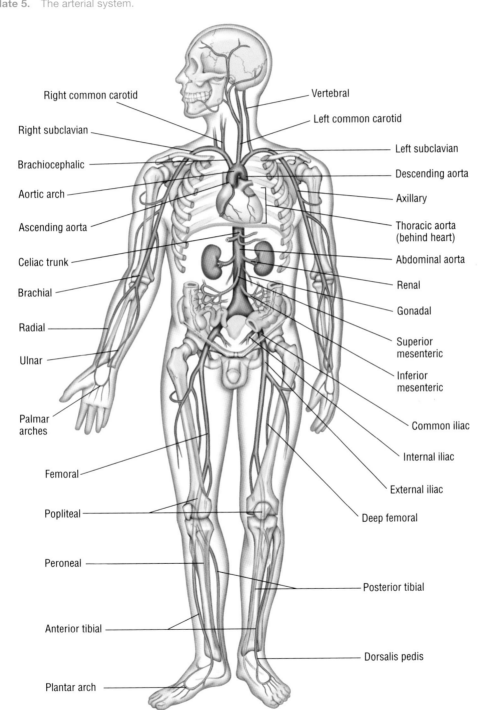

Right common carotid

Right subclavian

Brachiocephalic

Aortic arch

Ascending aorta

Celiac trunk

Brachial

Radial

Ulnar

Palmar arches

Femoral

Popliteal

Peroneal

Anterior tibial

Plantar arch

Vertebral

Left common carotid

Left subclavian

Descending aorta

Axillary

Thoracic aorta (behind heart)

Abdominal aorta

Renal

Gonadal

Superior mesenteric

Inferior mesenteric

Common iliac

Internal iliac

External iliac

Deep femoral

Posterior tibial

Dorsalis pedis

Plate 6. An overview of the venous system.

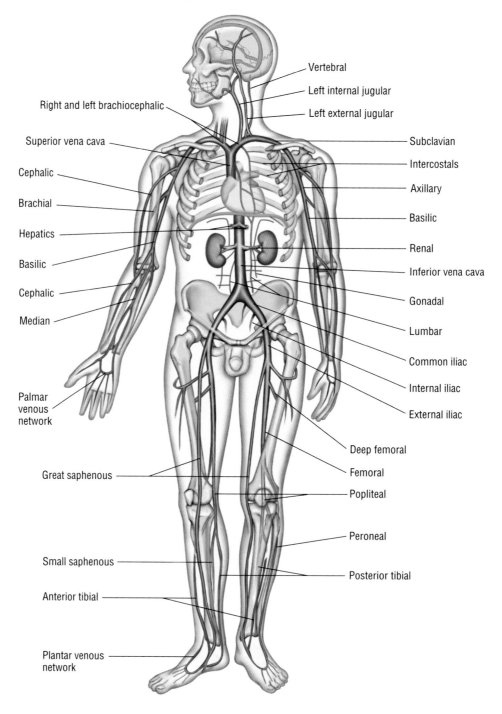

Vertebral

Left internal jugular

Left external jugular

Right and left brachiocephalic

Superior vena cava

Subclavian

Cephalic

Intercostals

Brachial

Axillary

Hepatics

Basilic

Basilic

Renal

Cephalic

Inferior vena cava

Median

Gonadal

Lumbar

Common iliac

Internal iliac

Palmar
venous
network

External iliac

Deep femoral

Great saphenous

Femoral

Popliteal

Peroneal

Small saphenous

Posterior tibial

Anterior tibial

Plantar venous
network

Plate 7. Venous drainage of the abdomen and chest.

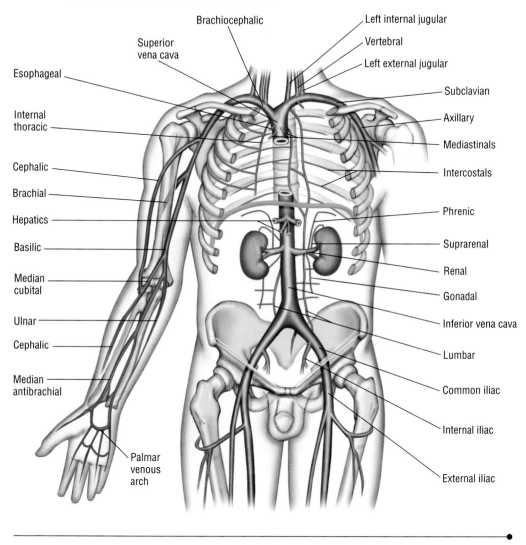

Brachiocephalic

Superior vena cava

Left internal jugular

Vertebral

Left external jugular

Esophageal

Internal thoracic

Subclavian

Axillary

Mediastinals

Cephalic

Intercostals

Brachial

Hepatics

Phrenic

Basilic

Suprarenal

Median cubital

Renal

Ulnar

Gonadal

Cephalic

Inferior vena cava

Median antibrachial

Lumbar

Common iliac

Internal iliac

Palmar venous arch

External iliac

Plate 8.   Circulation through vessels of the forearm in warm and cold environments. **A.** Circulation through the blood vessels of the forearm in a warm environment. Blood enters the limb in a deep artery and returns to the trunk in a network of superficial veins. These veins radiate heat into the environment through the overlying skin. **B.** Circulation through the blood vessels of the forearm in a cold environment. Blood now returns to the trunk via a network of deep veins that flow around the artery. The amount of heat loss is reduced, as is indicated in C. **C.** Countercurrent heat exchange occurs as heat radiates from the warm arterial blood to the cool venous blood flowing in the opposite direction. By the time the arterial blood reaches the distal capillaries, where most of the heat loss to the environment occurs, it is substantially cooler than it was when it left the trunk. This mechanism reduces the rate of heat loss while conserving body heat. In effect, the countercurrent exchange traps heat near the trunk.

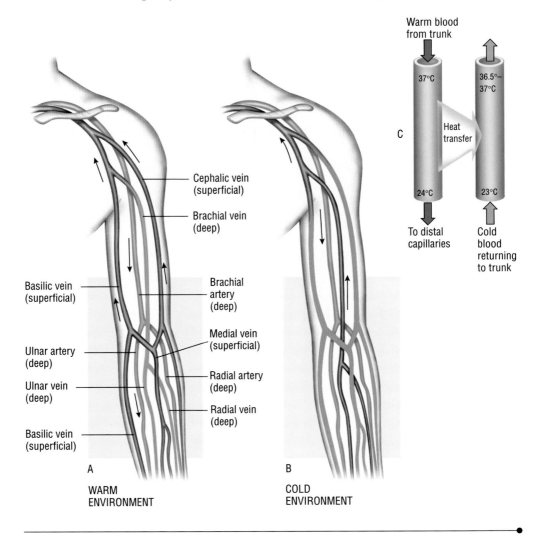

cord or the brain. Both the brain and the spinal cord are covered by protective membranes (**meninges**). Between these protective membrane layers are CSF-filled spaces that provide a cushion for the brain and the spinal cord. Furthermore, the brain and spinal cord are protected by the skull and vertebral column respectively. The bony segments of the vertebral canal are divided into regions (cervical, thoracic, and lumbar vertebrae). There are seven cervical vertebrae (C1–C7) that extend from the head to the thorax, twelve thoracic vertebrae (T1–T12) that extend from the chest to the back, and five lumbar vertebrae (L1–L5) that extend to the lower back. At the lower end of the vertebral column the sacrum (S1–S5) and coccyx are fused elements of the sacral and coccygeal vertebrae.

The brain has many vitally important areas. Along with the cranial nerves, its functions include all mental processes and many essential motor, sensory, and visceral responses. The spinal cord and the spinal nerves control sensory (touch), motor (voluntary movement), and reflex (knee-jerk) functions. Reflexes are responses to stimuli that do not require communication with the brain. A simple reflex, such as moving a finger from something hot, occurs even before the brain realizes the pain. Specific cranial and spinal nerves control all complex or simple action processes in the body. There are 31 pairs of spinal nerves (nerves that branch off of the spinal cord), each of which is identified by its location to the nearest vertebrae. Nerves that branch from the spinal cord (C5 through T1) and extend into the arm region (the brachial plexus) are the axillary, radial, musculocutaneous, median, and ulnar nerves. Refer to the front cover sheet in the Color Atlas. These nerves control all muscle movement of the shoulder, arm, and hand, and also control sensations of the skin of the entire shoulder, arm, and hand. In summary, the nervous system is the primary communication and regulatory system in the body (Box 2–4).

BOX 2–4. NERVOUS SYSTEM

Components:

- Brain
- Spinal cord
- Nerves
- Sense organs: eyes, ears, tongue, and sensory receptor in the skin

Functions:

- Allows communication throughout the body and regulates body functions
- Detects sensations (pain, pressure)
- Controls movements and physiological functions
- Controls intellectual processes

Disorders:

- Amyotrophic lateral sclerosis (ALS)
- Encephalitis
- Epilepsy
- Hydrocephaly
- Meningitis
- Multiple sclerosis (MS)
- Neuralgia
- Parkinson's disease
- Shingles

Diagnostic Tests:

- Acetylcholine receptor antibody
- Cerebrospinal fluid (CSF) analysis
- Cholinesterase
- Drug levels

⚠️ **Clinical Alert**

Nerve damage has also been known to occur as a result of accidental injury during phlebotomy procedures. Injury may be the result of excessive probing with the venipuncture needle, sticking the needle in a poor site for venipuncture, deep needle penetration all the way to the nerve, and/or if the patient suddenly jerks his arm during the venipuncture procedure causing the needle to puncture a nerve. The front cover sheet indicates the proximity of nerves to arteries and veins. Health care professionals should choose sites that are least likely to cause nerve damage (refer to Chapter 8) and take precautions to have the patient's movements stabilized as much as possible. Under no circumstances should phlebotomists use the anterior or palmar side of the wrist to collect a blood specimen because the risk of hitting a nerve is high due to nerve location close to the skin surface.

Nervous system disorders include infectious conditions, such as encephalitis, meningitis, tetanus, herpes, and poliomyelitis, and conditions such as amyotrophic lateral sclerosis (ALS), MS, Parkinson's disease, cerebral palsy (CP), tumors, epilepsy, hydrocephaly, neuralgia, and headaches.

Laboratory diagnosis of nervous system disorders is not very specific. Chemical assays can reveal drug interactions, as well as hormonal, protein, and enzyme alterations. Infections can be detected by bacterial, viral, or fungal cultures or by the presence of specific antibodies in the CSF.

RESPIRATORY SYSTEM

Respiration allows for the exchange of gases between blood and air. Once gases enter the blood, the circulatory system transports them between lungs and tissues. Together, the respiratory and circulatory systems carry O_2 to the cells and remove CO_2 from the tissue cells. Oxygen allows the body to burn its fuel from the nutrients eaten. It makes up about one fifth of the air around us. The average person inhales and exhales about 15 times per minute or approximately 20,000 times per day. As a person breathes in, the O_2 travels through air passages to the lungs. In the lungs, the exchange of gases occurs. Oxygen is exchanged for CO_2, which is then breathed out as the person exhales.

The main components of the **respiratory system** are in the head, the neck, and the thoracic cavity and include the nose, the pharynx, the larynx, the trachea, the bronchi, and the lungs (Box 2–5).

Receptors in the nose provide the sense of smell and allow for changes in voice. The nose also functions as the primary filter for air entering the body. It catches impurities and chemical substances that may irritate the respiratory system. In the nose, the throat, and the bronchial tree, mucus is continuously produced to trap unwanted particles and prevent them from entering the lungs or vocal cords. Tiny hairlike cilia line the passageways and sweep the mucus to the nose and mouth so that it can be coughed up, sneezed, or swallowed. The pharynx is a tubelike passageway for both food and air. Along with the larynx

> ## BOX 2–5.   RESPIRATORY SYSTEM
>
> ### Components:
>
> - Nasal cavity
> - Pharynx
> - Larynx
> - Trachea
> - Bronchi
> - Lungs
>
> ### Functions:
>
> - Filters air, exchanges gases
> - Supplies oxygen and removes carbon dioxide
> - Helps regulate blood pH
> - Protects vocal cords
>
> ### Disorders:
>
> - Asthma
> - Bronchitis
> - Cystic fibrosis
> - Emphysema
> - Pleurisy
> - Pneumonia
> - Respiratory distress syndrome
> - Respiratory syncytial virus
> - Respiratory tract infections
> - Rhinitis
> - Tonsillitis
> - Tuberculosis
>
> ### Diagnostic Tests:
>
> - Alkaline phosphatase (ALP)
> - Arterial blood gases
> - Complete blood cell (CBC) count
> - Bronchial washings
> - Drug levels
> - Electrolytes
> - Microbiological cultures
> - Pleuracentesis
> - Sputum cultures
> - Tuberculin skin test

(voice box), it determines the quality of voice. The trachea and the bronchial passages provide openings for outside air to reach the lungs. Within the bronchi are grapelike **alveolar sacs** that are enveloped by capillaries and allow diffusion between air and blood. The lungs are structured into millions of branches of alveoli with surrounding capillaries and therefore can quickly take in large amounts of O_2 and release large amounts of CO_2 if they are functioning properly. (Refer to Plate 4 in the Color Atlas.) The lungs are soft and spongy and reach from just above the collarbone down to the diaphragm. They have no muscles; consequently, the diaphragm and other surrounding muscles help enlarge and contract the chest cavity as respiration occurs. Humans have two lungs; the right lung has three lobes, and the left lung has only two, to allow room for the heart. An adult's lungs hold 3 to 4 qt (approximately 3 to 4 L) of air, depending on how vigorously the person is moving or exercising. In patients with pneumonia, the alveolar sacs become inflamed, and fluid or waste products block the minute air spaces, thus normal O_2 and CO_2 exchange is difficult.

Red blood cells transport O_2 and CO_2 as part of a molecule called *hemoglobin.* After O_2 crosses the respiratory membranes (in the lung) into the blood, about 97 percent of the O_2 combines with the iron-containing heme portion of hemoglobin. The remaining 3 percent dissolves in plasma. Hemoglobin carries O_2 from the alveolar capillaries through the blood vessels to the tissue capillaries. Oxygen and CO_2 rapidly combine with hemoglobin to form oxyhemoglobin and carbaminohemoglobin, respectively (Fig. 2–7). (Refer to Plate 4 in the Color Atlas.)

Figure 2–7. Oxygen (O_2) and carbon dioxide (CO_2) are transported by hemoglobin inside red blood cells. Red blood cells move from the lungs (where they pick up O_2) to the tissues (where O_2 is needed). When the hemoglobin releases the O_2 in the tissues, it picks up CO_2, and the red blood cells transport it back to the lungs. CO_2 is released in the lungs and is replaced by more O_2. Thus the cycle continues, and the body has enough oxygen to function normally.

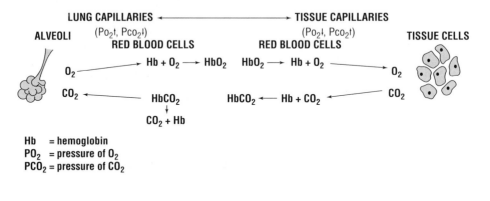

Association (chemical combination) and dissociation (chemical release) with hemoglobin depends on the gaseous pressure. In lung capillaries, O_2 pressure (partial pressure of oxygen [Po_2]) increases and CO_2 (partial pressure of carbon dioxide [Pco_2]) decreases, which allows O_2 to rapidly associate, or combine chemically, with hemoglobin, and CO_2 to dissociate, or be released, from carbaminohemoglobin. Thus, humans inhale O_2 into the lungs and exhale CO_2 from the lungs. In tissue capillaries, the opposite occurs: O_2 pressure decreases and CO_2 pressure increases, which allows O_2 to dissociate from oxyhemoglobin and CO_2 to combine with hemoglobin. Thus, O_2 is released into tissues and muscles, and CO_2 is picked up, taken to the lungs, and exhaled (Fig. 2–8).

Carbon dioxide has an important effect on the pH (acidity) of the blood. Normal body pH has a narrow range of between 7.35 and 7.45. Deviations from the normal or reference range can be dangerous and deadly. As CO_2 levels increase, the blood pH decreases (becomes more acidic). As the CO_2 level in the blood increases, chemoreceptors in the brain cause a faster and deeper rate of respiration (**hyperventilation**) in order to blow off excess CO_2 from the body. (The urinary system also plays a role in maintaining body pH, as described later in this chapter.) Gas pressure and blood pH levels can be measured in the clinical laboratory from appropriate blood samples.

Respiratory system disorders include infectious conditions, such as tuberculosis, laryngitis, bronchitis, whooping cough, pneumonia, and influenza; conditions such as asthma, emphysema, and cystic fibrosis; and tumors. Laboratory blood tests for chemical constituents (sodium, chloride, bicarbonate, ALP, and potassium) often indicate respiratory abnormalities. Lung biopsies, throat swabs, sputum cultures, and bronchial washings can be examined microscopically or cultured for pathogenic microorganisms, such as fungi; bacteria, such as acid-fast bacilli; and parasites. Pathogenic microorganisms can cause respiratory infections, such as the common cold, sore throats, tonsillitis, rhinitis, coughs, sneez-

Figure 2–8. Enclosed circulatory system. Oxygenated blood (red) comes from the lungs and is pumped by the heart to the organs and tissues. After O$_2$ is released, the blood becomes deoxygenated (blue) and is pumped through the heart back to the lungs.

ing, runny noses, bronchitis, and more serious diseases, such as tuberculosis, *Pneumocystis carinii* pneumonia, Legionnaires' disease, pleurisy, respiratory distress syndrome, respiratory syncytial virus, and other types of pneumonia. Tuberculosis (TB) is caused by acid-fast bacilli that destroy lung tissue. It can be caught early using a TB skin test. In cases of pneumonia, the air sacs in the lungs fill with fluid, and gaseous exchanges cannot occur. *Pneumocystis* infections are considered opportunistic infections (i.e., they become pathogenic when the patient is immunosuppressed) and are associated with acquired immunodeficiency syndrome (AIDS).

DIGESTIVE SYSTEM

The **digestive system** functions, first, to break down food chemically and physically into nutrients that can be absorbed and used by body cells, and, second, to eliminate the waste products of digestion. The gastrointestinal (GI) tract is made up of the following components: mouth, pharynx, esophagus, stomach, intestines, and some vital accessory organs, such as salivary glands, teeth, liver, gallbladder, pancreas, and appendix (Box 2–6). Many proteins, enzymes, and juices are released by these components to facilitate digestion, absorption, and movement through the GI tract. The passageway of the GI tract through

BOX 2–6.   DIGESTIVE SYSTEM

Components:

- Mouth
- Salivary glands
- Esophagus
- Stomach
- Intestines
- Liver and gallbladder
- Pancreas
- Teeth
- Appendix
- Pharynx

Functions:

- Breaks down food physically and chemically
- Absorbs nutrients
- Removes solid waste

Disorders:

- Cancer
- Parasitic infections
- Polyps
- Ulcers

Diagnostic Tests:

- Occult blood test
- Ova and parasite analysis

---

which food travels is known as the *alimentary canal.* It begins at the mouth and ends at the anus. In an adult, the average length of the alimentary canal is 27 feet. Circular muscles that surround the intestines contract to assist the movement of food through the body. These wavelike contractions are called **peristalsis.** One meal can take 15 hours to 2 days to pass through the alimentary canal. Peristalsis is such an effective process that a person can even swallow upside down. If the process is reversed, vomiting enables the body to reject food. Saliva moistens food and contains an enzyme that helps begin the breakdown of carbohydrates into simple sugars such as glucose. (If a salt cracker is chewed a long time, saliva begins the breakdown process so it may taste sweet.) Also, the liver secretes bile, which aids in fat digestion and absorption. In addition, it is involved in carbohydrate metabolism, protein and fat catabolism, and synthesis of many vital blood proteins for clotting and regulatory purposes. Each component functions either mechanically or chemically to keep the body in homeostasis.

The digestive system helps regulate the intake and output of essential proteins, carbohydrates, fats, minerals, vitamins, and water. The body can then use these substances by catabolizing them for stored energy or by anabolizing them to build other complex compounds, such as hormones, other tissue proteins, and enzymes. Levels of these constituents can be clinically measured in the laboratory from blood specimens and other body fluids. Materials that are not digested in the alimentary canal are eliminated from the body as fecal material or urine.

Disorders of the oral cavity can consist of dental caries or tooth decay, and periodontal disease, which is an inflammation and degeneration of the gums, ligaments, and bone around the teeth. Stomach disorders can include hiatial hernias (protrusion through the diaphragm), vomiting, and ulcers. Intestinal disorders (affecting small and large intestines) include polyps, maldigestion, malabsorption, cancer, appendicitis, constipation, diarrhea, dysentery, and hemorrhoids. Liver inflammation is referred to as *hepatitis* and can be caused by various agents, such as excessive alcohol consumption and viral hepatitis. A common disorder of the gallbladder is gallstones, which can cause blockage of the bile duct, pain, and inflammation. Numerous bacterial and parasitic infections can also affect the digestive tract. Examples include staphylococcal food poisoning, salmonellosis, typhoid fever, cholera, giardiasis, tapeworms, pinworms, hookworms, and ascariasis (roundworm). Specific diagnostic tests may include tissue biopsies, an occult blood test, bacterial cultures, and analysis for ova and parasites.

URINARY SYSTEM

The primary purpose of the **urinary system** is to produce and eliminate urine. This system consists of two kidneys, two ureters, one bladder, and one urethra (Box 2–7). The kidneys' main function is to regulate the amount of water, electrolytes (sodium, potassium, chloride, calcium, phosphate, magnesium), and nitrogenous waste products (urea) from protein metabolism. The proper concentration of these blood constituents is vital to life. Electrolytes function to maintain the body's acid–base balance. The normal ratio of acid (carbonic acid) to base (bicarbonate) is 1 : 20. Blood pH and blood gas determinations provide useful information about acid–base balance in the body. Normal blood pH is within a range of 7.35 to 7.45. As blood passes through the specialized kidney cells, called *glomeruli,* water and solutes are filtered out. Only the necessary amounts of these substances are reabsorbed into the blood. The rest are excreted as waste products in the urine. Ureters collect urine as it forms and transport it to the bladder, which serves as a reservoir until the urine can be voided. The urethra is the terminal component of the urinary system. In women, it is merely a passageway from the bladder, whereas in men, it eliminates both urine and semen from the body.

BOX 2–7.   URINARY SYSTEM

Components:

- Kidneys
- Ureters
- Bladder
- Urethra

Functions:

- Filters blood to eliminate waste
- Helps maintain blood pH
- Regulates water balance

Disorders:

- Cystitis
- Kidney stones
- Nephritis
- Renal failure
- Uremia
- Urinary tract infection (UTI)

Diagnostic Tests:

- Albumin
- Ammonia
- Blood urea nitrogen (BUN)
- Creatinine clearance
- Electrolytes
- Osmolality
- Urinalysis
- Urine cultures

Two thirds of human body weight is water. About 60 percent of the body's water is inside cells, and the rest is in the bloodstream or tissue fluids. The salt content of the body's water is extremely important for survival. When excess salt is in the tissues, the kidneys eliminate it; if there is excess water, the kidneys eliminate it. If the kidneys are not functioning properly, a mechanical filtering process (dialysis) must be used or one of the kidneys must be replaced with a transplant.

Acidosis occurs when the blood pH decreases to less than 7.35. If the condition worsens, the individual can become comatose. **Respiratory acidosis** results when the respiratory system is unable to eliminate adequate amounts of CO_2 (in conditions such as a collapsed lung or blockage of respiratory passages). **Metabolic acidosis** occurs when the kidneys cannot eliminate acidic substances (in conditions such as diabetes mellitus). Such acidosis can result in kidney (renal) failure and death.

Alkalosis results when the blood pH increases to more than 7.45. **Respiratory alkalosis** results from hyperventilation or the loss of too much CO_2 from the lungs. **Metabolic alkalosis** usually results from excessive vomiting or an abnormal secretion of certain hormones that cause excess elimination of hydrogen ions (from CO_2). The kidneys are vitally important in compensating for *respiratory* acidosis or alkalosis. Conversely, the respiratory system is vitally important in compensating for *metabolic* acidosis or alkalosis.

Laboratory assessment of urinary function includes the detection of osmolality, chemical constituents, such as proteins, blood, microorganisms, and cells in the urine, as well as chemical analysis of albumin, ammonia, blood urea nitrogen, blood pH, blood gases, and electrolytes in the blood. Various urine collection techniques and preservatives are available. The creatinine clearance test evaluates the degree to which kidneys are filtering out waste products of metabolism.

REPRODUCTIVE SYSTEM

Male reproductive structures include the testes, the seminal vesicles, the prostate gland, the epididymis, the seminal ducts, the urethra, the scrotum, the penis, and the spermatic cords. The primary functions of this system are spermatogenesis (sperm production); storage, maintenance, and excretion of seminal fluid; and secretion of hormones (the most important of which is testosterone). Female reproductive structures include the ovaries, the fallopian tubes, the uterus, the vagina, the vulva, and the mammary glands. These structures play a role in ovulation, fertilization, menstruation, pregnancy, labor, lactation, and secretion of hormones (estrogens and progesterone) (Box 2–8).

A sperm is one of the smallest cells in the body, whereas the mature egg is the largest. Each of these cells contains a nucleus with 23 chromosomes. Because a mother's egg and a father's sperm contain different sets of DNA, various genetic characteristics are paired. One of the pairs of chromosomes determines the sex of the fetus. The egg contains only an X chromosome; however, the sperm may contain an X or a Y chromosome. Therefore, if an X sperm fertilizes the egg, an XX pair of chromosomes forms, and the neonate will be a girl. If a Y sperm fertilizes the egg, an XY pair forms, and the neonate will be a boy. The 46 combined chromosomes contain the DNA-coded blueprint for the newborn. The DNA controls not only the sex, but all characteristics, such as height; eye, hair, and skin color; immunity to diseases; allergies; and many other factors.

BOX 2–8.   REPRODUCTIVE SYSTEM

Components:

- Male: testes, penis, duct system, glands
- Female: ovaries, uterine tubes, uterus, vagina, external genitalia
  Accessory organs: mammary glands

Functions:

- Secretes hormones
- Produces germ cells for reproduction (sperm and ova)
- In the female, maintains fetus and produces milk for nourishment of neonate

Disorders:

- Cervical, ovarian, uterine cancer
- Infertility
- Ovarian cyst
- Prostate, testicular cancer
- Sexually transmitted diseases (STDs)

Diagnostic Tests:

- Acid phosphatase
- Estrogen
- Follicle-stimulating hormone (FSH)
- Human chorionic gonadotropin (HCG)
- Luteinizing hormone (LH)
- Microbiological cultures
- Pap smear
- Rapid plasma reagin (RPR)
- Testosterone
- Tissue analysis

Disorders of the **reproductive system** include cancers, infertility, cysts, and **sexually transmitted diseases (STDs),** such as gonorrhea, genital herpes, syphilis, and **human immunodeficiency virus (HIV).** Diagnostic tests for such disorders include semen and cytogenetic analysis, as well as biopsies, Pap smears, and microbiological and viral cultures of infected areas. Blood tests include hormonal analysis (e.g., estrogen, follicle-stimulating hormone [FSH], luteinizing hormone [LH], human chorionic gonadotropin [HCG], testosterone) the rapid plasma reagin [RPR] test for syphilis, and acid phosphatase and prostatic specific antigen (PSA) for diagnosing and monitoring of prostate cancer.

ENDOCRINE SYSTEM

The human body has two types of glands. **Exocrine glands** secrete fluids, such as sweat, saliva, mucus, and digestive juices, which are transported through channels or ducts. **Endocrine glands,** or ductless glands, release their secretions (hormones) directly into the bloodstream. This glandular system has the same functions as those of the nervous system: communication, control, and integration. **Hormones** play an important role in metabolic regulation that influences growth and development, in fluid and electrolyte balance, in energy balance, and in acid-base balance. Hormonal imbalances can lead to severe disorders, such as dwarfism, gigantism, and sterility.

Endocrine glands include pituitary, thyroid, parathyroid, thymus, and adrenal glands, as well as ovaries and testes (Box 2–9). The **pituitary gland,** or *master gland,* as it is sometimes called, stimulates the other glands to produce hormones as needed. It controls and

BOX 2–9.   ENDOCRINE SYSTEM

Components:

- Hormone-producing structures: pituitary, pineal, thyroid, parathyroid, thymus, and adrenal glands
- Ovaries, testes, and pancreas

Functions:

- Composes a communications system that uses hormones as chemical messengers
- Helps maintain homeostasis
- Regulates body activities, such as metabolism and reproduction

Disorders:

- Acromegaly
- Addison's disease
- Cretinism
- Cushing's syndrome
- Diabetes insipidus
- Diabetes mellitus
- Dwarfism
- Gigantism
- Goiter
- Hyperinsulinism
- Hypoglycemia
- Hypo- and hyperthyroidism

Diagnostic Tests:

- Adrenocorticotropic hormone (ACTH)
- Aldosterone
- Antidiuretic hormone (ADH)
- Cortisol
- Erythropoietin
- Glucagon
- Glucose tolerance tests (GTTs)
- Growth hormone (GH)
- Insulin
- Renin
- Serotonin
- Thyroid function: triiodothyronine (T_3), thyroxine (T_4), thyroid-stimulating hormone (TSH)

regulates hormone production through chemical feedback. The pituitary hormones also regulate retention of water by the kidneys, cause uterine contractions during childbirth, stimulate breast milk production, and produce growth hormone (GH). This hormone controls growth by regulating the nutrients that are taken into cells. It also works with insulin to control blood sugar levels. If blood sugar is not controlled, diabetes mellitus, the most common disorder of the endocrine system, can result. The thyroid gland produces a hormone that affects cell metabolism and growth rate. Parathyroid glands regulate calcium and phosphorus in the blood and the bones. The thymus gland affects the lymphoid system. The **adrenals** (two glands) produce hormones as a result of emotions like fright or anger. This hormone production causes an increase in blood pressure, widened pupils, and heart stimulation. The adrenals also produce hormones that regulate carbohydrate metabolism and electrolyte balance.[1] As mentioned earlier, ovaries and testes produce estrogens and progesterone, and testosterone, respectively. The pineal gland secretes melatonin, a regulatory hormone. The pancreas contains exocrine tissue, which secretes pancreatic juice to aid in digestion, and endocrine tissue to secrete hormones, such as insulin and glucagon.

Disorders are frequently inherited and result in excessive or insufficient hormone production. Diseases of this system include Addison's disease, Cushing's syndrome, dwarfism, acromegaly, gigantism, diabetes insipidus, diabetes mellitus, hypo- or hyperthyroidism, hyperinsulinism, hypoglycemia, goiter, and creatinism.

BOX 2-10.   LYMPHATIC SYSTEM

Components:

- Lymph vessels and nodes
- Spleen
- Thymus gland
- Tonsils
- Bone marrow

Functions:

- Maintains tissue fluid balance
- Filters blood and lymph
- Produces white blood cells to protect the body from disease
- Absorbs fats

Disorders:

- Immune disorders
- Infectious processes
- Tumors (Lymphoma, Hodgkin's disease)

Diagnostic Tests:

- Bone marrow analysis
- Cell surface markers

Because hormones are transported by the bloodstream, abnormalities are easily detected by analyzing blood samples. Chemical assays are available for all types of hormones and provide very specific and sensitive results. In addition, specific thyroid function tests (tri-iodothyronine [T_3], thyroxine [T_4], and thyroid-stimulating hormone [TSH]) are available.

LYMPHATIC SYSTEM

The **lymphatic system** consists of lymph, lymphocytes, lymph vessels, lymph nodes, tonsils, the spleen, bone marrow, and the thymus gland (Box 2–10). Three main functions of the system are to maintain fluid balance in the tissues by filtering blood and lymph fluid, to provide a defense against disease, and to absorb fats and other substances from the digestive tract. About 30 L of fluid passes from the blood to the tissue spaces each day. If more than 3 L were retained in the tissue, edema (swelling) would result. The lymph nodes filter lymph fluid, and the spleen filters blood, removing microorganisms or other foreign substances. Enlarged or swollen lymph nodes are common after infections. Lymphatic organs contain lymphocytes, macrophages, and other cells that provide immunity and protection against infections from microorganisms.

Disorders involving the lymphatic system are tumors (such as lymphoma and Hodgkin's disease), immune disorders, and infectious processes. Some immune disorders can be analyzed from blood samples, bone marrow, or both. Lymph nodes, however, are often surgically removed or aspirated so that cells can be analyzed or cultures performed. Analysis of markers on the surface of the cellular material is also diagnostically valuable.

CARDIOVASCULAR SYSTEM

For study purposes and to complete the overview of all organ systems, the **circulatory system** is briefly summarized in Box 2–11. This system is reviewed in greater depth and scope in Chapter 3.

BOX 2–11.   CIRCULATORY OR CARDIOVASCULAR SYSTEM

Components:

- Heart
- Blood vessels
- Blood

Functions:

- Transports oxygen and nutrients to the cells and transports carbon dioxide and wastes away
- Transports hormones and other substances throughout the body
- Regulates body temperature
- Helps defend against diseases

Disorders:

- Anemia
- Angina pectoris
- Aortic stenosis
- Bacterial endocarditis
- Congestive heart failure
- Embolus
- Hemophilia
- Leukemia
- Myocardial infarction (MI)
- Pericarditis
- Phlebitis
- Polycythemia
- Thrombocytopenia
- Thrombophlebitis
- Thrombus
- Varicose veins

Diagnostic Tests:

- Arterial blood gases
- AST
- Bone marrow analysis
- Cholesterol
- Coagulation studies: bleeding time, prothrombin time (PT), partial thromboplastin time (PTT), fibrin degradation product
- Complete blood cell (CBC) count and differential
- Creatine phosphokinase (CPK)
- Erythrocyte sedimentation rate (ESR)
- Ferritin
- Hemoglobin and hematocrit (H&H)
- Indices (MCH, MCV, MCHC)
- Iron
- Lactic dehydrogenase (LDH)
- Potassium
- Total iron-building capacity (TIBC)
- Triglycerides

SELF STUDY

KEY TERMS

Acidosis
Adrenals
Alkalosis
Alveolar Sacs
Anabolism
Anatomy
Anterior
Body Planes
Cardiac (Striated Involuntary)
    Muscles
Cartilage
Catabolism
Centriole
Circulatory System
Cytoplasm
Deoxyribonucleic Acid (DNA)
Digestive System
Dorsal
Endocrine Glands
Endoplasmic Reticulum
Exocrine Glands
Frontal Plane
Genes
Golgi Apparatus
Hematopoiesis
Homeostasis
Hormones
Human Immunodeficiency Virus
    (HIV)
Hyperventilation
Integumentary System
Lateral
Lymphatic System
Lysosomes

Medial
Melanin
Meninges
Metabolic Acidosis
Metabolic Alkalosis
Metabolism
Mitochondria
Muscular System
Nervous System
Neurons
Nucleolus
Nucleus
Pathology
Peristalsis
Physiology
Pituitary Gland
Posterior
Reproductive System
Respiratory Acidosis
Respiratory Alkalosis
Respiratory System
Ribosomes
Sagittal Plane
Sexually Transmitted Diseases
    (STDs)
Skeletal (Striated Voluntary)
    Muscles
Skeletal System
Steady State
Transverse Plane
Urinary System
Ventral
Visceral (Nonstriated, Smooth,
    Involuntary) Muscles

STUDY QUESTIONS

The following may have *one* or *more* answers:

1. Which of the following body systems provide protection and support, and allow the body to move?

   a. integumentary
   b. skeletal
   c. muscular

   d. lymphatic
   e. digestive

2. Which of the following body systems provides for CO_2 and O_2 exchange?

   a. nervous
   b. muscular
   c. respiratory

   d. reproductive
   e. endocrine

3. Which of the following body systems is the primary regulator of hormones?

   a. digestive
   b. endocrine
   c. urinary

   d. integumentary
   e. nervous

4. The skeletal system provides which of the body's functions?

   a. support
   b. protection of tissues
   c. calcium storage

   d. blood cell formation
   e. leverage and movement

5. Germ cells are defined as

   a. sperm
   b. ova
   c. mammary glands

   d. neurons
   e. hair follicles

6. Which of the following pairs of words describe opposite regions or planes of the body?

   a. anterior/posterior
   b. distal/proximal

   c. anterior/ventral
   d. lateral/medial

7. The pituitary gland is often referred to as which of the following?

   a. respiratory control gland
   b. master gland

   c. lymph tissue
   d. germ cells

8. How many chromosomes are contained in human cells?

   a. 25
   b. 50
   c. 46

   d. 100
   e. 1000

9. What portion of human body weight is water?

   a. ninety percent
   b. one half

   c. one fourth
   d. two thirds

10. Homeostasis refers to which of the following?
    a. chemical imbalance
    b. steady-state condition
    c. balanced chemistry
    d. thousands of genes
    e. anabolism

References

1. Guy, JF: *Learning Human Anatomy: A Laboratory Text and Workbook.* Norwalk, CT; Appleton & Lange: 1992.
2. Martini, F: *Fundamentals of Anatomy and Physiology,* 3rd ed. Englewood Cliffs, NJ; Prentice Hall: 1995.

THREE

■

The Circulatory System

CHAPTER OUTLINE

CHAPTER OBJECTIVES

Upon completion of Chapter 3, the learner is responsible for the following:

1. Identify and describe the structures and functions of the heart.

2. Trace the flow of blood through the cardiovascular system.

3. Identify and describe the structures and functions of different types of blood vessels.

4. Identify and describe the cellular and noncellular components of blood.

5. Locate and name the veins most commonly used for phlebotomy procedures.

6. Describe the phases of hemostasis.

7. Describe how to take a person's blood pressure and pulse rate.

All body systems are linked by the **cardiovascular system,** a transport network that can affect every cell, tissue, and organ within seconds. To maintain homeostasis, the cardiovascular system must provide for the rapid transport of water, nutrients, electrolytes, hormones, enzymes, antibodies, cells, and gases to all cells. In addition, it contributes to body defenses and the coagulation process and controls body temperature, much like the cooling system in a car. The primary components of the cardiovascular system include circulating fluid (**blood**), a pump (the **heart**), and numerous connected tubes (the **circulatory system,** or **blood vessels**). This chapter discusses these three main components of the cardiovascular system and the processes by which they function.

An important point to remember is that the lymphatic system, which was covered in Chapter 2, is closely integrated with the cardiovascular system. Both systems share transport vessels and empty their cells and contents into the bloodstream; however, the main purpose of the lymphatic system is to circulate lymph fluid to and from the tissues and to produce blood cells that aid in body defenses. Lymph tissue is found in lymph nodes, the thymus, the spleen, the intestine, the bone marrow, the liver, and the tonsils.

■ THE BLOOD

Circulating blood provides nutrients, oxygen, chemical substances, and waste removal for each of the billions of individual cells in the body. These functions, which are summarized in Box 3–1, are essential to homeostasis and life. Any region of the body that is deprived of blood may die with minutes.

Whole blood is composed of water, solutes, and cells. In general, humans have approximately 5 qt (4.73 L) of whole blood. The volume varies according to body weight, however. For instance, adult men usually have 5 to 6 L of whole blood, whereas adult women usually have 4 to 5 L. Abnormally low or high blood volumes can seriously affect other parts of the cardiovascular system. For example, a high blood volume (hypervolemia) can place stress on the heart because the heart must push extra fluids around the body. [1,2]

Whole blood is composed of approximately 3 qt (2.84 L, or about 60 percent) of plasma and 2 qt (1.89 L, or about 40 percent) of cells. Plasma contains 92 percent water and 8 percent solutes. Solutes include proteins, such as albumin, globulins, and fibrinogen; metabo-

BOX 3–1.   FUNCTIONS OF THE BLOOD

Transportation	Carry gases
	Carry oxygen from the lungs to the tissues
	Carry carbon dioxide from the tissues to the lungs
	Transport waste products to sites such as the kidneys for excretion
	Transport antibodies and white blood cells to defend against pathogenic microbes and viruses
Disburse nutrients	Distribute nutrients absorbed in the digestive tract to all organs of the body
	Take nutrients released from fat, muscle, or tissues for use in other parts of the body
Regulation	Regulate the blood pH in all parts of the body
	Regulate electrolyte balance to maintain a "steady state" condition
Hemostasis	Restrict fluid loss when blood vessels are damaged
	Formation of blood clots to prevent bleeding
Regulation	Control body temperature by redistribution of heat

lites, such as lipids, glucose, nitrogen wastes, and amino acids; and ions, such as sodium (Na), potassium (K), calcium (Ca), magnesium (Mg), and chloride (Cl).

Circulating blood cells are classified as **red blood cells (RBCs, or erythrocytes), white blood cells (WBCs, or leukocytes),** and **platelets (thrombocytes).** Approximately 99 percent of the circulating cells are RBCs. White blood cells are divided further into cell lines called **granulocytes (basophils, neutrophils, eosinophils), lymphocytes,** and **monocytes.** (Refer to Table 3–1.)

All blood cells develop from undifferentiated stem cells in the **hematopoietic** (blood-forming) tissues, such as the bone marrow. Stem cells are considered immature cells because they have not developed into their functional state. As the stem cells mature, they differentiate into the different cell lines mentioned in the preceding paragraph. The maturing cells are given specific names on the basis of the cell type that they will produce. The cells undergo changes in the nucleus and cytoplasm so that when they reach the circulating blood, they become fully mature and functional. These changes are clearly visible when staining techniques and light microscopy are used, or they can be distinguished by specialized hematology instruments.

ERYTHROCYTES

Red blood cells measure about 7 μm in diameter with a thickness of 2 μm. Normally, when in the circulating blood, RBCs have no nuclei. Prior to reaching maturity in the bone marrow, RBCs lose their nuclei and simultaneously become biconcaved disks. Their flexible shape enables them to pass through very narrow capillaries and provides for maximum surface area to transfer oxygen and carbon dioxide. Within each mature RBC are millions of hemoglobin

Table 3–1. Blood Cells

CELLS	NUMBER/ SIZE	FUNCTION	FORMATION	DESTRUCTION
Erythrocytes (RBCs)	4.5–5.5 million/ mm^3; size 6–7 μm	Transport O_2 and CO_2	Bone marrow	Fragmentation and removal in spleen, liver, and bone marrow; life span, $\cong$ 120 days
Leukocytes (WBCs)	5000–9000/mm^3; size 9–16 μm	Defense	Granulocytes in bone marrow; nongranular WBCs in all lymphatic tissue	Removed in spleen, liver, bone marrow; life span—1 day to year
Thrombocytes (platelets)	250,000–450,000/ mm^3; size 1–4 μm	Clotting	Bone marrow	Removed in spleen; life span—9 to 12 days

Abbreviations: RBCs, red blood cells; WBCs, white blood cells.

molecules; each molecule is capable of carrying four oxygen (O_2) molecules. As mentioned in Chapter 2, **hemoglobin** can also carry carbon dioxide (CO_2).

Red blood cells are formed in the bone marrow from nucleated stem cells. Once the stem cell becomes committed to being an RBC, it matures through several stages, all of which are morphologically different if viewed under a microscope. The process occurs during several days, and the stages are called *rubriblast, prorubricyte, rubricyte, metarubricyte, reticulocyte,* and *mature RBC.* Because nomenclature differs among laboratories, however, the terms *pronormoblast, basophilic normoblast, polychromatic normoblast,* and *orthochromatic normoblast* can also be used for the first four stages.

The life span of RBCs is approximately 120 days in the circulating bloodstream. After this time, they begin to fragment and rupture. Cells in the liver, spleen, and bone marrow phagocytize the destroyed RBCs and begin to break down the hemoglobin into iron-containing pigments (hemosiderin) and bile pigments (bilirubin and biliverdin). The bone marrow reuses the iron for new RBCs, and the liver excretes the bile pigments into the intestines.[2]

The term **erythropoiesis** means the production of red cells. It is initiated by a hormone produced in the kidney called **erythropoietin.** When body tissues are not receiving enough oxygen it is called **hypoxia** and kidneys are stimulated to produce erythropoietin, which in turn, activates stem cells in the bone marrow to begin producing more red blood cells.[3]

Millions of RBCs are continuously being formed and destroyed daily. So that it can maintain a normal supply of these cells, the bone marrow must have an adequate supply of several substances, including amino acids, vitamin B complexes, and minerals, such as iron. Deficiencies of any of these substances or failure of the bone marrow to function properly may result in anemia.

An important and commonly ordered laboratory test, the **hematocrit** (Hct or crit), is the percentage of whole blood that is occupied by red cells. It describes the concentration of the red blood cells and therefore provides an indirect measure of the oxygen-carrying capacity of the blood. For normal adults, the Hct is between 0.38 and 0.54 (38%–54%), e.g., whole blood is made up of this percentage of red blood cells. (White cells and platelets make up only 0.01 of the Hct.)[3] Refer to Figure 3–1 for a basic depiction of the hematocrit.

! Clinical Alert

Blood transfused into a patient must never contain antibodies to the patient's blood group antigens on the red cells because such antibodies can cross-react with specific RBC antigens and destroy the red cells. When this type of cross-reaction occurs, the RBCs clump together (or agglutinate) and may rupture (hemolyze). Red blood cell clumps and fragments can clog small blood vessels and cause damage to the kidneys, lungs, heart, or brain. One situation in which a cross-reaction may occur is when a patient is transfused with blood that has been accidentally mistyped or confused with another patient's. Such a reaction can be rapidly fatal to the inappropriately transfused patient. (See Table 3–2 for a list of antibodies present in various blood types.)

Figure 3–1. A graphic representation of three hematocrits. Tube A shows a hematocrit that might indicate that the patient is anemic because of too few RBCs. Tube B shows a normal hematocrit, and Tube C shows a hematocrit from a patient with too many RBCs, a condition called polycythemia.

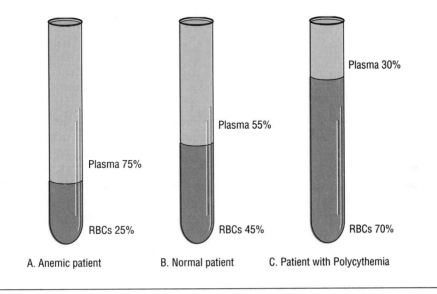

A. Anemic patient   B. Normal patient   C. Patient with Polycythemia

The surface membranes of RBCs contain antigens that designate the individual's blood type. Red blood cells with A antigen are type A, cells with B antigen are type B, RBCs containing both A and B antigens are type AB, and RBCs with neither A nor B antigens are type O. These antigens constitute the **ABO blood group system.** ABO antibodies (also called *agglutinins*) are present in plasma and provide protection and cross-reactions with opposing antigens. For example, type A blood contains anti-B, which will attack type B RBCs. Conversely, type B blood contains anti-A, which will cross-react with type A blood cells. Type O whole blood contains anti-A and anti-B, and type AB does not contain A or B antibodies. Type O is the most common blood type (46 percent of the U.S. population), followed by types A (40 percent), B (10 percent), and AB (4 percent).

Another commonly recognized blood group system contains the **Rh factor.** If the RBCs contain the antigen for Rh factor, the individual is considered Rh positive. Rh-negative people do not have the Rh-factor antigen on their RBCs. In contrast to the ABO system, in the Rh system, the plasma of Rh-negative people does not have anti-Rh agglutinins. Rh antibodies are present only if the body has been exposed to Rh-positive RBCs. This situation may occur accidentally by transfusion or during pregnancy. When an Rh-negative mother is carrying an Rh-positive fetus (the Rh-positive gene comes from the father), she becomes sensitized to the Rh-positive blood during delivery when the placental connection breaks down and when bleeding occurs. The mother then develops Rh antibodies. If she becomes pregnant again, the Rh antibodies will cross-react with the Rh-positive blood of the fetus. This condition can result in hemolytic disease of the newborn (HDN). It is preventable by administration of RhoGam (anti-Rh agglutinins) during and after the first pregnancy.[2]

Table 3–2. ABO Blood Types

BLOOD TYPE	ANTIGENS ON RBC	ANTIBODIES IN IN SERUM PLASMA
A	A	Anti-B
B	B	Anti-A
AB	AB	Neither anti-A nor anti-B
O	None	Anti-A and anti-B

Abbreviations: RBC, red blood cell.

To prevent a cross-reaction, physicians often request **cross-match testing,** which involves exposing a blood donor's blood to the patient's (recipient) blood. This procedure detects cross-reactivity. In addition to ABO and Rh, at least 48 possible cross-reactions can occur because of numerous antigens on the blood cells and antibodies in sera.

Type O individuals are called *universal donors.* Their RBCs can be transfused into a person with any ABO type because their RBCs do not contain A or B antigens to react with either the anti-A or the anti-B present in type B or type A blood, respectively.

LEUKOCYTES

White blood cells (leukocytes) differ in color, size, shape, and nuclear formation, and they are divided into two major groups: granular (with granules in the cytoplasm) and agranular (without cytoplasmic granules). **Neutrophils, eosinophils,** and **basophils** are **granulocytes.** Neutrophilic granules stain bluish with neutral dyes, and their nuclei generally have two or more lobes. These granulocytes are often referred to as *polymorphonuclear (PMN) leukocytes.* Eosinophilic granules stain orange-red with acidic dyes. Their nuclei normally have two lobes. Basophilic granules stain dark purple or black with basic dyes, and their nuclei are often S-shaped. Agranular leukocytes, lymphocytes, and monocytes have relatively large nuclei (see Fig. 3–2 and the Color Atlas).

Leukocytes function primarily as part of the body's defense mechanism. The cells phagocytize or ingest pathogenic microorganisms. Consequently, lymphocytes play a role in immunity and in the production of antibodies.

White blood cells are formed in bone marrow and lymphatic tissues. The exact life span of a cell varies with cell type from 1 day to several years. Normally, blood contains 5000 to 9000 leukocytes/mm^3, with designated percentages for each cell line. The morphological characteristics of leukocytes and erythrocytes are routinely analyzed by using special staining techniques and visualizing the cells under the microscope. Categorization of cells and abnormalities are noted on the test report called a **differential,** which can be performed manually or by using specialized instrumentation. Hematology instruments are able to produce automated differentials at a high speed in a cost-effective manner, whereas manual readings require significant expertise and time to interpret microscopic analysis.

Leukocytes contain specific cell surface antigens that are expressed at certain times during the development of the various WBC types. These antigens can be characterized with sophisticated techniques, such as flow cytometry and monoclonal antibodies, in the clinical

Figure 3–2. Human blood cells.

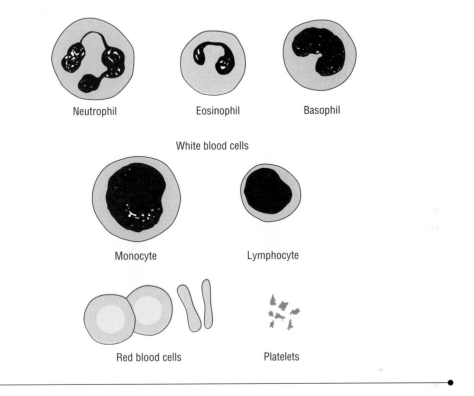

Neutrophil   Eosinophil   Basophil

White blood cells

Monocyte   Lymphocyte

Red blood cells   Platelets

laboratory. Using these laboratory techniques, clinicians can tell more precisely how mature or immature the WBCs are in the bone marrow, peripheral blood, or both.

THROMBOCYTES OR PLATELETS

Platelets are much smaller than other blood cells. They are fragments of **megakaryocytes** (*mega* means big), which are located in the bone. Normally, there are 250,000 to 450,000 platelets/mm^3. Platelets help in the clotting process by transporting needed chemicals for clotting, forming a temporary patch or plug to slow blood loss, and contracting after the blood clot has formed. Their life span is 9 to 12 days.

Abnormalities in the quality or quantity of platelets results in platelet disorders. Two tests are commonly used to test for a bleeding disorders, the bleeding time tests platelet quality, and the platelet count checks the quantity of platelets in the blood. Platelet disorders involving low counts or dysfunctional platelets are often treated by platelet transfusions to restore normal clotting capacity. Phlebotomists must be particularly cautious about patients on anticoagulant therapy such as aspirin, heparin, coumadin, and dextran because a simple venipuncture may cause excessive bleeding. On the contrary, thrombocytosis is a disease characterized by too many platelets. Patients with this condition may exhibit increased clot formation.

Figure 3–3.   Blood specimens with and without anticoagulant, respectively.

Plasma (contains fibrinogen)

White blood cells and platelets

Red blood cells

Serum (minus clotting elements)

Clot (blood cells in fibrin clot)

PLASMA

The liquid portion of the blood is called **plasma.** Blood cells are suspended in plasma. If a chemical agent called an **anticoagulant** is added to prevent clotting, a blood sample can be separated by centrifugation into the cells and the plasma (Fig. 3–3).

Plasma is composed of 90 percent water and 10 percent dissolved solutes, which include nutrients, such as glucose, amino acids, fats, metabolic wastes (urea, uric acid, creatinine, and lactic acid), respiratory gases (O_2 and CO_2), regulatory substances (hormones, enzymes) electrolytes (sodium, potassium, calcium, and chloride) and protective substances (antibodies). The cellular portion of the specimen contains WBCs, platelets, and RBCs. If the specimen is centrifuged or allowed to settle, the RBCs (the heaviest) will sink to the bottom of the tube. The WBCs and platelets form a thin white layer above the RBCs called the **buffy coat.** The fluid plasma portion is straw colored and remains on the top.

Some of plasma's substances, such as proteins, cannot pass through the capillary pores because of their large molecular size. The majority of proteins stay in the vascular space, where they exert osmotic pressure. This pressure keeps fluid (blood volume) levels in balance. Proteins in the plasma perform other functions, such as providing energy when the body is not getting enough from regular food intake. In conjunction with electrolytes, proteins help "buffer" the blood. *Buffering* is a term used to describe the body's ability to control the pH of the blood. The pH describes the degree of acidity or alkalinity of a solution on a pH scale between 1 and 14. An "acidic" pH is low (1–7), and a "basic" pH is high (7–14). The normal range of blood pH is slightly basic, from 7.35–7.45. Refer to Fig. 3–4 on the following

Figure 3–4. The pH Scale.

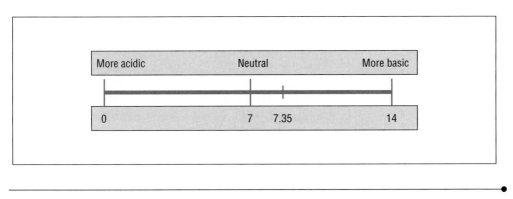

page. If the pH becomes too acidic or too basic serious complications can result for the patient. In acidosis, carbon dioxide (CO_2) and organic acids build up in the blood causing it to become acidic. If it is not detected by laboratory testing, blood and tissues can be damaged. Keep in mind that the lungs and kidneys also aid in the regulation of pH.[3]

Electrolytes in the plasma function in normal physiologic processes, including nerve conduction, muscle contractions, and maintenance of fluid levels in cells. Plasma glucose (sugar) is a vital source of energy for all body tissues. Insulin, a hormone produced in the pancreas, enables glucose to penetrate other cellular membranes. Patients with diabetes are unable to produce insulin, so they must take insulin injections.[3]

SERUM

If a blood specimen is allowed to clot, the result is **serum** plus blood cells meshed in a fibrin clot. Serum contains essentially the same chemical constituents as plasma, except the clotting factors and the blood cells are contained within the fibrin clot (see Fig. 3–3). Serum is also straw colored.

■ THE HEART

The human heart is a muscular organ about the size of a man's closed fist. (Refer to the color atlas for detailed representations of the structural and anatomic components of the heart.) The heart contains four chambers and is located slightly left of the midline in the thoracic cavity. The two **atria** are separated by the interatrial septum (wall), and the interventricular septum divides the two **ventricles.** Each atrium shares a valve with the ventricle on the same side. Heart valves are positioned for blood to flow in one direction only and to prevent backflow.

The right atrium of the heart receives blood from two large veins, the **superior vena cava** and the **inferior vena cava.** The superior vena cava brings blood from the head, neck, arms, and chest; the inferior vena cava carries O_2-poor blood from the rest of the trunk and the legs. Once the blood enters the right atrium, it passes through the heart valve (right atrioventricular, or tricuspid, valve) into the right ventricle. When blood exits the right ventricle, it begins the **pulmonary circuit,** where it enters the right and left pulmonary arteries. Arteries of the pulmonary circuit differ from those of the systemic circuit because they carry deoxygenated blood. Like veins, they are usually shown in blue on color-coded charts. These vessels branch into smaller arterioles and capillaries within the lungs, where gaseous exchange occurs (O_2 is picked up, and CO_2 is released). (Refer to Chapter 2 for more information about respiratory gas exchange.) From the respiratory capillaries, blood flows into the left and right pulmonary veins and then into the left atrium. The left atrium also has a valve (left atrioventricular, or bicuspid, or mitral, valve). Blood flows through the mitral valve into the left ventricle. When blood exits the left ventricle, it passes through the aortic semilunar valve and into the **systemic circuit** by means of the ascending aorta. The systemic circuit carries blood to the tissues of the body. If a valve malfunctions, blood flows backward and a heart murmur results. The right side of the heart pumps O_2-poor blood to the lungs to pick up more O_2; the left side pumps O_2-rich blood toward the legs, head, and organs.

The heart's function is to pump sufficient amounts of blood to all cells of the body by contraction (systole) and relaxation (diastole). Because the lungs are close to the heart, and the pulmonary arteries and veins are short and wide, the right ventricle does not need to pump very hard to propel blood through the pulmonary circuit. Thus, the heart wall of the right ventricle is relatively thin. On the other hand, the left ventricle must push blood around the systemic circuit, which covers the entire body. As a result, the left ventricle has a thick, muscular wall and a powerful contraction.

Blood pressure increases during ventricular systole and decreases during ventricular diastole. Blood pressure not only forces blood through vessels, but also pushes it against the walls of the vessels like air in a balloon. Therefore, it can be measured by how forcefully it presses against vascular walls. The instrument used for such measurements is called a *sphygmomanometer,* or a *blood pressure cuff* (Fig. 3–5). When blood pressure is reported, **systolic pressure** and **diastolic pressure** are written with a slash between the two numbers (e.g., 120/80) (Figs. 3–6 and 3–7, and Box 3–2).

The average heart beats 60 to 80 times per minute. Children have faster heart rates than adults, and athletes have slower rates because more blood can be pumped with each beat. During exercise, the heart beats faster to supply muscles with more blood; during and after meals, it also beats faster to pump blood to the digestive system; and during fever, the heart pumps more blood to the skin surface to release heat. The heart rate (pulse rate) is measured by feeling for a pulse and counting the pulses per minute (Fig. 3–7 and Box 3–2).

■ THE VESSELS AND CIRCULATION

Three kinds of blood vessels exist in the human body: **arteries, veins,** and **capillaries.** The largest artery (**aorta**) and veins (**venae cavae**) are approximately 1-in. wide. Normally, blood vessels have smooth, flexible walls. With age, however, arterial walls may "harden" (called *hardening of the arteries* or *arteriosclerosis*). The inner walls of the vessels become

Figure 3–5. Sphygmomanometer.

rough because of cholesterol or calcium deposits. As the deposits build, blood clots may form that clog the artery further, and the blood supply to tissues is reduced. In serious cases, this lack of blood results in a stroke (if the blood supply in the brain is reduced) or a heart attack (if the blood supply in the coronary, or heart, vessels is reduced).

ARTERIES

Arteries are highly oxygenated vessels that carry blood away from the heart (efferent vessels). They branch into smaller vessels, called **arterioles,** and into capillaries. The principal arteries of the body are indicated in the Color Atlas. Arteries are normally bright red in color, have thicker elastic walls than veins do, and have a pulse.

VEINS

Blood is carried toward the heart by the veins (afferent vessels). Because the blood in veins flows against gravity in many areas of the body, these vessels have one-way valves and rely on weak muscular action to move blood cells. The one-way valves prevent backflow of blood. All veins except the pulmonary veins contain deoxygenated blood, are normally dark red in

Figure 3–6. The pressure points indicated may be used to check a patient's pulse. Blood pressure is commonly measured using a sphygmomanometer at the site of the brachial artery.

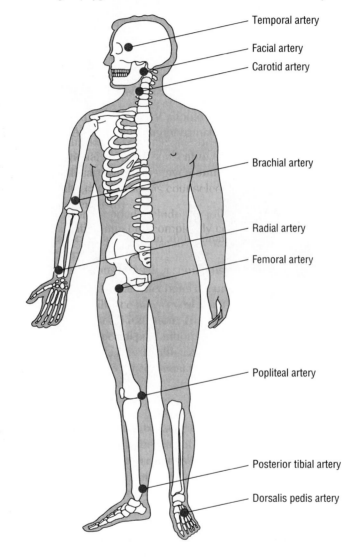

Temporal artery

Facial artery

Carotid artery

Brachial artery

Radial artery

Femoral artery

Popliteal artery

Posterior tibial artery

Dorsalis pedis artery

Figure 3–7. Major arm veins. Note that the *cephalic vein* extends almost the entire length of the arm. The superficial *median cubital vein* serves as a connection between the cephalic and basilic veins. The subclavian, brachial, and axillary veins are deeper veins.

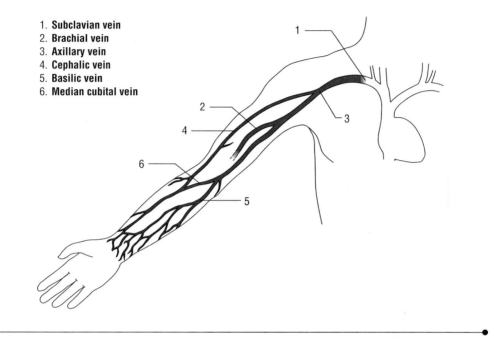

1. **Subclavian vein**
2. **Brachial vein**
3. **Axillary vein**
4. **Cephalic vein**
5. **Basilic vein**
6. **Median cubital vein**

color, and have thinner walls than arteries. The principal veins of the body are also indicated in the Color Atlas.

Phlebotomists should be familiar with the principal veins of the arms and legs (Figs. 3–7 to 3–10). The forearm vein most commonly used for venipuncture is the **median cubital vein** because it is generally the largest and best anchored vein. Others that are acceptable are the **basilic vein** and the **cephalic vein.**

CAPILLARIES

Microscopic vessels that carry blood and link arterioles to **venules** (minute veins) are called *capillaries.* Capillaries may be so small in diameter as to allow only one blood cell to pass through at any given time. Gas exchange occurs in the capillaries of tissues.

■ HEMOSTASIS AND COAGULATION

Hemostasis (not to be confused with homeostasis) is the maintenance of circulating blood in the liquid state and retention of blood in the vascular system by preventing blood loss. When a small blood vessel is injured, the hemostatic process repairs the break and stops the hemorrhage. The first (vascular) phase in this process is **vasoconstriction,** a rapid

BOX 3–2. PULSE RATE AND BLOOD PRESSURE MEASUREMENT

Pulse Rate

1. To take a pulse measurement, begin by pressing two fingertips (usually the second and third fingers, not the thumb) on an artery. Choose an artery that lies against a solid mass, such as a bone; the most common site is the radial artery of the wrist (at the base of the thumb). Other possible sites include the temporal, facial, carotid, brachial, femoral, popliteal, posterior tibial, and dorsalis pedis arteries. The pulse is felt as a pressure against the fingertips.

2. Measure the pulse rate by counting the pulses for 60 seconds. The normal adult pulse rate is about 75 per minute.

Blood Pressure

Blood pressure is measured by an instrument called a *sphygmomanometer,* or *blood pressure cuff.* Values on the instrument relate to millimeters of mercury (mm Hg) in a tube at certain points. Systolic pressure, the highest, is measured when the artery receives blood. Diastolic pressure, the lowest, is measured when the heart's ventricles relax. Blood pressure is reported with two numbers, one for the systolic pressure and one for the diastolic pressure (e.g., the normal average adult reading of 120/80 means that the systolic pressure measures 120 mm Hg and the diastolic pressure measures 80 mm Hg).

1. Place the inflatable cuff around the patient's upper arm so that the cuff squeezes the brachial artery.

2. Place a stethoscope over the artery distal to the cuff, then inflate the cuff until the pressure reads approximately 30 mm Hg. At this point, the brachial artery collapses, the flow of blood stops, and the sound of the pulse disappears.

3. Slowly let the air out of the cuff. At first, blood enters only at peak systolic pressure, and the stethoscope picks up the sound of blood pulsing through the artery. As air is removed from the cuff, the sounds change because the artery is remaining more open. When the cuff pressure decreases to less than diastolic pressure, blood flow becomes continuous, and the sound of the pulse becomes muffled or disappears completely. The pressure reading when the pulse appears corresponds to the peak systolic pressure (the first number reported). When the pulse fades, the pressure reading (the second number reported) has reached diastolic levels.

Note: Blood pressure changes frequently. For this reason, ambulatory pressure-monitoring devices are available that provide a continual printout of the patient's blood pressure. Normal blood pressure fluctuates from lows around 2:00 A.M. to peak values during the day.

---

constriction of the vessel, which decreases the blood flow to the surrounding vascular bed. In the second (platelet) phase, platelets degranulate, clump together, and adhere to the injured vessel in order to form a plug and inhibit bleeding. In phase three (**coagulation**), many specific coagulation factors are released and interact to form a **fibrin** meshwork or blood clot. This clot seals off the damaged portion of the vessel. Phase four (clot retraction) occurs when the bleeding has stopped. The entire clot retracts to bring torn edges closer together. In phase five (**fibrinolysis**), final repair and regeneration of the injured vessel occurs, and the clot slowly begins to break up (lysis) and dissolve as other cells carry out further repair.

The coagulation process (phase three) is a result of numerous coagulation factors. For simplicity, it is divided into two systems: intrinsic and extrinsic. All coagulation factors required for the **intrinsic system** are contained in the blood, whereas the **extrinsic**

Figure 3–8. Major arm veins. Since all individuals are unique, the exact location of veins may vary from one to another. This figure depicts variations in venous patterns in the arms of two individuals.

factors are stimulated when tissue damage occurs. For example, blood vessels are lined with a single layer of flat endothelial cells and are supported by subendothelial cells and collagen fibers. Normally, endothelial cells do not react or attract platelets; however, they do produce and store some clotting factors. When the clotting sequence is initiated by vessel injury, endothelial cells react with degranulated platelets in forming the fibrin plug (Fig. 3–11).[2]

Large- or medium-sized veins and arteries require rapid surgical intervention to prevent bleeding. Bleeding of small arteries and veins can, however, be controlled by the hemostatic process.

Disorders of the hemostatic process are serious. Overactive clotting can cause clots within the body, such as an embolus or a thrombus, or disseminated intravascular coagulation (DIC) disease. Drugs such as heparin and Coumadin (warfarin), which suppress clotting factors, can be used to prevent such problems. On the other hand, if clotting factors are not produced by the body, excessive bleeding may occur, as in hemophilia.

Figure 3–9.   Major leg veins. The *femoral vein* is a deep vein. Note that the *greater saphenous vein* is the longest vein in the body. It ascends up the medial side of the leg and the medial thigh and empties into the femoral vein in the groin area. The *lesser saphenous vein* comes up the lateral side of the ankle and enters the deeper *popliteal vein* behind the knee.

1. **Femoral vein**
2. **Greater saphenous vein**
3. **Popliteal vein**
4. **Lesser saphenous vein**

◼ DIAGNOSTIC ASSESSMENT

The number of RBCs, their morphological traits, and their hemoglobin content can be determined from an anticoagulated blood specimen in the clinical hematology laboratory. Platelets and WBCs can be assessed on the basis of number and morphological features. The results of a WBC differential count enumerate specific cell lines in percentages. Platelet function, as well as each coagulation factor, can be measured from anticoagulated blood specimens in the coagulation section of the clinical hematology laboratory. In addition, bone marrow, which is removed by a physician from the iliac crest of the hip, can be stained and studied microscopically in the hematology laboratory for the detection of abnormal numbers and morphological characteristics of blood cells.

Tests for blood types and cross-matches for donor blood are done in an immunohematology, a transfusion, or a blood banking laboratory. Serum and plasma constituents, including

Figure 3–10. Overview of the pattern of circulation. Venous blood flow is on the left side of the diagram, and arterial flow is on the right side. RA, right atrium; RV, right ventricle; LA, left atrium; LV, left ventricle.

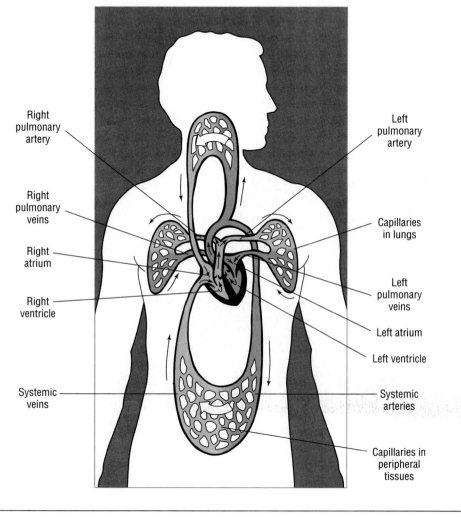

nutrients, metabolic wastes, respiratory gases, regulatory substances, and protective substances, can all be evaluated in the clinical chemistry laboratory.

Blood pressure and **pulse rate** measurements are performed as part of routine physical assessments (Figs. 3–6 to 3–9). High blood pressure can cause a stroke when a vessel ruptures in the brain. Having slightly low blood pressure is generally considered to be a healthier state than having high blood pressure; however, if a person's pressure is too low, blood will not flow to the head, and a faint feeling may result. In these cases, the best response is to lower the head to restore and increase blood flow to the head.

Figure 3–11. Clotting response.

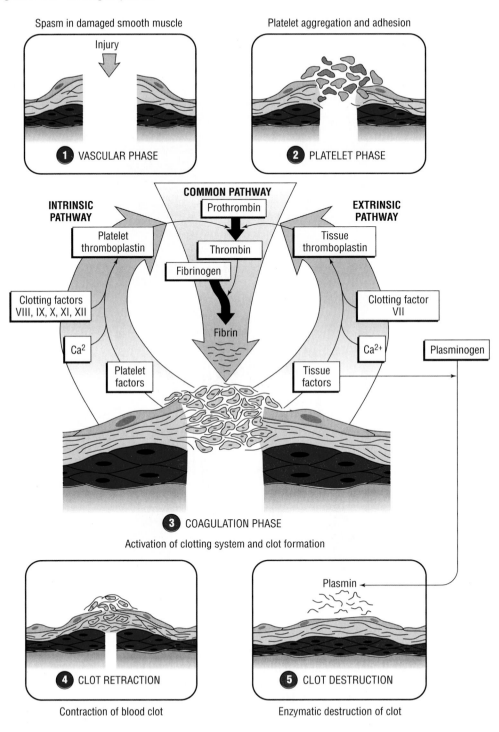

Spasm in damaged smooth muscle

Injury

1 VASCULAR PHASE

Platelet aggregation and adhesion

2 PLATELET PHASE

INTRINSIC PATHWAY

COMMON PATHWAY

Prothrombin

Thrombin

Fibrinogen

Fibrin

Platelet thromboplastin

Clotting factors VIII, IX, X, XI, XII

Ca^2

Platelet factors

EXTRINSIC PATHWAY

Tissue thromboplastin

Clotting factor VII

Ca^{2+}

Tissue factors

Plasminogen

3 COAGULATION PHASE

Activation of clotting system and clot formation

4 CLOT RETRACTION

Contraction of blood clot

5 CLOT DESTRUCTION

Plasmin

Enzymatic destruction of clot

SELF STUDY

KEY TERMS

ABO Blood Group System
Anticoagulant
Aorta
Arteries
Arterioles
Atria
Basilic Vein
Basophils
Blood
Blood Pressure
Blood Vessels
Buffy Coat
Capillaries
Cardiovascular System
Cephalic Vein
Circulatory System
Coagulation
Cross-Match Testing
Diastolic Pressure
Differential
Eosinophils
Erythropoiesis
Erythropoietin
Extrinsic Factors
Fibrin
Fibrinolysis
Granulocytes (Basophils, Neutrophils, Eosinophils)
Heart
Hematocrit

Hematopoietic
Hemoglobin
Hemostasis
Hypoxia
Inferior Vena Cava
Intrinsic System
Lymphocytes
Median Cubital Vein
Megakaryocytes
Monocytes
Neutrophils
Plasma
Platelets (Thrombocytes)
Pulmonary Circuit
Pulse Rate
Red Blood Cells (RBCs or Erythrocytes)
Rh Factor
Serum
Superior Vena Cava
Systemic Circuit
Systolic Pressure
Vasoconstriction
Veins
Venae Cavae
Ventricles
Venules
White Blood Cells (WBCs or Leukocytes)

STUDY QUESTIONS

The following questions may have *one* or *more* answers.

1. Whole blood consists of which of the following?

    a. water

    b. solutes

    c. cells

    d. tissue

2. Which type of blood cell is most numerous in the circulating blood?

   a. red blood cell
   b. white blood cell
   c. platelet
   d. macrophage

3. Identify the four chambers of the heart.

   a. right atrium, right ventricle
   b. superior vena cava, inferior vena cava
   c. left atrium, left ventricle
   d. ascending aorta, descending aorta

4. The liquid portion of an anticoagulated blood specimen is called

   a. plasma
   b. serum
   c. cellular components
   d. oxygenated blood

5. Which of the following veins are most commonly used for venipuncture procedures?

   a. popliteal
   b. brachial
   c. median cubital
   d. cephalic
   e. basilic

6. Functions of the blood include which of the following?

   a. transportation of gases, enzymes, and hormones
   b. regulation of pH and electrolytes
   c. regulation of body temperature
   d. transportation of waste products

7. Blood pressure is reported in which of the following ways?

   a. diastolic pressure only
   b. diastolic pressure/systolic pressure
   c. systolic pressure/diastolic pressure
   d. systolic pressure only

8. Which of the listed circulating blood cells have no nuclei?

   a. neutrophils
   b. erythrocytes
   c. basophils
   d. eosinophils

9. The most common blood type is

   a. A
   b. B
   c. AB
   d. O

10. The coagulation process occurs in phases that include the

   a. vascular phase
   b. platelet phase
   c. coagulation phase
   d. clot-retraction phase

References

1. Guy, JF: *Learning Human Anatomy: A Laboratory Text and Workbook.* Norwalk, CT: Appleton & Lange: 1992.

2. Martini, F: *Fundamentals of Anatomy and Physiology,* 3rd ed. Englewood Cliffs, NJ: Prentice Hall: 1995.

3. Dailey, JF: *Dailey's Notes on Blood,* 3rd ed. Arlington, MA; Medical Consulting Group: 1996.

PHLEBOTOMY CASE STUDY

■

Changing Roles in Phlebotomy Practice

Ms. Sanborn had been working in the hospital clinical laboratory for 4 years as a phlebotomist. She was highly regarded by her laboratory colleagues because of her efficiency in blood collection on three different units of the hospital, her assistance with specimen processing, and overall attention to details. She was recognized by her department as outstanding in her ability to communicate effectively with patients. Outside of work she routinely socialized with her co-workers on weekends. As part of the hospital restructuring plan, she was reassigned to report to a nursing director on a surgical unit of the hospital. Her new work duties included phlebotomy, glucose bedside testing, clerical functions on the unit, and occasional patient transportation from the unit to other parts of the hospital as needed. She was very reluctant to leave her friends and old job duties in the laboratory to be relocated to the surgical unit. Ms. Sanborn knew that all the phlebotomists' positions in the hospital were being reassigned, and she did not want to work anywhere else because she felt loyal to the hospital. She was too proud to complain about her unhappiness with the situation.

QUESTIONS

1. Name three trends in the health care industry that might be contributing to the hospital's changes. How could Ms. Sanborn learn more about these changes?

2. List four character traits that Ms. Sanborn should remember about working with health care teams.

3. Describe the positive professional character traits exhibited by Ms. Sanborn and how they may be beneficial in her new job assignment.

See Answers in Appendix.

PHLEBOTOMY CASE STUDY
■

Collection from the Dorsal Side of the Hand

Mr. Whitefield, a phlebotomist who recently completed his training program at Amber Community College, acquired a position at Oakhaven Hospital on the early morning shift. One morning, he was informed by the nurse on the orthopedic floor that any blood collections from Patient Davis should be taken while Mr. Davis is in the supine position and that all collections should be taken from the left dorsal hand.

QUESTIONS

1. Is the dorsal area the same as the proximal area? Explain the similarities or differences.
2. Should Mr. Davis sit up or lie down during the blood collection?
3. *Orthopedic* refers to what type of specialty?

See Answers in Appendix.

PHLEBOTOMY CASE STUDY

■

Communication and Cultural Sensitivity: Keys to Success

———————————————————————————————————— ●

Mrs. Rodriguez is pregnant and has come to see her obstetrician for a routine prenatal visit. She is accompanied by her 8-year-old daughter, her mother, and her 2 sisters. None of them speak English very well. Her examination includes laboratory tests and urinalysis. She also needs to be screened for gestational diabetes. Elizabeth, an experienced health care worker who cannot speak Spanish, is assigned to collect the specimens from Mrs. Rodriguez.

———————————————————————————————————— ●

QUESTIONS

1. Describe possible barriers to the effective communication between Mrs. Rodriguez and Elizabeth.

2. Even though there is limited information presented here, what characteristics seem important to Mrs. Rodriguez?

3. Describe at least five communication strategies that Elizabeth might use during her encounter with Mrs. Rodriquez?

4. What role(s) can the family members play in this situation?

5. Describe career development strategies that Elizabeth might consider to improve her ability to communicate effectively with patients like Mrs. Rodriguez.

See Answers in Appendix.

SAFETY
PROCEDURES

PART II PROVIDES A DETAILED LOOK at safety and regulatory factors that affect the health care professional in practicing phlebotomy and associated procedures. The chapters cover methods for protecting patients and providers from the risks of infections and hazardous situations, ways to document information about phlebotomy practices, and procedures for proper transportation of specimens and documentation essentials.

Chapter 4, Infection Control, describes the essentials of infection control, which include surveillance, knowledge of the chain of infection, and isolation protocol. Detailed procedures are presented that are designed to protect the patient from infections and to protect the employee from being exposed. Infection control programs designed for various hospital units are also described.

Chapter 5, Safety and First Aid, provides basic procedures for safe handling of specimens, equipment , and reagents in the work setting. Topics covered include fire, electrical, radiation, mechanical, and chemical safety and emergency care procedures and exposure control issues.

Chapter 6, Specimen Documentation and Transportation, provides the essentials of documentation for the clinical or medical record. Special components that relate to phlebotomy practice are highlighted, such as specimen requisition forms, labels, and reports. Specimen transportation and delivery procedures are also described for settings within a hospital and ambulatory sites. Manual and computerized processes are also discussed.

FOUR

■

Infection Control

CHAPTER OUTLINE

Chapter Objectives
Surveillance
Chain of Infection
- Source
- Mode of Transmission
- Susceptible Host
- Breaking the Chain

OSHA Standards for Occupational
Exposure to Blood-Borne Pathogens
- OSHA Needlestick Safety and
Prevention Act
- Isolation Procedures

Standard Precautions
- OSHA Standards for the Health
Care Employer
- Blood-Borne Exposure Procedures
- Isolation for Hospital Outbreaks
- Protective, or Reverse, Isolation
- Infection Control in Hospital Units
- Infection Control in a Nursery Unit
- Infection Control in a Burn Unit

- Infection Control in an ICU or a
Postoperative Care Unit
- Infection Control in a Dialysis Unit
- Infection Control in the Clinical
Laboratory

Specific Isolation Techniques
- Hand Washing
- Gowning
- Masking
- Gloving
- Entering and Exiting the Room
- Disposing of Contaminated Items

Prevention of Laboratory-Acquired
Infections

Sterile Technique for Health Care
Workers
- Disinfectants and Antiseptics

Self Study
- Key Terms
- Study Questions

CHAPTER OBJECTIVES

Upon completion of Chapter 4, the learner is responsible for the following:

1. Define the term *nosocomial infection*.

2. Identify the basic programs for infection control.

3. Explain the proper techniques for hand washing, gowning, gloving, masking, double bagging, and entering and exiting the various isolation areas.

4. Identify the potential routes of infection and methods for preventing transmission of microorganisms through these routes.

5. Identify steps to avoid transmission of blood-borne pathogens.

6. Describe the various isolation procedures and reasons for their use.

The condition in which the body is invaded with pathogenic (causing disease) bacteria, fungi, viruses, or parasites is called *infection*. **Nosocomial infections** are those that are acquired after admission to a health care facility, such as a hospital, clinic, nursing home, or psychiatric institution. Approximately 5 percent of all hospitalized patients in the United States acquire nosocomial infections and account for 88,000 deaths yearly.[1,2] These infections are often harmful to the patient and costly to both patients and insurers; each year, billions of dollars are spent on nosocomial infections. In an attempt to control them, **infection control programs** have been developed. Using guidelines established by the Centers for Disease Control and Prevention (CDC), the Joint Commission on Accreditation of Healthcare Organizations (JCAHO), and state regulatory agencies, managers of each health care institution are responsible for developing and implementing an infection control program. These programs usually address the issues of **surveillance,** reporting, **isolation procedures,** education, and management of community-acquired infections, as well as health care–associated infections. An infection control nurse or practitioner usually works closely with or in the clinical microbiology laboratory and communicates with personnel in the health care facility and home health care providers to make the necessary assessments.

The **Centers for Disease Control and Prevention (CDC),** as part of the U.S. Public Health Service, oversees the investigation and control of various diseases, especially those that are communicable and threaten the U.S. population. CDC provides infection control and safety guidelines to protect health care workers and patients from infection.

There are many different guidelines for the isolation of patients and the protection of health care workers (e.g., category-specific isolation, blood and body fluid precautions, body substance isolation, and/or standard or universal and transmission-based precautions) that are discussed in this chapter. Whatever the system in place, the main issues for health care workers are to understand what pathogens can infect them, how such pathogens are transmitted, and how to protect themselves in the workplace.

The cornerstones for infection protection of the health care worker, particularly phlebotomists are as follows:

- Frequent hand washing.
- Use of barrier garments and personal protective equipment.
- Waste management of contaminated materials.

These protective procedures must become part of a phlebotomist's routine procedures and standards for practice. These practices are also discussed in Chapters 7 and 8.

■ SURVEILLANCE

In most health care institutions, the infection control program involves monitoring and collecting data on several specific populations, such as (1) patients at a high risk of infection;

(2) patients with previously acquired infections; (3) personnel or patients accidentally exposed to a communicable disease, contaminated equipment, or hazardous reagents; (4) patients in certain areas of the hospital or in certain rooms; and (5) patients in ambulatory settings, such as home or long-term care facilities. The health care worker should be aware of these special circumstances for two reasons. First, the phlebotomist can take the necessary precautions to prevent infecting him- or herself or the patient. Second, he or she can mentally prepare to deal with these special patients in a professional and humanistic manner. Because each health care facility has its own infection control program and policy manual, the health care worker should read and be familiar with both.

If the phlebotomist works for a home health care agency, it is imperative to have knowledge of infection control protocols for home health care because the home is an uncontrolled, unpredictable environment in which to provide care.

Infection control surveillance also involves the classification of infections according to prevalence rates. The prevalence rates of commonly identified nosocomial infections are represented in Figure 4–1. Each of the infections cited in this figure can be transmitted in a variety of ways, and each health care worker should realize that he or she can be a potential recipient or transmitter of infectious agents. Table 4–1 lists causative agents for nosocomial infections.

Infection control programs also monitor employee health programs. The primary objective is to minimize the risk of infection or hazardous circumstances for employees and patients. Most employees are screened for the following diseases prior to employment: measles, mumps, tuberculosis, hepatitis, diarrheal disease, syphilis, and skin diseases. Immunization for a variety of diseases is often made available initially and throughout employment, free of charge. Often, the hospital stipulates policies for employees with specific infections or employees who have been exposed to certain infections, such as those listed in Table 4–2.

For the employee's protection, many types of warning labels are used. Among these are isolation signs and radiation hazard signs. Radiation signs may be posted on the hospital doors of patients treated with radioactive isotopes. In general, a short period of contact with these patients is not significant.

■ CHAIN OF INFECTION

Nosocomial infections result when the **chain of infection** is complete. The three components that make up the chain are the **source, mode of transmission,** and **susceptible host.**[3]

SOURCE

In a normal environment, relatively few things are sterile; therefore, potential sources of infection cover a wide range. Inanimate objects, as well as people, are colonized with various microorganisms, many of which help carry out normal body functions. Some of these microorganisms, however, are more pathogenic than others. For example, relatively few *Shigella* organisms need to be ingested before a diarrheal infection occurs. With *Salmonella,* however, large numbers of the organisms must be ingested before symptoms appear. Conversely, numerous anaerobic and aerobic bacteria must be present in the gastrointestinal (GI) tract for normal metabolism to occur.

Figure 4–1. Prevalence of nosocomial infections.

(From Castle M, Ajemian E. *Hospital Infection Control.* New York: John Wiley & Sons: 1987, with permission.)

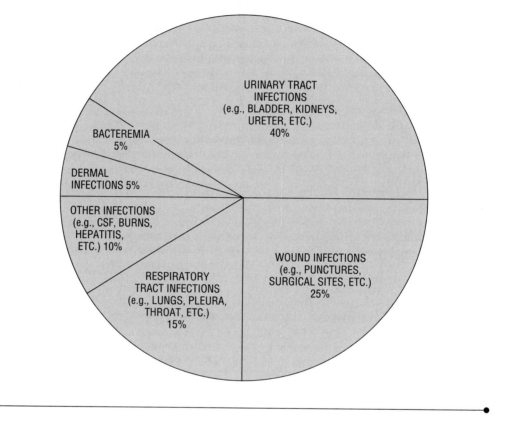

Regarding the sources of nosocomial infections, infection control practitioners must consider the amount of contamination, viability of the infectious agent, virulence of the agent, length of time from contamination to contact, and the manner in which the agent is transmitted from the source. Sources of nosocomial infection are numerous in the health care environment (Table 4–3). For instance, human hands provide a warm, moist environment for microorganisms. Therefore a physician, phlebotomist, or nurse can transmit organisms from themselves or an infected patient to another potential host. Uniforms or other clothing that comes in contact with infectious agents and is then worn around other patients is another potential source of infection. Likewise, medical instruments that come into contact with open wounds, mucous membranes, or organs can transmit microorganisms. For example, an instrument, such as a fiber-optic bronchoscope, may be used repeatedly only if thoroughly decontaminated after each use. Otherwise, it may be implicated in transmitting bacterial pneumonia. Although many other pieces of invasive equipment are also potential

Table 4–1. Pathogenic Agents Causing Nosocomial Infections

BODY AREAS OR HOSPITAL AREAS	COMMONLY IDENTIFIED PATHOGENIC AGENTS
Blood and cerebrospinal fluid	Any microorganisms
Burn unit	All Gram-negative bacilli
	Gram-positive rods
	Fungi
Dialysis unit	Hepatitis and other viruses
	Bacteria
	Fungi
Ear	*Pseudomonas aeruginosa*
	Streptococcus pneumoniae
	Gram-negative bacilli
Eye	*Staphylococcus aureus*
	Neisseria gonorrhoeae
	Gram-negative bacilli
	Moraxella lacunata
	Haemophilus influenzae
	S. pneumoniae
	P. aeruginosa
Gastrointestinal tract	*Salmonella* sp.
	Shigella sp.
	Clostridium difficile
	Enteropathogenic *Escherichia coli*
	Vibrio cholerae
	Campylobacter sp.
	Parasitic protozoans
	Candida albicans
	Some viruses (i.e.,Rotavirus)
Genital tract	*N. gonorrhoeae*
	Haemophilus vaginalis
	C. albicans (yeast)
Intensive care or postoperative care unit	Any microorganisms
Nursery unit	*S. aureus*
	Group B *Streptococcus*
	E. coli
	S. pneumoniae
	Other Gram-negative bacilli
	Viruses (i.e., Rotavirus)
Respiratory tract	*Streptococcus pyogenes*
	Corynebacterium diphtheriae
	Bordatella pertussis
	Staphylococcus epidermidis

(continued)

Table 4–1. (continued)

BODY AREAS OR HOSPITAL AREAS	COMMONLY IDENTIFIED PATHOGENIC AGENTS
Respiratory tract (continued)	
	Acinebacter spp.
	S. aureus
	S. pneumoniae
	H. influenzae
	Any Gram-negative bacilli
	Fungi
	Certain viruses (i.e., Influenza A2 and B; Parainfluenza; Rhinovirus)
Skin	S. aureus
	S. pyogenes
	C. albicans
	Smallpox
	Herpes virus
	Enterovirus
	Measles
Urinary tract	Any microorganism in sufficient numbers
Wounds and abscesses	Any microorganisms

Table 4–2. Employee Infections or Special Circumstances*

DISEASE	WORK STATUS	DURATION OF WORK OR WORK LIMITATIONS
Conjunctivitis, infectious	Off	Until discharge ceases
Diarrheal diseases	Off	Until symptoms resolve
Draining abscess, boils, and so forth	Off	Until drainage stops, if employee has patient contact
Chicken pox (varicella)	Off	For 7 days after eruption first appears in normal host, provided lesions are dry and crusted when he or she returns
Diarrhea Shigella Salmonella	Variable	Individual, depending on extent of symptoms, cultures, and evaluation by Personnel Health Services
Gonorrhea	May Work	
Hepatitis A	Off	Until 7 days after onset of jaundice (must bring note from private physician upon return)

Table 4–2. *(continued)*

DISEASE	WORK STATUS	DURATION OF WORK OR WORK LIMITATIONS
Hepatitis B	Off	Must bring note from private physician upon return
Hepatitis C	May Work	Period of infectivity has not been determined
Herpes simplex	May Work	Evaluation by Personnel Health Services, depending on work area
Herpes zoster (shingles)	No patient contact	If able to work, may do so
Human immunodeficiency virus	May work with restriction	Evaluated by Employee Health Physician
Influenza and upper respiratory infections	Variable	Until acute symptoms resolve
Impetigo	Off	No patient contact until crusts
German measles (rubella)	Off	Until rash clears (minimum of 5 days)
Measles	Off	Until rash clears (minimum of 4 days)
Mononucleosis	Off	At discretion of private physician
Positive PPD Conversion	May Work	Evaluation by chest x-ray and follow-up by Personnel Health Services
Pregnancy (first or second trimester)	May Work	Avoid contact with patients having viral or rickettsial infections, tuberculosis, or those being treated with radioactive material
Pregnancy (third trimester)	May Work	Avoid contact with patients in any type of isolation
Active TB	Off	Until under treatment and smears are negative for 2 weeks
TB PPD converter	No restriction	
Scabies	Off until treated	
Strep throat (Group A)	Off	May work 24 hours after being placed on appropriate antibiotic therapy and symptom free
Weeping dermatitis	No patient contact	No patient contact until acute symptoms resolve

Abbreviations: PPD, purified protein derivative; TB, tuberculosis.

*Sample guideline for employees with infection; their work status and when they can return to work.

(References: Castle M, Ajemian E. *Hospital Infection Control.* New York: John Wiley & Sons; 1987, Bennett J, Brachman P. *Hospital Infections.* 3rd ed. Boston: Little, Brown & Co.; 1992, and Bolyard B, Tablan O, *Am J Infect Control,* 1998; 26(3): 299–301.)

Table 4–3.   Considerations for Sources of Nosocomial Infections

Health care personnel (e.g., lack of hand washing between patients)

Visitors

Medical instruments (e.g., contaminated needles, intravenous [IV] catheters, Foley catheters, bronchoscopes, respiratory therapy equipment)

Medical reagents (e.g., IV fluid)

Other patients (e.g., those having severe wound drainage

---

transmitters unless adequately sterilized, some pieces of equipment that can become contaminated with bacteria are less likely to cause infection. As an example, tourniquets come in contact with intact skin but are less likely to be sources of infection. They should, however, also be decontaminated after each use.

MODE OF TRANSMISSION

The second link in the chain of infection involves transmission from the source to the next host. **Pathogenic agents** may be transmitted by five modes: (1) direct contact, (2) air, (3) medical instruments, (4) other objects, and (5) other vectors. Direct contact involves close or intimate contact with an infected person. For example, some patients acquire staphylococcal infections, chickenpox, hepatitis, or diarrhea after touching other infected individuals. During contact, the infective microorganism rubs off one person onto another. Hand washing is the best means of preventing infections transmitted by this route.

Microscopic airborne droplets may carry infectious agents, such as the causative agent of tuberculosis and Legionnaire's disease. Droplets may become airborne in the following instances: when an individual coughs or sneezes, when linens are shaken, when dust is stirred by sweeping, or when ventilation is inadequate. Preventative measures include wearing a mask, isolating specific patients, and ensuring good ventilation.

As mentioned previously, invasive medical instruments may expose a susceptible patient to pathogenic agents. To prevent instrument-induced infections, health care personnel should change or decontaminate instruments, such as tourniquets and catheters, after each use. Needles should be used only once, then disposed of in appropriate containers.

Other inanimate objects, such as toys in the pediatric areas, common toilets and sinks, linens, and water fountains are all potential modes of transmission. Objects that can harbor infectious agents and transmit infection are called **fomites**. Fomites that are found in health care settings are listed in Table 4–4. Preventing transmission by fomites can be accomplished by following isolation techniques, using **sterile technique** for injections or venipuncture, wearing gloves during equipment handling, and restricting the use of common toys or facilities.

Many insects (mosquitoes, ticks, fleas, mites) and rodents act as vectors in transmitting infectious diseases, such as plague, rabies, and malaria. Patients may be exposed to these vectors in unsanitary conditions in a home setting or in areas where the diseases are prevalent.

SUSCEPTIBLE HOST

The third link in the chain of infection is the susceptible host. Factors that affect a host's susceptibility are age, drug use, the degree and nature of the illness, and the status of the

Table 4–4. Fomites Found in Health Care Facilities

Computer keyboards

Door knobs

Telephones

Countertops

Scrub suits

Phlebotomy trays

Eyeglasses

Pens and pencils

Water-faucet handles

Laboratory coats

Manuals and books

Phlebotomy supplies and equipment

IV equipment

immune system. The patient's progress in the hospital significantly affects his or her chances of acquiring an infection. Underlying diseases, such as diabetes, acquired immune deficiency syndrome (AIDS), and cancer, as well as therapeutic measures (chemotherapy, radiation therapy, antibiotics), all change the status of the body and make it a potential host for infection.

BREAKING THE CHAIN

Infection control programs aim at breaking the infection chain at one or more links, as shown in Figure 4–2. Hand-washing procedures for sterile technique, proper waste disposal, appropriate laundry services, and housekeeping are ways of controlling the sources. Isolation techniques, control of insects and rodents, and use of disposable equipment and supplies help interrupt the modes of transmission. Host susceptibility is controlled by speeding the patient's recovery. Immunizations, transfusions, proper nutrition, medication, and adequate exercise all help the patient to regain health.

■ OSHA STANDARDS FOR OCCUPATIONAL EXPOSURE TO BLOOD-BORNE PATHOGENS

Patients who are infected with blood-borne pathogens, such as hepatitis or HIV, cannot always be readily detected. Therefore the CDC states that "under **universal precautions,** all patients should be assumed to be infectious for HIV and other blood-borne pathogens."[4] Other blood-borne pathogens include viruses, and other microorganisms that cause malaria, syphilis and Creutzfeldt-Jakob disease (CJD). The term "blood-borne pathogens" can be used for any infectious microorganism present in blood and other body fluids and tissues.

Occupational Safety and Health Administration (OSHA), an agency of the U.S. Department of Labor, requires employers to provide measures that will protect workers exposed to biological hazards. On December 6, 1991, OSHA standards for occupational exposure to blood-borne pathogens (29 CFR 1930.1030), based mainly on the use of the

Figure 4–2. The chain of nosocomial infection can be interrupted by infection control procedures.

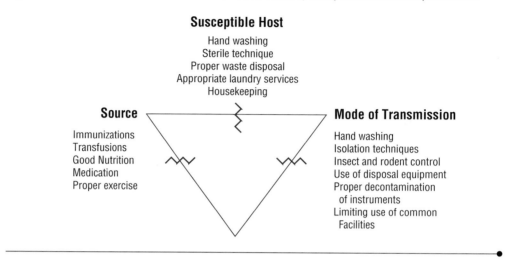

hepatitis B vaccine and the previously described CDC recommendations regarding universal precautions, were published.[5] These federal standards are intended to decrease, if not eliminate, occupational exposure to the viruses that cause hepatitis, AIDS and other blood-borne pathogens.

OSHA NEEDLESTICK SAFETY AND PREVENTION ACT

On November 6, 2000, the Needlestick Safety and Prevention Act became law. It amended the 1991 OSHA standard—29 CFR 1930.1030.[6] The federal act is significant to those performing blood collection because it requires that employers identify, evaluate, and make use of effective safer medical devices. The definition of safety devices in the standard is "a non-needle sharp or a needle device used for withdrawing body fluids, accessing a vein or artery, or administering medications or other fluids, *with a built-in safety feature or mechanism that effectively reduces the risk of an exposure incident.* In addition, the amended standard *requires* employers to involve "frontline" blood collectors in the evaluation and selection of safer blood collection devices. A new type of sharps injury log must be maintained that includes detailed information on the injury, including the "type and brand" of device involved in the incident, the department or work area where the exposure incident occurred, and an explanation of how the incident occurred. Unfortunately, it does not provide a mechanism for covering state and municipal employees in federal OSHA states. States with state OSHA plans are required to have regulations that are "at least as effective" as federal OSHA's standards.

ISOLATION PROCEDURES

Isolation procedures, methods of removing diseased individuals from society, date to antiquity. Although the supplies for and methods of isolation have been updated, the fear of being

Figure 4–3.   Isolation sign.

ISOLATION

STANDARD PRECAUTIONS

MUST BE FOLLOWED PLUS

RESPIRATOR MASK MUST BE WORN

NOTE: DOOR MUST BE CLOSED AT
ALL TIMES

contaminated and the stigma associated with a patient in isolation are still present. The psychological effects of being a patient in isolation are profound. Therefore the health care provider should make an effort to reduce the patient's anxiety by communicating in a calm, professional, and reassuring manner.

■ STANDARD PRECAUTIONS

In the past, isolation procedures were established in varying degrees. They ranged from sterile rooms or wards to isolation procedures for one disease only. Isolation techniques were formally divided into two types by the CDC: category-specific precautions and disease-specific precautions.[3] Under a newer guideline, standard precautions are combined with isolation practices for moist and potentially infectious body substances (BSI practices) into a single set of safeguards, which are to be used for the care of all patients. These precautions apply to blood, *all* body fluids, nonintact skin, and mucous membranes. **Standard precautions** are designed to reduce the risk of transmission of microorganisms (see example of isolation sign in Fig. 4–3) from both recognized and unrecognized sources of infection in health care facilities. All the steps of the universal precautions apply to the standard precautions for health care workers involved in blood collection. The old categories of isolation and disease-specific precautions have been collapsed into three sets of precautions based on the route of transmission: airborne, droplet, and contact as shown in Figure 4–4 with listings of specific syndromes in both adult and pediatric patients that are highly suggestive of infection.[7]

Use of Standard Precautions

1. All health care workers should routinely use appropriate barrier precautions to prevent skin and mucous membrane exposure when contact with blood or other bloody fluids of any patient is anticipated. Barriers (e.g., gloves, facial masks, respirators, gowns, shields) are also referred to as personal protective equipment (PPE). Gloves should be worn (a) for touching blood and body fluids, mucous membranes, or nonintact skin of all patients; (b) for handling items or surfaces soiled with blood or body fluids; and (c) for performing venipunctures and other vascular access procedures. Gloves should be changed after contact with each patient. Masks and protective eyewear or face shields should be worn to prevent exposure of mucous membranes of the mouth, nose, and eyes during procedures that are likely to generate droplets of blood or other body fluids or fluid-resistant splashes of blood or other body fluids. A personal respirator should be used if the risk of aerosolized *Mycobacterium tuberculosis* is present.

2. Hands and other skin surfaces should be washed immediately and thoroughly if contaminated with blood or other body fluids. Hands should be washed immediately after gloves are removed.

3. All health care workers should take precautions to prevent injuries caused by needles, scalpels, and other sharp instruments or devices (a) during procedures, (b) when cleaning used instruments, (c) during disposal of used needles, and (d) when handling sharp instruments after procedures. To prevent needlestick injuries, health care workers should not recap needles, purposely bend or break them by hand, remove them from disposable syringes, or otherwise manipulate them by hand. After they are used, disposable syringes and needles, scalpel blades, and other sharp items should be placed in puncture-resistant containers for transport to the reprocessing area.

4. Although saliva has not been implicated in HIV transmission, to minimize the need for emergency mouth-to-mouth resuscitation, health care workers should ensure that mouthpieces, resuscitation bags, or other ventilation devices are available for use in areas in which the need for resuscitation is predictable.

5. Health care workers who have exudation lesions or weeping dermatitis should refrain from all direct patient care and from handling patient care equipment until the condition resolves.

6. Pregnant health care workers are not known to be at greater risk of contracting a viral (i.e., HIV, hepatitis C, etc.) infection than health care workers who are not pregnant; however, if a health care worker develops a viral (i.e., HIV) infection during pregnancy, the infant is at risk of infection resulting from perinatal transmission. Because of this risk, pregnant health care workers should be especially familiar with and strictly adhere to precautions to minimize the risk of a viral (i.e., HIV) transmission.

Figure 4–4. Types of precautions and patients requiring them.

Standard Precautions
Use standard precautions for the care of all patients.

Airborne Precautions
In addition to standard precautions, use airborne precautions for patients known or suspected to have serious illnesses transmitted by large particle droplets:

1. Invasive *Haemophilus influenzae* type b disease, including meningitis, pneumonia, epiglottitis, and sepsis
2. Invasive *Neisseria meningitidis* disease, including meningitis, pneumonia, and sepsis
3. Other serious bacterial respiratory infections spread by droplet transmission:
   * Diphtheria (pharyngeal)
   * Mycoplasma pneumonia
   * Pertusis
   * Pneumonic plague
   * Streptococcal (group A) pharyngitis, pneumonia, or scarlet fever in infants and young children
4. Serious viral infections spread by droplet transmission:
   * Adenovirus*
   * Influenza
   * Mumps
   * Parovirus B19
   * Rubella

Contact Precautions
In addition to standard precautions, use contact precautions for patients known or suspected to have serious illnesses easily transmitted by direct patient contact or by contact with items in the patient's environment:

1. Gastrointestinal, respiratory, skin, or wound infections or colonization with multidrug-resistant bacteria judged by the infection control program, based on current state, regional, or national recommendations, to be of special clinical and epidemiologic significance.
2. Enteric infections with a low infectious dose or prolonged environmental survival:
   * *Clostridium difficile* infection
   * For diapered or incontinent patients, enterohemorrhagic *Escherichia coli* 0157:H7, *Shigella,* hepatitis A, or rotavirus infection
3. Respiratory syncytial virus, parainfluenza virus, or enteroviral infections in infants and young children

(continued)

Figure 4–4. Types of precautions and patients requiring them. (*continued*)

4. Skin infections that are highly contagious or that may occur on dry skin:
   - Diptheria (cutaneous)
   - Herpes simplex virus (neonatal or mucocutaneous)
   - Impetigo
   - Major (noncontained) abscesses, cellulitis, or decubiti
   - Pediculosis
   - Scabies
   - *Staphylococcus furunculosis* in infants and young children
   - Zoster (disseminated or in the immunocompromised host)*
5. Viral hemorragic conjunctivities
6. Viral hemorragic infectious (Ebola, Lassa, or Marburg)

*Certain infections require more than one type of precaution.

†See the CDC's *Guidelines for Preventing the Transmission of Tuberculosis in Health-Care Facilities,* http://www.cdc.gov/epo/mmwr/preview/rr4313.html

Source: Reprinted with permission from J. S. Garner, Guideline for Isolation Precautions in Hospitals, *Infection Control and Hospital Epidemiology,* Vol. 17, No. 1, pp. 53–80, © 1996, Slack, Inc.

OSHA STANDARDS FOR THE HEALTH CARE EMPLOYER

❗ Clinical Alert

1. An implementation and compliance program requiring all employers and employees to observe universal standard precautions.
2. PPE devices to minimize the risk of infection from blood-borne pathogens (e.g., fluid-resistant gowns, goggles, respirators).
3. Engineering practice controls that isolate or remove the blood-borne pathogen hazard from the health care facility (e.g., sharps disposal containers, self-sheathing needles. Also, employers should **not** tell blood collectors to reuse blood tube holders!
4. Work practice controls that change the manner in which a blood collection task is performed to reduce the likelihood of exposure (e.g., prohibiting needle recapping; prohibiting eating, drinking, or smoking in the clinical laboratory).
5. Appropriate cleaning methods in blood and other body fluid collection areas to prevent exposure to infectious agents (e.g., use of 10 percent solution of household bleach as a disinfectant for the area).

Clinical Alert

6. The hepatitis B virus (HBV) vaccine available at no cost to employees. The HBV vaccine protects against HBV, as well as delta hepatitis. The hepatitis virus is the most frequently occurring laboratory-associated infectious agent. It attacks the liver and is a life-threatening blood-borne pathogen.

7. Postexposure follow up for employees exposed to HBV, HIV, or other blood-borne pathogens. The follow up must involve an immediate confidential medical evaluation of the employee with continued evaluation and counseling at periodic intervals. The employee's medical record must include the employee's name, social security number, and HBV vaccination dates. Health care workers are concerned about HIV and hepatitis C virus (HCV) because they are blood-borne pathogens that lead to a poor prognosis if workers are exposed by needle stick or another method. Although the incidence of HIV and/or hepatitis C viral infections occurring as a result of on-the-job exposure is relative low, caution must be used because no vaccine is available for protection.

8. Training and educational information on blood-borne pathogens (e.g., HIV, HCV, and HBV) available for employees at no cost and accessible during the employees' working hours. These training sessions must occur at the beginning of task assignments involving occupational exposure to blood-borne pathogens. Each employee must have annual training on this topic, and each employer must maintain an accessible copy of OSHA's blood-borne pathogen standards with statements that relate these standards to the specific health facility's environments.

9. Labels and signs that warn of biological hazards and contaminated waste. These labels and signs must be affixed to appropriate refrigerators, freezers, waste containers, and storage cabinets containing infectious materials. The labels must be fluorescent orange or orange-red, bearing the word *biohazard* in English and other predominant languages spoken in the region (e.g., *peligro biologico* in Spanish). In addition, the biohazard symbols shown in Chapter 5. Figure 5–5 should be on the label. Alternatively, red or orange bags may be substituted for labels.

BLOOD-BORNE EXPOSURE PROCEDURES

OSHA requires managers at health care facilities to provide a confidential medical evaluation, treatment, and follow-up for any employee who has had a blood-borne exposure incident (e.g., needle stick). Immediately after an exposure incident, the employee must (1) decontaminate the needle-stick site with an appropriate antiseptic (e.g., iodine) for 30 seconds or (2) flush the exposed mucous membrane site (e.g., eyes) with water for 10 minutes. Then, he or she should report the incident to his or her supervisor, who will direct the employee to the appropriate clinic for medical evaluation, treatment, and counseling.

The medical evaluation involves the following five steps[5]:

1. The exposed health care worker's blood is tested for HIV in an accredited laboratory.
2. The source individual is identified and tested for HIV and HBV, if the person gives permission. For possible exposure to hepatitis C, it is recommended to test the source for anti-HCV.[8]
3. If the source individual tests positive for HIV, the exposed health care worker is given counseling and evaluated for HIV infection immediately and 6 weeks, 12 weeks, and 6 months later. Also, azidothymidine (AZT) therapy is provided to the exposed employee as soon as possible, preferably within 1 hour of exposure.

The health care worker exposed to HCV should have the baseline and 6-month follow-up testing for anti-HCV and ALT (alanine aminotransferase) activity.[8]

4. If the source individual does not consent to testing and is in a high-risk category, the exposed health care worker is given immune globulin or an HBV vaccination;
5. The exposed health care worker is counseled to be alert for acute viral symptoms within 12 weeks of exposure.

This entire medical evaluation must be completely confidential.

ISOLATION FOR HOSPITAL OUTBREAKS

Occasionally, outbreaks of particular infections occur in one or more hospital areas. For example, infection control surveillance may reveal that the nursery unit is having an excessive number of cases of staphylococcal infection. To control the outbreak, the infection control staff may dictate the need for special precautions, isolation procedures, or employee screening for staphylococcal carriers. Any health care worker entering or exiting these areas should be made aware of the special circumstances.

PROTECTIVE, OR REVERSE, ISOLATION

Many patients are put in isolation not because they have an infection, but because they are highly susceptible to infection and need to be protected from the external environment. Therefore, this type of isolation is referred to as **protective (reverse) isolation.** In general, keeping the patient in a private room and using good hand-washing techniques are sufficient precautions for health care workers caring for patients in protective isolation, but additional precautions, such as gowns, gloves, and masks, may also be used. Articles may be removed from the room and do not need to be double bagged because these patients do not have infections. Articles *entering* the room, however, must be sterile or carefully decontaminated.

A few hospitals in the United States have large protective isolation facilities for patients with combined immunodeficiencies who must live in an environment that is completely sterile. All food and articles are sterilized before they are taken into the patient's room. Some patients must live their entire lives in such a protected environment.

INFECTION CONTROL IN HOSPITAL UNITS

Other areas where patients are at a high risk of infection are the nursery, the burn unit, the postoperative care unit, the intensive care unit (ICU), and the dialysis unit. The clinical laboratory plays an important role in infection control in these hospital units and is also subject to specific infection control procedures.

INFECTION CONTROL IN A NURSERY UNIT

Newborns are easy targets for infections of all sorts because their immune systems are not fully developed at birth. Neonates may pick up pathogens from their mothers, other babies, or hospital personnel. The best way to minimize infection is to use gloves and an antiseptic for hand washing. Special clothing may be worn by nursery personnel, changed daily, and limited to the unit. Bibs should be used and discarded after contact with only one baby. Often, a baby is assigned a single nurse to limit the possible sources of infection transmission. Babies whose mothers have genital herpes must be isolated from other infants. Mothers with genital herpes must also be isolated. All individuals having contact with either the mothers or the children must be gowned and gloved, and double-bagging procedures must be used for disposal of contaminated articles in the patient's room.

INFECTION CONTROL IN A BURN UNIT

Patients with burns are also highly susceptible to infection. In some institutions, infection rates for burn patients are lower because of the availability of a completely isolated environment for each patient. Each bed is surrounded by a plastic curtain with sleeves. Hospital personnel use these sleeves when having contact with the patient. All supplies and equipment are kept outside the curtain.[1]

In hospitals lacking these facilities, burn patients are housed in private rooms. Gowning, gloving, **double bagging** (as described later in this chapter), and strict hand-washing procedures should be used. All articles in the room, as well as the room itself, should be disinfected or sterilized frequently.

INFECTION CONTROL IN AN ICU OR A POSTOPERATIVE CARE UNIT

Patients in ICUs are more critically ill and, by nature, more susceptible to infections. In most hospitals, ICUs are open areas, with numerous patients in one large room so as to be more easily monitored. Patients with known infections should be isolated according to the types of infections they have, and strict hand-washing and gloving policies are necessary in all ICUs.

Postoperative patients are susceptible to infection because surgical wounds or drains enable bacteria to gain easy access to deeper tissues. Again, each patient who becomes infected should be isolated and dealt with according to the type of infection acquired.

INFECTION CONTROL IN A DIALYSIS UNIT

Patients needing dialysis are most often immunosuppressed, which makes them a high-risk group for contracting infection, especially hepatitis. Protective gowns and gloves may be worn in the unit, and strict hand-washing and gloving techniques should be adhered to.

Table 4–5.   Infection Control Responsibilities Required in Blood Collection

Frequent handwashing

Use of personal protection equipment

Use of appropriate waste disposal practices

Maintaining good personal hygiene, including wearing clean clothes, keeping hair clean and tied back if necessary, keeping fingernails clean, and washing hands frequently

Maintaining good health by eating balanced meals in the designated areas, getting enough sleep, and getting enough exercise

Reporting personal illnesses to supervisors

Becoming familiar with and observing *all* isolation policies

Learning about the job-related aspects of infection control, and sharing this information with others

Cautioning all personnel working with known hazardous material (this can be done with proper warning labels)

Reporting violations of the policies

Reporting potential candidates for infection control (e.g., patients who are jaundiced)

INFECTION CONTROL IN THE CLINICAL LABORATORY

The clinical laboratory contributes to infection control programs in the following manner:

1. Maintaining laboratory records for surveillance purposes.
2. Reporting on infectious agents, drug-resistant microorganisms, and outbreaks.
3. Evaluating the effectiveness of sterilization or decontamination procedures.

Laboratory personnel must be cautious because they often handle specimens with infectious agents. Laboratorians have a higher incidence of hepatitis antigen, tuberculosis, tularemia, and Rocky Mountain spotted fever than that of other hospital personnel.[1] Many of these infections are acquired by aerosol spray, needle sticks, spills, mouth pipetting, and eating, drinking, or smoking in the laboratory. Such danger can easily be prevented or minimized by adhering to policies that prohibit mouth pipetting, eating, drinking, and smoking in the laboratory. Other useful procedures include hand washing; gloving; wearing protective clothing such as laboratory coats, scrubs, and face shields, if appropriate; surface decontamination; and careful disposal of needles.

The health care worker should remember that the quality of laboratory test results is only as good as the specimen collected. If the specimen is contaminated or improperly collected, laboratory test results reflect this fact and may be misleading. If sloppy techniques are used, the potential for mistakes and infection is greater. Table 4–5 details the infection control policies that health care workers must follow during blood collection.

■ SPECIFIC ISOLATION TECHNIQUES

In most hospitals, all supplies required for isolation procedures are located in an area or on a cart just outside the patient's room. After washing their hands, health care personnel may put on the appropriate PPE just prior to entering the room.

HAND WASHING

Hand washing is the most important procedure in the prevention of disease transmission in hospitals. It should be the first and last step of any isolation procedure (Fig. 4–5A–C). Scrubbing for surgery requires a different procedure than washing hands for general patient care. For general purposes, hand washing usually removes potential pathogens but does not necessarily sterilize the hands. Good technique involves soap, warm running water, and friction.[1] Soap removes oils that may hold bacteria to the skin. Many varieties of soap are available for general purposes; however, health care personnel who purchase supplies should choose soaps that are mild, easy to use, and form a good lather. In health care environments with high rates of antibiotic-resistant organisms, medicated hand-washing agents (i.e., chlorhexidine) instead of bland soap should be used.[9] Rubbing action with soap and water should continue for at least 10 seconds to create a lather over the entire hand surface. Warm running water washes away loosened debris and lathers the soap. Friction from rubbing the hands together loosens and removes dead skin, oil, and microorganisms. The health care worker should thoroughly rub both sides of each hand and between each finger. Hands should be rinsed in a downward position. After rinsing, the faucet should be turned off by grasping the handles with paper towels to prevent reinoculation of microorganisms onto the hands. Drying of hands should be with single-use or disposable towels or with an air dryer.

GOWNING

After hand washing, a sterile gown should be put on by touching only its inside surface. It should have long sleeves and be large and long enough to cover all clothing (Fig. 4–5D). Gowns are generally made of cloth or paper. The health care worker's back must be completely covered, the belt tied, and the sleeves pulled all the way to the wrists.

MASKING

After gowning, a mask (if necessary) may be put over the nose and mouth (Fig. 4–5E). Masks protect the health care worker from small-particle droplets that may carry infectious agents. Often, a small metal band on the mask can be shaped to fit the nose. Two ties are usually made, the first around the upper portion of the head and the second around the upper portion of the neck. Most masks become ineffective after prolonged use (20 minutes) or if they become wet.[1]

GLOVING

Chemically clean disposable gloves may be used for most isolation procedures. The exception is protective isolation procedures, for which *sterile* disposable gloves should be used.

Figure 4–5. Specific isolation techniques: hand washing, gowning, masking, gloving, and double bagging. A. Hand-washing techniques should involve soap lather, friction between hands, and thorough washing between fingers. B. Washing should include the wrist areas.

A

B

Figure 4–5. C. Lather should be rinsed. Rinsing should continue until all soap is removed. If the water must be turned off by hand, a clean paper towel should be used to grab the faucet. D. Gowns should be large enough to cover all clothing. Sleeves should be pulled down and the back covered. E. The mask should be tied in two places and should fit comfortably. F. Gloves should be pulled over the ends of gown sleeves.

C

D

E

F

(continued)

Figure 4–5. *(continued)*   G–I. After specimen collection, the gown should be removed from inside out. J. Double bagging involves two individuals, one inside the room and one outside.

G

H

I

J

Gloves should be pulled over the ends of gown sleeves (Fig. 4–5F). Rings and other pieces of jewelry should not be worn because they may puncture a glove during patient contact. Gloves are also discussed in Chapter 8.

ENTERING AND EXITING THE ROOM

Isolation bags for transporting specimens are often available. The bag may be turned halfway inside out and left near the door outside the room, or someone may be available to hold the bag outside the door. Only the needed supplies should be taken into the room. Phlebotomy requisitions may be left outside the room on the isolation cart. If drawing a blood specimen, the health care provider may use a tourniquet in the room or leave the one brought in. The specimen should be labeled at the bedside and the pen left in the room. Used needles, swabs, and so forth should be put in appropriate containers inside the room.

Any blood on the outside of the specimen container should be removed with a paper towel. While standing in the doorway, and touching only the inside of the isolation bag, the health care worker should place the specimen inside the bag. Gloved hands should be washed in the room. The faucet may be turned off with a paper towel.

The mask, if used, can be removed by carefully untying the lower tie first, then the upper one. Only the ends of the ties should be held. The mask should then be properly disposed of inside the room. In some cases, a special container for masks is placed just outside the room to prevent exposure of hospital personnel to airborne diseases while inside.

The gown is removed by first breaking the paper tie or untying the sash. It should be removed and folded with the contaminated side turned inside and with care taken not to touch the uniform (Fig. 4–5G–I). One glove may be removed, and the second one can be slipped off by sliding the index finger of the ungloved hand between the glove and the hand.

Just before leaving the room, however, hands must be washed again and a paper towel used to turn off the faucet. A clean paper towel should be used to open the door. The door should be held open with one foot and the used paper towels discarded in the wastebasket directly inside the patient's room.

Once outside the room, the requisition forms may be checked again, placed carefully in the isolation bag, and sealed. Care must be taken to avoid touching the inside of the bag holding the specimen. Personnel should wash their hands again before proceeding with other duties.

DISPOSING OF CONTAMINATED ITEMS

Trash, linens, and other articles in an isolation room may be removed by using one sturdy biohazardous bag or the double-bagging procedure. Double bagging involves putting contaminated material in one bag and sealing it inside the room. A different person should stand outside the doorway with another opened, clean, impermeable bag (Fig. 4–5J). The person standing outside the room should have the ends of the bag folded over the hands to shield them from possible contamination. The sealed bag from the room may then be placed inside the clean bag. The person outside the room can then fold over the edges, expel the air, and seal the outer bag. The bag must be labeled with biohazard warnings.

■ PREVENTION OF LABORATORY-ACQUIRED INFECTIONS

As mentioned previously, health care workers must be extremely cautious with biohazardous specimens. Policies and procedures for handling such specimens should be defined in the laboratory policy manual and should be reviewed periodically by health care workers who collect and transport specimens. Infections from these specimens may be spread during collection and handling by means of several routes. The actual occurrence of an infection from a biohazardous specimen depends on the virulence of the infecting agent and the host's susceptibility.

■ STERILE TECHNIQUE FOR HEALTH CARE WORKERS

All health care personnel should realize that bacteria and other microorganisms can be found everywhere. For example, human skin is covered with bacteria. Because of this fact, all health care personnel should be responsible for cleanliness and maintaining sterility when handling instruments, catheters, IV supplies, or other devices that come into contact with patients.

! Clinical Alert

The following are possible routes of infection from collected specimens and therefore should be considered when health care personnel must collect or process specimens for laboratory assays:

1. *Skin contact.* Virulent organisms can enter through skin abrasions and cuts or through the conjunctiva of the eye. Thus, scratches from needles and broken glass must be avoided. If the health care worker has a cut or an abrasion, he or she should always wear a laboratory coat, gloves, and protective adhesive tape over the cut or abrasion to prevent possible inoculation from infectious specimens. He or she must also avoid rubbing the eyes.
2. *Ingestion.* Failure to wash contaminated hands and subsequent handling of cigarettes, gum, food, or drinks can result in an infection from a biohazardous specimen. Each employee must comply with the safety rules of the laboratory to prevent transmission of infections.
3. *Airborne.* Aerosol spray created from patient's specimens by careless splashing or centrifugation must be prevented. Dangerous, infectious aerosol spray can be caused from popping tops off blood specimen vacuum tubes and centrifugating the blood specimens. To protect against blood exposure during this hazardous step, cover the tube with a gauze pad while removing the top. Also, manufacturers recently developed different types of items that minimize airborne transmissions (see Chapter 7, Blood Collection Equipment). Prior to centrifugation, vacuum tubes should be inspected for cracks, and tubes with wet rims should be wiped dry. The centrifuge brake should not be applied to save time because braking can cause infectious aerosol formation. Centrifuged infectious specimens must not be poured because of the potential hazards from aerosol formation. Instead, the contents should be transferred by using a disposable pipette with a rubber bulb or its equivalent and gently transferring the contents down the wall of the aliquot tube or tubes.

The health care worker is responsible for using sterile supplies for skin punctures and venipunctures and antiseptics for patient preparation. Alcohol pads are often used to cleanse skin sites for venipuncture. Although rubbing with alcohol pads destroys most of the bacteria, it does not destroy all microorganisms. A special decontamination procedure is required to obtain a sterile site. Venipuncture for blood cultures requires this type of preparation, as discussed thoroughly in Chapter 12.

New needles and most blood collection tubes are sterilized by the manufacturers. Once the covering of a needle or a lancet is removed, the needle or lancet should not touch anything until it punctures the skin. If it accidentally touches *anything* prior to contact with the skin site, it must be discarded appropriately and replaced with a new one. If a needle is used for an unsuccessful venipuncture, it too *must* be discarded and replaced with a new one before another puncture is attempted.

Sterile technique and isolation procedures may require sterile gloves. If this is the case, the health care worker must make sure that the package of gloves indicates that they are sterile. Some manufacturers produce gloves that are *chemically clean* but not necessarily *sterile*. Most sterile gloves are available in various hand sizes. If the gloves do not fit properly, they may interfere with the procedure. Use of gloves is also discussed in Chapter 7 on Blood Collection Equipment.

DISINFECTANTS AND ANTISEPTICS

Disinfectants are chemical compounds used to remove or kill pathogenic microorganisms.[10] Chemical disinfectants are regulated by the Environmental Protection Agency (EPA). A list of EPA-registered products may be obtained by contacting the National Antimicrobial Information Network at 800.447.6349 or http://www.ace.orst.edu/info/nain/index/htm. **Antiseptics** are chemicals used to inhibit the growth and development of microorganisms but do not necessarily kill them. Antiseptics may be used on human skin, whereas disinfectants are generally used on surfaces and instruments because they are too corrosive for direct use on skin. A disinfectant with a product label claiming that the disinfectant is HIVcidal or tuberculocidal, or a disinfectant having a chlorine bleach dilution of 1:10, should be used to disinfect tourniquets and items contaminated with blood or other body fluids. A more diluted solution of chlorine bleach (1:100) can be used for routine cleaning of surfaces.[11] Gloves and gowns should be worn when performing decontamination procedures. The *minimal* contact time for disinfectants to be effective is 10 minutes.[12] Table 4–6 lists some of the more common hospital disinfectants and antiseptics used.

Table 4–6. Common Antiseptics and Disinfectants for the Health Care Setting

COMPOUND	USES AND RESTRICTIONS
Alcohols	
Ethyl (70%)	Antiseptic for skin
Isopropyl (70%)	Antiseptic for skin
Chlorine	
Chloramine	Disinfectant for wounds
Hypochlorite solutions	Disinfectant
Ethylene oxide	Disinfectant (toxic)
Formaldehyde	Disinfectant (noxious fumes)
Glutaraldehyde	Disinfectant (toxic)
Hydrogen peroxide	Antiseptic for skin
Iodine	
Tincture	Antiseptic for skin (can be irritating)
Iodophors	Antiseptic for skin (less stable)
Phenolic compounds	
1–2% phenols	Disinfectant
Chlorophenol	Disinfectant (toxic)
Hexachlorophene	Antiseptic for skin (used in surgery)
Chlorhexidine	Antiseptic for skin
Hexylresorcinol	Antiseptic for skin
Quaternary ammonium compounds	Antiseptic for skin (ingredient in many soaps)

SELF STUDY

KEY TERMS

Antiseptics
Centers for Disease Control and
 Prevention (CDC)
Chain of Infection
Disinfectants
Double Bagging
Fomites
Infection Control Programs
Isolation Procedures
Mode of Transmission
Nosocomial Infections

Occupational Safety and Health
 Administration (OSHA)
Pathogenic Agents
Protective (Reverse) Isolation
Source
Standard Precautions
Sterile Technique
Surveillance
Susceptible Host
Universal Precautions

STUDY QUESTIONS

The following may have *one* or *more* answers:

1. Which of the following types of nosocomial infections are most prevalent?

   a. dermal infections
   b. wound infections

   c. respiratory tract infections
   d. urinary tract infections

2. Name the links in the chain of infection.

   a. poor isolation technique
   b. susceptible host

   c. source
   d. mode of transmission

3. What is/are the primary function(s) of isolation procedures?

   a. keep the hospital clean
   b. prevent transmission of
      communicable diseases
      environments

   c. protect the general public
      from disease
   d. provide protective

4. Nurses, physicians, and other health care workers are responsible for knowing the
   procedures of which type(s) of isolation?

   a. strict
   b. drainage/secretion
   c. enteric

   d. droplet
   e. airborne
   f. universal precautions

5. Which of the following precautions prevents infectious aerosol spray?
    a. popping the cap on a vacuum collection tube rather than twisting it
    b. inspecting vacuum tubes for cracks prior to centrifugation
    c. applying the centrifuge brake to save time during centrifugation of specimens
    d. pouring the specimens into the required aliquot tubes

6. Protective isolation is generally used for
    a. an adult patient with active tuberculosis
    b. a pediatric patient who has an immunodeficiency
    c. an adult patient with meningitis
    d. a pediatric patient who has whooping cough

7. Which of the following laboratory-acquired infections is most prevalent?
    a. HIV infection
    b. Rocky Mountain spotted fever
    c. HBV infection
    d. tuberculosis

8. Airborne precautions may be required for patients with infections such as
    a. tuberculosis
    b. whooping cough
    c. *Salmonella*
    d. Rocky Mountain spotted fever

9. According to the OSHA standards for occupational exposure to blood-borne pathogens, which of the following is a PPE?
    a. 10 percent household bleach
    b. fluid-resistant gown
    c. goggles
    d. respirator

10. In Spanish, *peligro biologico* refers to the English term
    a. hepatitis
    b. biohazardous
    c. blood-borne pathogen
    d. *Salmonella*

References

1. Bennett, JV, Brachman, PS (eds.): *Hospital Infections,* 3rd ed. Boston; Little, Brown & Co: 1992.
2. Jasny, BR, Bloom, FE: It's not rocket science—but it can save lives. *Science* 1998; 280:1507.
3. Castle, M, Ajemian, E: *Hospital Infection Control.* New York; John Wiley & Sons: 1987.
4. Guidelines for prevention of transmission of human immunodeficiency virus and hepatitis B virus to health-care and public-safety workers. *MMWR* 1989; 38(S-6).
5. US Department of Labor and Occupational Safety and Health Administration (OSHA): Occupational exposure to bloodborne pathogens; final rule (29 CFR 1910.1030). *Federal Register* 1991; Dec 6: 6404-64182.
6. Needlestick Safety and Prevention Bill (11/2000). HR 5178 www.thomas.loc.gov
7. Garner, JS: Guideline for Isolation Precautions in Hospitals. *Infection Control and Hospital Epidemiology* 17(1):53–60.
8. Department of Health and Human Services, Centers for Disease Control and Prevention: *Hepatitis Surveillance: Issues and Answers.* Report No. 56, April, 1996.

9. Wade, JJ, Pesai, N, Casewell, MW. Hygienic hand disinfection for the removal of epidemic vancomycin-resistant *Enterococcus Faecium* and gentamicin-resistant *Enterobacter cloacae*. *J. Hosp Infect* 1991; 18:211–218.

10. Luebbert, P. Choosing the appropriate disinfectant. *Lab Med.* 1992; 23 (2):126.

11. National Committee for Clinical Laboratory Standards (NCCLS): *Protection of Laboratory Workers from Instrument Biohazards and Infectious Disease Transmitted by Blood, Body Fluids and Tissue.* NCCLS Document M29-A. Villanova, PA; 1997.

12. Sattar, SA, Springthorpe, VS. Survival and disinfection inactivation of HIV. A Critical Review. *Rev Infect Dis* 1991; 13:430–447.

FIVE

■

Safety and First Aid

CHAPTER OUTLINE

CHAPTER OBJECTIVES

Upon completion of Chapter 5, the learner is responsible for the following:

1. Discuss safety awareness for health care workers.
2. Explain the measures that should be taken for fire, electrical, radiation, mechanical, and chemical safety in a health care facility.
3. Describe the essential elements of a disaster emergency plan for a health care facility.

4. Explain the safety policies and procedures that must be followed in all phases of specimen collection and transportation.

5. Describe the safe use of equipment in health care facilities.

The goal of safety in the health care institution is to recognize and eliminate hazards and provide information on safety education so that employees can work in a healthy environment. Safe working conditions must be ensured by the employer and have been mandated by law under the **Occupational Safety and Health Administration (OSHA)** standards (1910.1030).[1] Knowledge of OSHA requirements and cooperation between the employer and employee concerning these requirements are necessary in all health care facilities, including home health care agencies (Box 5–1). The health care worker involved in blood collection needs to become aware of safety policies and procedures in his or her health care facility and to receive proper instruction on safety requirements. These safety policies and procedures must follow *Universal Precautions* as discussed in Chapter 4. The NCCLS has also published a similar set of recommendations for the prevention of blood-borne exposure.[2]

■ SAFETY IN SPECIMEN HANDLING

Patients' specimens should be handled with caution to prevent the possibility of acquiring an infection, such as hepatitis or one associated with acquired immunodeficiency syndrome (AIDS). Health care workers who are routinely exposed to blood and body fluids must take the simple precaution of wearing gloves to protect themselves from infection. Further discussion of precautionary measures for specimen handling can be found in Chapter 4, Infection Control.

BOX 5–1.   SAFETY PRECAUTIONS FOR THE HEALTH CARE WORKER

1. Gloves must be worn during *all* phases of blood collection procedures (at inpatient and outpatient facilities). Health care workers should make every effort to avoid contact with blood, body fluids, nonintact skin, and mucous membranes.

2. Gloves must be changed between patient collections, and hands must be washed after gloves are removed.

3. A laboratory coat, a smock, or a gown must be worn during blood collection procedures and left at the laboratory or clinic when the health care worker leaves the work area. The laboratory coat must be cleaned at the health care facility.

4. A personal respirator should be used if exposure to aerosolized *Mycobacterium tuberculosis* is possible.

5. Facial protection must be provided at the health care facility and used by the health care worker if any possibility of body fluid or blood splashing exists.

6. Needles should *never* be recapped by hand.

7. All sharps, including needles and lancets, must be disposed of *carefully* in a rigid needle container.

8. Blood collection items must be disposed of according to the proper procedure for biohazardous waste disposal.

9. Blood collection devices and surfaces must be decontaminated. Work surfaces must be cleaned at least once a day as well as after contact with blood or other potentially infectious materials with *freshly* prepared 10% solution of household bleach (5.25% sodium hypochloride).

OSHA Revised Directive for Safer Medical Devices

On November 5, 1999, OSHA issued a revised compliance directive (CPL2-2.44D) for the Bloodborne Pathogens Standard that provides an expanded definition of "engineering controls," emphasizing the use of safer medical devices as a primary means of reducing needlesticks and other sharps injuries.[3] The following recommendations have been provided for both the health care facility employer and the health care worker.

Recommendations for Employers
- Eliminate the use of needle devices where safe and effective alternatives are available.
- Implement the use of needle devices with safety features and evaluate their use to determine which are most effective and acceptable.
- Analyze needlestick and other sharps-related injuries in your workplace to identify hazards and injury trends.
- Set priorities and prevention strategies by examining local and national information about risk factors for needlestick injuries and successful intervention efforts.
- Ensure that health care workers are properly trained in the safe disposal of needles.
- Modify work practices that pose a needlestick injury hazard to make them safer.
- Promote safety awareness in the work environment.
- Establish procedures for and encourage the reporting and timely follow up of all needlestick and other sharps-related injuries.
- Evaluate the effectiveness of prevention efforts and provide feedback on performance.

Recommendations for Health Care Workers
- Avoid the use of needles where safe and effective alternatives are available.
- Help your employer select and evaluate devices with safety features.
- Use devices with safety features provided by your employer.
- Avoid recapping needles.
- Plan safe handling and disposal before beginning any procedure using needles.
- Dispose of used needle devices promptly in appropriate sharps disposal containers.
- Report all needlestick and other sharps-related injuries promptly to ensure that you receive appropriate follow-up care.
- Tell your employer about hazards from needles that you observe in your work environment.
- Participate in bloodborne pathogen training and follow recommended infection prevention practices, including Hepatitis B vaccination.

From " NIOSH Alert: Preventing Needlestick Injuries in Health Care Settings," November, 1999. Available on the Web at: www.cdc.gov/niosh

Safety Advisory Issued for Glass Capillary Tubes

The Food and Drug Administration (FDA), the National Institute for Occupational Safety and Health (NIOSH) of the Centers for Disease Control and Prevention (CDC), and the Occupational Safety and Health Administration (OSHA) issued a safety advisory on the potential risk of injury or infection from blood-borne pathogens—including HIV, hepatitis B, and hepatitis C—from breakage of glass capillary tubes containing blood specimens.[4] Glass capillary tubes have been used for the collection of blood in a variety of health care settings, including hospitals, ambulatory care facilities, physicians' offices, blood donation facilities, and blood testing centers. Accidental breakage of these slender, fragile tubes has been reported when the tubes are inserted into putty to be sealed and during centrifugation.

To reduce the risk of injury due to breakage of capillary tubes, FDA, NIOSH, and OSHA recommend that users consider blood collection devices less prone to accidental breakage, including:

1. Capillary tubes that are not made of glass.
2. Glass capillary tubes wrapped in puncture-resistant film.
3. Products that use a method of sealing that does not require manually pushing one end of the tube into putty to form a plug.
4. Products that allow the blood hematocrit to be measured without centrifugation. Additional information on this advisory can be found at the FDA Web site: www.fda.gov/cdrh/safety.html or NIOSH at phone number 800.35.NIOSH.

■ EXPOSURE CONTROL

! Clinical Alert

Any incident of exposure to potentially harmful or infectious substances should be reported immediately to Employee or Personnel Health, or in the absence of a separate department, to a supervisor. Each health care worker should know who to contact, where to go, and what to do if inadvertently exposed. This information is included in an **Exposure Control Plan** that is designed for that health care facility. This is important because the health care worker should seek advice about medical treatment or prophylaxis, depending on the type of exposure. Also, reporting work-related exposures is required for worker's compensation documentation. If exposures are not reported, it is difficult to prove retrospectively that an exposure was work-related.

■ PERSONAL HYGIENE

! Clinical Alert

While on the job, nothing should be inserted into one's mouth (e.g., food, pencils). Hands should be washed frequently during the day; before and after contact with patients or patients' specimens; before and after eating, drinking, or smoking; and before and after using restrooms. Cosmetics should not be applied while on the job. The health care worker should avoid biting his or her fingernails and rubbing the eyes. Eating, drinking, or smoking within the specimen control section and other laboratory sections must be avoided (Fig. 5–1). No food should be placed in any laboratory refrigerator unless the refrigerator is designated "FOR FOOD ONLY." A laboratory coat should be worn completely buttoned while collecting specimens and removed prior to coffee

Clinical Alert (*continued*) ❗

breaks or lunch. Loose clothing, such as scarves, which might become entangled in the centrifuge, should never be worn. Long hair must be tied so that it cannot come in contact with specimens or become entangled in the centrifuge. Open-toed shoes are usually prohibited in most clinical laboratories because of potential chemical and glassware hazards.

Figure 5–1. Required safety precautions during specimen collection and specimen processing.

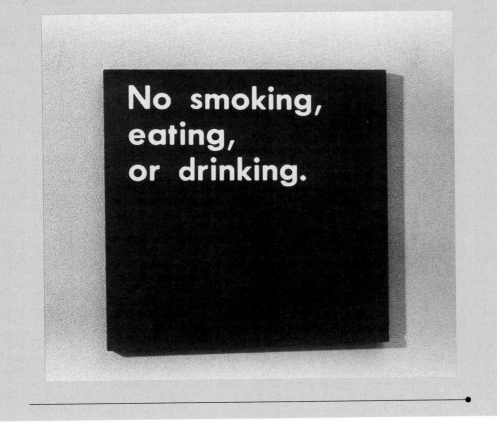

■ LABORATORY SAFETY

Laboratory safety includes a variety of policies. All health care workers, however, should remember a few key safety rules at all times.

- Patients' specimens should be covered at all times during transportation and centrifugation.

- Centrifugation of specimens should be performed within a biohazard safety hood.
- All wastes from specimen collections must be disposed of in the correct containers.
- Needles should not be recapped, bent, or broken.

Specific **Environmental Protection Agency (EPA)** and OSHA regulations, as well as state and local laws, regulate the disposal of wastes. Blood and body fluids should be disposed of through an approved biohazardous waste disposal company. Urine specimens are usually flushed down the drain with water or flushed down the toilet. These biological liquid wastes should be disposed of gently so that they do not splash onto other objects, and hand washing should not occur in sinks used for disposal of these wastes.

Needles *must not* be recapped before disposal (Fig. 5–2). Sharps, such as needles and lancets, should be disposed of in a special container that is spillproof, tamperproof, puncture resistant, and closable and that can be autoclaved. The sharps container must be labeled in red or orange, must be maintained upright, and must display the biohazard symbol (Fig. 5–3).

In addition, the specimen collection area should be decontaminated with a 1:10 bleach solution. Because a diluted bleach solution becomes unstable when exposed to oxygen, it must be prepared daily. Alternatively, a diluted bleach solution that is stable is available

Figure 5–2.   Universal precautions in patient care.

(Courtesy of United Ad Label [UAL] Co., Inc., Brea, CA.)

Includes blood and any body fluids

1. Wash hands BEFORE and AFTER patient care.

2. Wear gloves when likely to touch body substances, mucous membranes or non-intact skin.

3. Wear gown when clothing is likely to become soiled.

4. Wear mask and protective eyewear or a face shield when likely to be splashed with body fluids.

5. Place intact needle/syringe units and sharps in designated disposal container. DO NOT BREAK OR BEND NEEDLES.

Figure 5–3. Biohazard symbol.

commercially. If blood or other body fluids are spilled, encapsulating powder, which is available from manufacturers of safety products (e.g., United Ad Label Direct, Brea, CA), should be used to gel the liquid for safe cleanup.

Colored biohazard labels must be affixed to all containers of regulated waste, refrigerators and freezers containing blood or other body fluids, and other containers used to store, transport, or ship these materials.

If an accident occurs, such as a needle stick, the injured health care worker should immediately cleanse the area with isopropyl alcohol and apply a Band-Aid. Then, he or she should follow the exposure control plan for that facility (i.e., notify the immediate supervisor, fill out the necessary incident and medical forms, and undergo the appropriate laboratory tests). In addition, the health care worker should be counseled and evaluated for HIV and HCV infection at periodic intervals (see "OSHA Standards for Occupational Exposure to Blood-Borne Pathogens" in Chapter 4).

■ FIRE SAFETY

Fire safety is the responsibility of all employees in the health care institution. Health care workers should be familiar with not only the use and location of the fire extinguishers but also the procedures to follow during a fire. They should also be knowledgeable of the exact locations of fire extinguishers and fire blankets. The blankets should be available to smother burning clothes or to use as a fire shield if fire is blocking the exit. Health care institutions usually conduct periodic safety education programs in which the health care worker can participate and become skillful in and knowledgeable about the use of fire safety equipment.

CLASSIFICATION OF FIRES

The components of fire are fuel, oxygen, and heat, plus the necessary chain reaction. Four general classifications of fires have been adopted by the National Fire Protection Association (NFPA).[5] These classifications are as follows:

1. *Class A fires* occur with ordinary combustible material, such as wood, rubbish, paper, cloth, and many plastics.
2. *Class B fires* occur in a vapor–air mixture over flammable solvents, such as gasoline, oil, paint, lacquers, grease, and flammable gases.
3. *Class C fires* occur in or near electrical equipment.
4. *Class D fires* occur with combustible metals, such as magnesium, sodium, and lithium. These fires are infrequently encountered in health care institutions.

■ FIRE EXTINGUISHERS

Fire extinguishers are classified to correspond with each class of fire.

1. *Class A extinguishers* contain soda and acid or water and are used to cool the ordinary fire.
2. *Class B extinguishers* contain foam, dry chemicals, or carbon dioxide (CO_2) and are used to combat fires occurring in vapor–air mixtures over solvents.
3. *Class C extinguishers* contain dry chemicals, Halon (Allied Corporation, Morristown, NJ), or CO_2 (nonconducting extinguishing agents) and are used to combat electrical fires.
4. *Multipurpose (ABC) extinguishers* are frequently installed in health care institutions because they reduce the confusion associated with operating and maintaining different types of extinguishers.

As shown in Figure 5–4, the health care worker should learn how to use the various kinds of fire extinguishers in the workplace. Use of the wrong type of extinguisher may not only fail to put out the fire, but it can actually spread it.

In the event of a fire, the health care worker should *do* the following:

- Immediately pull the lever in the alarm box nearest the area he or she is in.
- Call the assigned fire number, which should be posted on or near each telephone.
- If the fire is small, attempt to extinguish it, using the proper extinguisher.
- If evacuation becomes necessary, use only the stairwells for exiting.
- Close all doors and windows before leaving the area.
- If clothing is on fire, drop to the ground and roll, preferably in a fire blanket.
- If caught in a fire, crawl to the exit. Because smoke rises, breathing is easier at floor level. Breathing through a wet towel is also helpful.

The health care worker should *not do* the following:

- Block entrances.
- Reenter the building.
- Panic.
- Run.

Figure 5–4. Proper use of fire extinguishers.

(Courtesy of Risk Analysis and Loss Control— Institutional Affairs, The University of Texas–Houston Health Science Center, Houston, TX.)

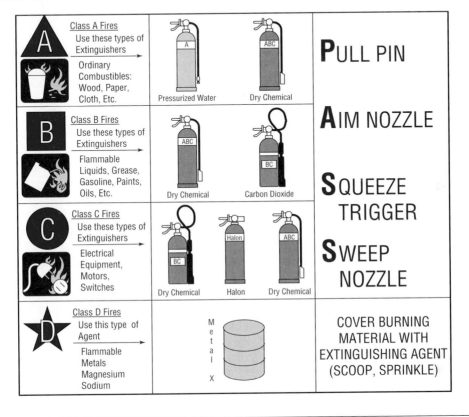

■ ELECTRICAL SAFETY

A major hazard in any area of a health care institution is the possibility of electrical current passing through a person. For example, in the clinical laboratory or physician office laboratory, the health care worker sometimes operates electrical equipment, such as a centrifuge. He or she should be aware of the location of the circuit breaker boxes in order to assure a fast response in the event of an electrical fire or an electrical shock.

The health care worker should not use electrical equipment if power cords are frayed or if control switches and thermostats are not in good working order. The centrifuge or other electrical equipment must be unplugged before maintenance is performed. Any electrical instrument that has had liquid spilled on or in it or has had liquid come in contact with the wiring should be immediately unplugged and dried prior to further use.

If an electrical accident occurs involving electrical shock to an employee or a patient, the health care worker should be aware of the following two points:

1. The electrical power source must be shut off. If this is impossible, carefully remove the electrical contact from the victim using something, such as asbestos gloves, that does not conduct electricity, or place your hand in a glass beaker and push the power supply away from the victim. The rescuer should not attempt to touch the victim without heeding these precautions.
2. Medical assistance should be called and **cardiopulmonary resuscitation (CPR)** started immediately. The victim should not be moved prior to the arrival of medical assistance. A fire blanket or other warm clothing should be put over the victim to keep him or her warm until medical help arrives.

■ RADIATION SAFETY

The three cardinal principles of self-protection from radiation exposure are time, shielding, and distance. Radiation exposure is cumulative; thus, limiting the length of exposure at any one time is a major factor in minimizing the hazard.

Areas where radioactive materials are in use and stored must have warning signs (Fig. 5–5) posted on the entrance doors. All radioactive specimens and reagents must also be properly labeled with the radioactive sign.

The health care worker will probably encounter potential hazards from radiation exposure only if he or she must collect specimens from patients in the nuclear medicine or x-ray department or must take specimens to the radioimmunoassay section in research or a clinical chemistry laboratory. Thus the health care worker should be cautious when entering an area posted with the radiation sign and should be knowledgeable of the institution's procedures pertaining to radiation safety. Health care workers who are pregnant should be aware of the potential hazard of radiation to the fetus.

Figure 5–5. Sign for possible radiation hazard.

■ MECHANICAL SAFETY

The centrifuge is a frequently used instrument for blood specimen preparation and testing. Thus a health care provider who collects and prepares blood specimens for testing should learn how to maintain this instrument and become familiar with its parts. For example, he or she should know if the carriers are in the correct position prior to use. If the carriers are not in the correct position, they can swing out of the holding disks into the side of the centrifuge. Also, the wrong head, the wrong cups, or imbalanced tubes can lead to the same dangerous problem. If this particular type of accident occurs, tubes containing patients' specimens or spinning chemicals may be propelled onto the side of the centrifuge, and broken, and a dangerous, hazardous problem created. Thus it is of utmost importance to abide by the preventive maintenance schedule and procedures for the centrifuge.

■ CHEMICAL SAFETY

Because a health care worker must sometimes pour preservatives, such as hydrochloric acid (HCl), into containers for 24-hour urine collections and transport these specimens to the patients' floor, he or she should be knowledgeable of chemical safety. Labeling may be the single most important step in the proper handling of chemicals. Laboratorians should be able to ascertain from appropriate labels not only the contents of the container but also the nature and extent of hazards posed by the chemicals. Carefully read the label before using any reagents.

CHEMICAL IDENTIFICATION

Various chemicals are needed in health care facilities, especially in the clinical laboratory department. Because chemicals may pose health or physical hazards, OSHA amended the *Hazard Communication Standard* (29 CFR 1910.1200, Right to Know/HCS Standard) to include health care facilities.[6,7] Thus labels for hazardous chemicals must (1) provide a warning (e.g., corrosive), (2) explain the nature of the hazard (e.g., flammable, combustible), (3) state special precautions to eliminate risks, and (4) explain first-aid treatment in the event of a chemical leak, a chemical spill, or other exposure to the chemical. In addition to mandating labels, the Right to Know law requires chemical manufacturers to supply **material safety data sheets (MSDSs)** for their chemicals. The MSDS is required for any chemical with a hazard warning label. An MSDS lists general information, precautionary measures, and emergency information.

The NFPA developed a labeling system for hazardous chemicals that is frequently used in health care facilities (Fig. 5–6). The system uses a diamond-shaped symbol, four colored quadrants, and a hazard rating scale of 0 to 4. The health hazard is shown in the blue quadrant, the flammability hazard is shown in the red quadrant, the instability hazard is indicated in the yellow quadrant, and the specific hazard is shown in the white quadrant.

PROTECTIVE MEASURES

The proper clothing must be worn when a health care worker is working with chemicals. A buttoned laboratory coat, safety glasses, and gloves provide protection and prevent skin contact. When transporting acids or alkalis, an *acid carrier* should be used. It is a specially designed container for carrying large quantities of hazardous solutions.

Figure 5–6. National Fire Protection Association (NFPA) 0 to 4 hazard rating system.

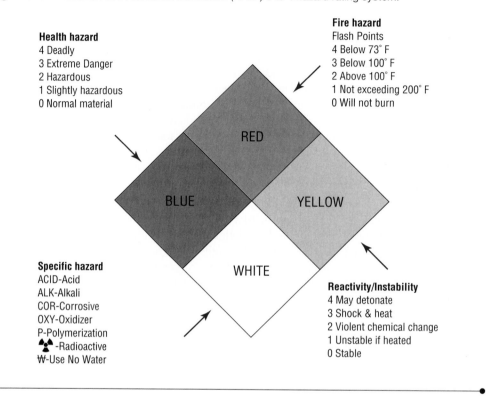

Health hazard
4 Deadly
3 Extreme Danger
2 Hazardous
1 Slightly hazardous
0 Normal material

Fire hazard
Flash Points
4 Below 73° F
3 Below 100° F
2 Above 100° F
1 Not exceeding 200° F
0 Will not burn

Specific hazard
ACID-Acid
ALK-Alkali
COR-Corrosive
OXY-Oxidizer
P-Polymerization
☢-Radioactive
W̶-Use No Water

Reactivity/Instability
4 May detonate
3 Shock & heat
2 Violent chemical change
1 Unstable if heated
0 Stable

The entrance of any room in which hazardous chemicals are in use or in storage must be posted with a caution sign specifying the types of chemicals present. No chemicals should be stored above eye level because of the danger of breakage or spillage involved in reaching. All explosives should be stored in an explosionproof or a fireproof room that is separate from the flammables.

SAFETY SHOWERS AND THE EYEWASH STATION

Safety showers should be nearby for use if an accidental chemical spill occurs. Because permanent damage to the skin can result from chemical burns, the victim of a chemical accident must immediately rinse for at least 15 minutes after removing contaminated clothing.

In case of a chemical spill in the eye, the victim should rinse his or her eyes at the eyewash station for a minimum of 15 minutes. Contact lenses must be removed prior to the rinsing in order to thoroughly cleanse the eyes. The victim should not rub the eyes because doing so may cause further injury. If someone is hurt in a chemical spill, it is preferable to take the victim to the emergency department for treatment after his or her eyes have been rinsed for 15 minutes.

CHEMICAL SPILL CLEANUP

If a chemical spill occurs, the health care worker should obtain a spill cleanup kit from the clinical chemistry section. The kit includes absorbents and neutralizers to clean up acid, alkali, mercury, and other spills. The absorbent and neutralizer used depend on the type of chemical spill and have an indicator system that identifies when the spill has been neutralized and can be considered safe for sweep up and disposal. The health care worker should become familiar with the procedures for cleaning up chemical spills in his or her place of employment.

DISPOSAL OF CHEMICALS

Chemical wastes that are water soluble, such as acids and alkalis, can be flushed down the sink with cold water; however, acids and alkalis should be poured into a large amount of water before flushing them down the sink. The acid *must* be added to the water and not vice versa to prevent a violent chemical reaction.

■ EQUIPMENT AND SAFETY IN PATIENTS' ROOMS

Each member of the health care team is responsible for the safety of the patient. All health care professionals are responsible for patient safety from the time the patient enters the health care setting until his or her departure. As a matter of general patient safety, the phlebotomist should do the following when in the patient's room:

1. Make certain that all specimen collection supplies, needles, and equipment are either properly disposed of or returned to the specimen collection tray after blood collection.
2. Check to see whether the bed rails are up or down. Always place bed rails up before leaving the patient if they were up when you entered the room.
3. Report unusual odors to the nursing station because a pipe may be broken and be leaking gas or liquid.
4. Check for food or liquid spilled on the floor, urine spills, or intravenous (IV) line leakage. Areas on which the patient and health care professionals walk must be dry. They should be free of obstacles and slipping hazards. Thus, in cases of spills, make certain that the area is cleaned and dried for the safety of the patient and hospital personnel.
5. During blood collection, be very cautious not to touch any electrical instrument located adjacent to the patient's bed because if the instrument malfunctions, the health care worker may ground the patient and, as a result, a microshock could pass through the health care worker and into the patient. A serious problem could result from such a shock if the patient has an electrolyte imbalance or is wet with perspiration or other fluid. Furthermore, the needle inserted in the patient's arm could produce ventricular fibrillation and death if the patient has a pacemaker or an unstable heart ailment.
6. Report the following problem immediately to the nursing station: If the patient has an IV line and the site is swollen and red, the IV needle is probably no longer in the vein and the IV solution is infiltrating into the surrounding tissues. Some chemicals

in IV solutions are toxic to body tissue, so gangrene could result from such infiltration. Also, if blood is backing up the IV line from the needle insertion to the IV drip container, the IV solution container is empty. Report this problem immediately.

7. If the patient's alarm for the IV drip is sounding, report this problem to the nursing station immediately.

8. If the patient is in unusual pain or is unresponsive, notify the nursing station immediately.

■ PATIENT SAFETY OUTSIDE THE ROOM

Health care workers should be aware of possible hazards to patients outside the patients' rooms. As a matter of general safety practice, the following guidelines should be followed:

1. Because trays, carts, and ladders may be placed around a hallway corner, the health care worker should be careful not to travel too quickly from one room to another and around corners.

2. Items lying on the floor, such as flower petals, may cause someone to slip and should be reported for cleanup.

3. Avoid running in a health care facility because patients and visitors may become alarmed and begin to run as well. Also, someone may be hurt if the health care worker runs into him or her (e.g., a cardiac patient walking in the hall with an inserted IV stand or another health care worker carrying a specimen collection tray).

■ PATIENT SAFETY RELATED TO LATEX PRODUCTS

Patients, as well as health care workers, may be allergic to latex products. The signs and symptoms of an allergic reaction to latex may include a skin rash; hives; nasal, eye, or sinus irritation, and sometimes, shock. Table 5–1 provides examples of items frequently used in the health care environment that contains Latex. Figure 5–7 shows an example of a "Latex Safe Environment Sign."

■ DISASTER EMERGENCY PLAN

Many health care institutions have developed procedures to be followed in case of a hurricane, flooding, earthquake, bomb threat, and other disasters. The health care worker should become familiar with these procedures because he or she must be prepared to take immediate action whenever conditions warrant such action.

■ EMERGENCY PROCEDURES

The health care worker should become knowledgeable of emergency care procedures because accidents do occur even though precautionary measures are in place. He or she must be able to detach him- or herself from the emergency situation to some degree in order to

Table 5–1. Products Containing Latex

MEDICAL EQUIPMENT	PERSONAL PROTECTIVE EQUIPMENT	OFFICE SUPPLIES	MEDICAL SUPPLIES
Tourniquets	Gloves	Adhesive tape	Condom-style
Syringes	Goggles	Erasers	urinary collection
Stethoscopes	Rubber aprons	Rubber bands	device
Oral and nasal	Surgical masks		Enema tubing tips
airways			Injection ports
IV tubing			Rubber tops of
Disposable gloves			stoppers on
Breathing circuits			multidose vials
Blood pressure cuffs			Urinary catheter
			Wound drains

Source: Reprinted from *Preventing Allergic Reactions to Natural Rubber Latex in the Workplace,* The Centers for Disease Control and Prevention, National Institute for Occupational Safety and Health Alert, Atlanta, GA, June 1997.

Figure 5–7. Latex-safe environment sign.

LATEX SAFE ENVIRONMENT

DOOR MUST
REMAINED CLOSED!

CHECK FOR LATEX
CONTENT of PRODUCTS &
EQUIPMENT BEFORE

perform well and deliver the best possible health care. In an emergency situation, the following objectives must be met for the victim: prevent severe bleeding, maintain breathing, prevent shock and further injury, and send for medical assistance.

BLEEDING AID

Severe bleeding from an open wound can be controlled by applying pressure directly over the wound. OSHA requires adherence to "Universal Precautions" when health care workers respond to emergencies that provide potential exposure to blood and other potentially infectious materials. "Universal precautions" stress that all patients should be assumed to be infectious for HIV and other blood-borne pathogens. Health care workers responding to an emergency should be protected from exposure to blood and other potentially infectious materials through the use of personal protective equipment (i.e., gloves, mask, etc.). A clean handkerchief or other clean cloth (compress) should be placed over the wound before applying pressure by the gloved hand. In an emergency in which a clean cloth is not available, the gloved hand should be used until a cloth compress can be located. Bleeding of a limb (i.e., an arm or a leg) can be decreased by elevation. The injured portion should be raised above the level of the victim's heart unless the injured portion is broken. Even with elevation, however, pressure should be maintained on the wound until medical assistance arrives. A tourniquet should not be used to control bleeding except for an amputated, mangled, or crushed arm or leg, or for profuse bleeding that cannot be stopped otherwise.

BREATHING AID

When a victim's breathing movements stop or his or her lips, tongue, and fingernails become blue, immediate mouth-to-mouth resuscitation is needed. Any delay in using this technique may cost the victim's life. To perform mouth-to-mouth breathing, include the following:

1. See if the victim is conscious by *gently* shaking the victim and yelling, "ARE YOU OKAY?" If any possibility of a neck injury exists, do not shake the victim! If there is no response to the gentle shaking and yelling, call out for help and start aid immediately.
2. Place the victim on his or her back on a firm, flat surface. Caution must be exercised if the person has a spinal or neck injury. No twisting should occur to the victim's body.
3. Open the airway passage by checking for obstructions: tongue, chewing gum, vomitus, and so on.
4. Place one hand on the victim's forehead and, applying firm, backward pressure with the palm, tilt the head back (Fig. 5–8). Place the fingers of the other hand under the bony part of the victim's lower jaw, near the chin, and lift to bring the chin forward with the teeth almost to occlusion. The jaw should be supported as the head is tilted back. This position is called the *head-tilt/chin-lift*.
5. Listen and feel for return of air from the victim's mouth and nose for approximately 3 to 5 seconds. Also, simultaneously, look for the victim's chest to rise and fall.
6. If there is no breathing, maintain the head-tilt/chin-lift and pinch the victim's nose shut with the hand to prevent air from escaping. Open mouth widely, take a deep breath, and seal mouth over the victim's mouth (Fig. 5–9). Blow into victim's mouth. Watch for the victim's chest to rise. (If it does not, the airway is blocked and must be cleared.)

Figure 5–8. Head-tilt/chin-lift for emergency care.

Figure 5–9. Breathing aid in emergency situation.

7. Give two full ventilations. If this still does not start an air exchange, reposition the head and try again. After two more ventilations, again look, listen, and feel for breathing. Improper chin and head positioning is the most common cause of difficulty with ventilation.

CIRCULATION AID

To maintain circulation in a victim, a health care provider must know the techniques of basic CPR. Thus, he or she should check with the supervisor about the availability of CPR classes at the health care institution because this emergency technique must be demonstrated so that the employee can learn the proper skills.

SHOCK PREVENTION

Shock usually accompanies severe injury. It may result from bleeding, extensive burns, an insufficient oxygen (O_2) supply, and other traumatic events. Early signs include pale, cold, clammy skin; weakness; a rapid pulse; an increased, shallow breathing rate; and, frequently, nausea and vomiting. The main objectives in treating a shock victim are to improve circulation, to provide sufficient O_2, and to maintain normal body temperature.

The following six actions are recommended if first aid is given to a shock victim:

1. Correct the cause of shock if possible (e.g., control bleeding).
2. Keep the victim lying down.
3. Keep the victim's airway open. If he or she vomits, turn head to the side so that the neck is arched.
4. In the absence of broken bones, elevate the victim's legs so that the head is lower than the trunk of the body.
5. Keep the victim warm.
6. Call for emergency assistance.

Actions that are *not* recommended include the following:

1. Given fluids to a victim who has an abdominal injury (the person is likely to require surgery or a general anesthetic).
2. Giving fluids to an unconscious or a semiconscious person.

SELF STUDY

KEY TERMS

Cardiopulmonary Resuscitation
(CPR)
Environmental Protection
Agency (EPA)
Exposure Control Plan

Material Safety Data Sheets
(MSDSs)
Occupational Safety and Health
Administration (OSHA)

STUDY QUESTIONS

The following may have *one* or *more* answers:

1. If a fire occurs in or near electrical equipment, which of the following fire extinguishers should be used?

   a. class A extinguisher

   b. class B extinguisher

   c. class C extinguisher

   d. ABC extinguisher

2. What are the major principles of self-protection from radiation exposure?

   a. distance

   b. time

   c. combustibility

   d. shielding

3. Which of the following safety rules should be maintained in patients' rooms?

   a. specimen collection supplies and needles are properly disposed of

   b. unusual odors in the patient's room should be reported to the nursing station

   c. health care providers should not touch electrical instruments located adjacent to the patient's bed

   d. if the patient has an IV line and the site is swollen and reddish, this problem should be reported to the nursing station

4. The main objectives of treating a shock victim are to

   a. improve circulation

   b. provide sufficient drinking water

   c. provide sufficient oxygen

   d. maintain normal body temperature

5. In an emergency situation, which of the following is/are objective(s) that must be met for the victim?

   a. prevent severe bleeding

   b. maintain breathing

   c. prevent shock

   d. send for medical assistance

6. Which of the following should occur first if a fire breaks out in the health care facility?

   a. run from the floor where the fire is located
   b. call the assigned fire number
   c. use the fastest elevator to escape from the floor where the fire is located
   d. close all windows before leaving the area of the fire

7. The Right to Know law originated with the

   a. CDC
   b. CAP
   c. OSHA
   d. NFPA

8. The hazardous labeling system developed by the NFPA has the blue quadrant of the diamond to indicate:

   a. flammability hazard
   b. health hazard
   c. instability hazard
   d. specific hazard

9. If an electrical accident occurs involving electrical shock to an employee or a patient, the *first* thing that the health care worker should do is

   a. move the victim
   b. shut off electrical power
   c. start CPR
   d. place a blanket over the victim

References

1. US Department of Labor, and Occupational Safety and Health Administration (OSHA): Occupational exposure to bloodborne pathogens; final rule (29 CFR 1910.1030). *Federal Register.* 1991; Dec 6: 64004-64182.

2. National Committee for Clinical Laboratory Standards: *Protection of Laboratory Workers from Instrument Biohazards and Infectious Disease Transmitted by Blood, Body Fluids, and Tissue; Approved Guideline.* NCCLS Document M29-A, Wayne, PA, National Committee for Clinical Laboratory Standards, 1997.

3. NIOSH: NIOSH ALERT: Preventing Needlestick Injuries in Health Care Settings. DHHS (NIOSH) Publication No. 2000-108. Cincinnati, OH: U.S. Department of Health and Human Services, Public Health Service, Centers for Disease Control and Prevention, National Institute for Occupational Safety and Health; 1999.

4. FDA, NIOSH, OSHA: Glass capillary tubes: joint safety advisory about potential risks. Rockville, MD: Food and Drug Administration. Web site: www.cdc.gov/niosh/capssa9.html; 1999.

5. National Fire Protection Association (NFPA): *National Fire Codes.* Vol. 1. Quincy, MA: NFPA; 1990.

6. Occupational Safety and Health Administration (OSHA): *Hazard Communication Standard.* 29 CFR 1910.1200. Washington, DC; OSHA: 1986.

7. Occupational Safety and Health Administration (OSHA): *Toxic and Hazardous Substances.* 29 CFR 1910.1001–1047. Washington, DC; OSHA: 1989.

■ ADDITIONAL SOURCES FOR SAFETY INFORMATION

Centers for Disease Control and Prevention (CDC)

Division of Biosafety
1600 Clifton Rd, NE
Atlanta, GA 30333
(404) 639-3883
http://www.cdc.gov

College of American Pathologists (CAP)
325 Waukegan Rd
Northfield, IL 60093-2750
(800) 323-4040 or (847) 832-7000
http://www.cap.org

Department of Transportation (DOT)
Materials, Transportation Bureau, Information Services Division
Washington, DC 20402
(202) 366-4000

Joint Commission on Accreditation of Healthcare Organizations (JCAHO)
One Renaissance
Oakbrook Terrace, IL 60181
(630) 792-5000
http://www.jcaho.org

National Committee for Clinical Laboratory Standards (NCCLS)
940 W. Valley Rd S-1400
Wayne, PA 19087-1898
(610) 525-2435
http://www.NCCLS.org

National Fire Protection Association (NFPA)
One Batterymarch Park
Quincy, MA 02269-9101
(617) 770-3000
http://www.NFPA.org

Occupational Safety and Health Administration (OSHA)
US Department of Labor
200 Constitution Ave, NW
Washington, DC 20210
(202) 523-8148
http://www.cdc.gov/niosh

PHLEBOTOMY CASE STUDY

∎

Accidental Injury

Sally Landers had been on the job for only 8 months. She was a phlebotomist at a rural hospital in the Southwest where she had been hired to do early morning blood collections and deliver specimens to the centralized laboratory. She was tired when she went to work one Friday morning. She drew blood from a frail middle-aged man, Mr. Johnson. She had trouble with the collection procedure in that she had to stick him twice before she acquired the blood specimen. She was relieved when she finally finished the procedure. As she began to clean up and discard the used equipment, she noticed that the biohazard container was full. She decided, however, that it could probably hold the needles she had used on Mr. Johnson. She used her fingers to push the used needles and needle holders into the container and she felt a sharp puncture. She realized that she had stuck herself with a contaminated sharp object. She gathered the specimens she had drawn and quickly left. She immediately reported the injury to her supervisor.

QUESTIONS

1. Describe what Sally did correctly and incorrectly?
2. What procedures would need to be reviewed with Sally?
3. What additional education would you recommend for Sally?

See Answers in Appendix.

PHLEBOTOMY CASE STUDY

■

Transporting Specimens from Homebound Patients to the Laboratory

The medical assistant, Larry Smith, works for Mackin Home Health Agency. His job is multifaceted because he performs history and physical assessments, and when required to, he draws blood for laboratory testing. One day he went to collect blood and urine samples on Mr. Gonzales, an 80-year-old man who spoke very little English. He greeted Mr. Gonzales and found the bathroom and a suitable spot to draw blood from him. He felt confident that Mr. Gonzales had understood his communication. He was successful on the first attempt to collect the blood sample, and he helped Mr. Gonzales to the bathroom to collect the urine. Mr. Gonzales followed directions except he did not close the urine bottle tightly because he lacked the strength. Larry did not notice that the lid was not on tightly. He placed all the specimens in the container he had brought. He decided to leave the lid open because he knew his next stop was just 1 block away. On the way to the next house, a car ran a stop sign so Larry had to jam on his brakes, and the container with specimens fell off the seat of the car. The urine specimen spilled all over the floor of his vehicle.

QUESTIONS

1. What could Larry have done to avoid the situation?
2. What should Larry do now?

See Answers in Appendix.

6

SIX

■

Specimen Documentation and Transportation

CHAPTER OUTLINE

CHAPTER OBJECTIVES

Upon completion of Chapter 6, the learner is responsible for the following:

1. Describe the basic components of a clinical, or medical, record.
2. List appropriate uses of the medical record.
3. Identify six ways to enhance the intralaboratory communication network.
4. Describe essential elements of requisition and report forms.
5. Name three methods commonly used to transport specimens.
6. Name areas or departments that usually receive laboratory reports.

■ FUNDAMENTALS OF DOCUMENTATION

All health care organizations have methods of documenting information related to each patient and procedure that include some common elements. One document that can be found in all health care settings is the **clinical (or medical) record** for each patient. It is the definitive legal document that provides a chronological log of the patient's care. Any information that is clinically significant should be included in the medical record, including laboratory results. Box 6–1 describes the components most likely to be found in a medical record. In addition, numerous other documents provide a record of actions and results of the procedures that occur in the daily processes of providing health care services. Documentation in any health care setting is important for the following seven reasons.[1,2]

1. *Quality of care.* Documentation is used to describe what has been done and how the patient responds.
2. *Coordination of care among health care providers.* Documentation is used to plan interventions, evaluate progress, and assist the health care team in making effective decisions. It provides a vehicle for communication among all health care providers involved with the patient.
3. *Accrediting and licensing.* The Joint Commission for Accreditation of Healthcare Organizations (JCAHO) and other such accrediting agencies require specific standards for documentation in each patient's clinical, or medical, record. They usually include some guidelines for containing an assessment, a plan of care, medical orders (e.g., laboratory, radiology, etc.), progress notes, and a discharge summary.
4. *Quality monitoring.* State and JCAHO regulations also mandate that ongoing quality assessment activities take place. For this purpose, the clinical record is used to collect objective, readily measurable indicators that allow these agencies to assess the structure, process, and outcomes of patient care.
5. *Peer review.* Similar to quality monitoring, peer review organizations (PROs) also use documentation in the clinical records to evaluate the quality of care for specific indicators, such as nosocomial infections, medical stability of patients, unnecessary procedures and tests, adequate discharge planning, and the occurrence of avoidable discomfort or death. PROs can impose fines, impose sanctions, or deny reimbursement for care if patient care is inappropriate.
6. *Legal protection.* Documentation in the clinical records can provide proof of the quality of care given. Documentation can serve as evidence in disability, personal

BOX 6–1.   COMPONENTS COMMONLY FOUND IN A MEDICAL/CLINICAL RECORD

The following components are commonly used in medical/clinical records. In some cases, these components are combined into one section. The format of the medical record may vary by setting, e.g., a hospital vs. a doctor's office, or by the amount of documentation that is required, e.g., open-ended forms vs. checklists. In larger hospitals, some or all of the medical record is kept and maintained via a computerized system.[1, 3]

PERSONAL INFORMATION: Includes patient's name, date of birth (DOB), social security number (SSN), address, marital status, closest relative, known allergies, and physician's name.

PERSONAL AND FAMILY MEDICAL HISTORY: Completed by the physician and the nurse; contains information about the initial assessment.

ORDERING DOCUMENTATION: Includes physician and/or other qualified providers' orders, (e.g., nurse practitioners (NP), clinical nurse specialists (CNS), physician assistants (PA),) for laboratory, radiology, pharmacy, etc.

CONSENT AND RELEASE FORMS: Includes consent forms for procedures performed, authorization forms for release of medical information, and other forms related to the patient's preferences, (e.g., do-not-resuscitate orders, etc.).

PATIENT'S PLAN OF CARE: Includes medical and nursing care diagnoses, interventions, and patient outcomes. This section often includes flowcharts or checklists indicating recordings of the patient's temperature, pulse rate, respiratory rate, blood pressure, glucose screening levels, weight, and other assessments.

DIAGNOSTIC TEST RESULTS: Includes results from all tests performed on the patient, e.g., laboratory, radiology, etc.

MEDICATION ADMINISTRATION RECORD: Includes information about medication dosage and timing, route of administration, site, and date.

PROGRESS NOTES: Includes notes from qualified health providers (MD, NP, CNS, PA) about the patient's progress, interventions used, and treatment effectiveness.

CONSULTATIONS: Includes evaluation summaries by clinical specialists, (e.g., infectious disease specialists, endocrinologists, etc.).

HEALTH CARE TEAM NOTES: Includes progress notes from other departments such as Nutrition, Physical Therapy, Occupational Therapy, Counseling, etc.

DISCHARGE PLAN OR SUMMARY: Includes plans for after discharge from a hospital, including special diets, medications, home health visits, and follow-up appointments.

injury, malpractice, and mental competency cases. Appropriate documentation is the key to winning or losing a case for individual members or employees of the health care facility.

7. *Research.* In teaching institutions, documentation can provide important data for clinical research on new therapies and procedures.

General guidelines for documentation are as follows:

- *Accuracy.* Record only the facts, not opinions or assumptions; and, clinical records should never be changed or falsified to cover a mistake.
- *Completion.* Notes should be made about each event, procedure, or problem that occurs. Writing the documentation as soon as possible with the exact time of a procedure and identifying other sources of information about the process can become vitally important. For example, if a phlebotomist is unable to identify a patient because of a missing armband, the notation should include the time, the date, the name of the nurse who positively identified the patient, and the phlebotomist's name.

- *Objectivity.* Documented comments should not assign blame (e.g., "blood was not collected from Mr. Jones because nurse Daly did not complete the proper requisition.") Likewise, comments about staffing shortages or working overtime should not be recorded because it would be confusing in a courtroom in that it may or may not have a direct influence on the patient's condition.
- *Timeliness.* Documentation must be made as soon as possible.

Every notation in the patient's record should be legibly written in blue or black ink on the appropriate forms and signed. Computerized notations should be done by authorized personnel and according to the organizations' policies. Chapter 17 addresses other legal aspects of documentation.

■ THE LABORATORY COMMUNICATION NETWORK

The major purpose of a clinical laboratory is the acquisition and determination of valid data by analytic procedures performed on patient specimens and the timely communication of those data to the physician. Specimen collection procedures are the first and most critical steps in this process. The number of persons and steps involved varies greatly depending on the size of the institution and the type of laboratory involved. Clinical laboratories may be centralized or may be decentralized, with satellites, or minilaboratories, in various locations. With each additional location or person involved, another potential source of error or delay is introduced into the system.

There are many ways to conceptualize the cycle of performing laboratory tests flowing from **preanalytical phases** of the initial test request to the specimen collection to the **analytic phase** to the final reporting of results. One example is shown in Figure 6–1.

Sources of error in laboratory testing can be related to variables in the preanalytic phase. Preanalytic variables include the following:

- *Patient variables.* Fasting versus nonfasting, diurnal variations, refusal to cooperate, patient is unavailable, stress or anxiety, etc.
- *Transportation variables.* Specimen leakage, tube breakage, excessive shaking, etc.
- *Specimen processing variables.* Centrifugation is inadequate, delays in processing, contamination of the specimen, exposure to heat or light, etc.
- *Specimen variables.* Hemolysis, inadequate volume in the tube, inadequate mixing of anticoagulant, etc.

The individual who performs the phlebotomy is a vital link in the preanalytic phase of laboratory testing. He or she should be knowledgeable about the procedures to help prevent these sources of errors and he or she should know how to react in case of unusual circumstances. Phlebotomists should anticipate potential variables and assist in writing protocols that minimize errors.[4] Furthermore, there should be a dependable communication link among laboratory staff, physicians, patients, and other members of the health care team.

In a relatively small laboratory, as in the case of a physician's office laboratory, the communication processes, both within the laboratory (intralaboratory) and with all others outside the laboratory (extralaboratory), are essentially the same. As the size of the institution increases, however, the requirements for effective and efficient intralaboratory and extralaboratory communication are expanded, and the use of computer technology is enhanced.

Figure 6–1. A patient-physician-laboratory network can be depicted in an analytic phase (A) and a preanalytic phase (PA). (QC, quality control.)

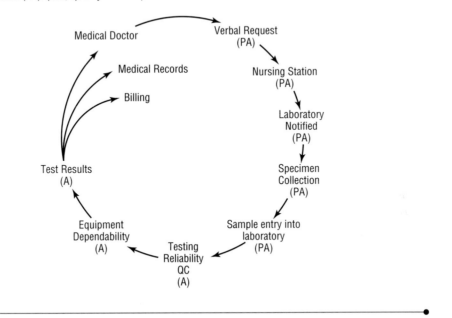

■ INTRALABORATORY COMMUNICATION NETWORK

Using well-written procedures in the clinical laboratory improves the communication network by ensuring continuity of methods; avoiding shortcuts; minimizing the chances of errors, specimen recollections, and reruns; preventing expensive substitutions of reagents; and enhancing quality control (QC), teaching, and safety. Overall, such procedures lead to more efficient data collection and reporting.

POLICIES AND PROCEDURES

All health care facilities have policy and procedure manuals that guide practices within the organization. Employees usually spend time during their orientation/training period to learn and practice the policies. Policy and procedure manuals cover technical, administrative, and safety/infection control procedures that are specific for the organization, a department such as the laboratory, and/or a smaller subunit of a larger organization such as the IV therapy team. Regardless of the facility, employees should be trained to practice accordingly. Phlebotomists commonly utilize the examples of manuals that are summarized below in a variety of settings.

Specimen Collection Manual

The College of American Pathologists (CAP), an accrediting agency for clinical laboratories, requires that a **specimen collection manual** (electronic or paper-based) be available to phlebotomists at all sites where specimens are collected. It must include instructions for the following[5]:

- Patient preparation
- Type of collection container and amount of specimen required
- Timing requirements (e.g., creatinine clearance, therapeutic drug monitoring, etc.)
- Type and amount of preservative or anticoagulant needed
- Special handling or transportation needs (e.g., refrigeration, immediate delivery, etc.)
- Proper labeling requirements
- Need for additional clinical data when indicated (e.g., fasting vs. non-fasting, etc.)

In addition to these requirements, many laboratories include procedures about specific situations or events related to the blood collection process. Examples of procedures that arise in phlebotomy situations are included in Box 6–2. In addition, clarification needs to be provided for phlebotomists about whether the documentation should be handwritten or entered via computer. According to the CAP, phlebotomists should be appropriately instructed and evaluated on competencies for all procedures.

BOX 6–2. SAMPLE PROCEDURES: HANDWRITTEN DOCUMENTATION OF SPECIFIC PHLEBOTOMY SITUATIONS

Logbook Verification Procedure

1. Requests on computer-generated labels that serve as requests for phlebotomy are checked against the logbook prior to the drawing of blood. Any discrepancy should be brought to the attention of the unit secretary or nurse for resolution of orders. Any test deleted from the log by request of a unit will be circled and an explanation of the deletion, along with requester's name, will be written in the log. Any tests added to requests also should be added to the logbook. If any tests are added but not requested on computer labels, a stamped request must be made by the nursing unit personnel.
2. After the appropriate specimens have been collected, each patient's collection that is complete will be initialed by the health care worker collecting the blood and time of draw will be entered in the appropriate box in the logbook. At the bottom of the list of patients, a line is drawn and "EOR," or End of Run, is written to signify that all is complete.

Inability to Draw Specimen

1. A maximum of two laboratory employees will attempt to obtain blood from a patient.
2. Any unsuccessful attempt to obtain blood *must* be documented in the logbook and on the request slip.

Patient Unavailable

1. If you are unable to obtain blood when requested because a patient is unavailable (gone to x-ray or surgery, out of room), hold these requisitions until you have completed all other patients on that nursing unit. Check the patient's room again before leaving unit.
2. If the patient is still unavailable, notify the primary nurse, if available, or unit clerk. Leave the requisitions at the desk, circle the orders, and write the following in the logbook:

    Reason patient is unavailable.

    Time and initials of collector.

    Name of nurse notified.

    The patient's blood will then be drawn on the next scheduled run.

BOX 6–2.   *(continued)*

Patient Refused to Have Blood Drawn

If the patient refuses to have blood drawn, notify his or her primary nurse. Often, the nurse can convince the patient to cooperate. If not, leave requisitions at the unit desk, with the following information written in the logbook:

Patient refused.

Time and initials of collector.

Name of nurse notified.

Patient Missed

If at any time the person collecting blood is unable to obtain the blood, he or she should check to see whether another collector is available to help. If no other health care worker is available, notify the patient's nurse that the patient was missed and that another person from the laboratory will try on the next run unless the nurse requests that the attempt be made sooner. Leave the requisitions at the desk, with the following information written in the logbook:

Unable to collect specimen.

Time and initials of collector.

Name of nurse notified.

Upon returning to the laboratory, notify the supervisor. If the second person is unable to obtain the specimen, a nurse is again notified, and the previous information is again documented on the requisitions and in the logbook. At this time, request that a physician draw the blood.

Combative Patient

In cases when an adult patient is combative or verbally abusive of laboratory personnel, and nursing staff is unavailable, the health care worker should notify the supervisor. If the health care worker is instructed by the supervisor to refuse to draw blood, the primary nurse should be notified of the refusal and it must be documented in the logbook, noting:

Reason for refusal.

Name of the nurse notified.

Unidentified Test Requested

If a test is requested that cannot be found in the specimen collection manual, the nurse should be asked to consult the doctor to clarify the request. Meanwhile, the health care worker can call the laboratory for a more familiar name for the test and test requirements. If no other name can be found and no clarification is offered, he or she *must* refuse to draw a specimen for the test. The logbook should be marked "no such test," the primary nurse notified, and his or her name recorded in the logbook. The supervisor of the laboratory also should be notified.

Administrative Procedures

While the following topics are generally covered in an administrative procedure manual for any department, they are particularly important for phlebotomists.

- Performance evaluation procedures and job descriptions
- Disciplinary policies
- Compensatory time, annual leave, and overtime policies
- Attendance and punctuality policies
- Holiday schedules

- Handling of employee accidents
- In-service requirements
- Vaccination policies (e.g., hepatitis)
- Telephone etiquette policies
- Translation procedures for non–English speaking patients
- Release of information policies
- Sexual harassment policies
- Quality improvement plan
- Patient billing methods
- Dress code (Box 6–3 includes a sample dress code policy)

Safety and Infection Control Procedures

Safety procedures should be distributed to all management staff and made known to all personnel. One book of safety procedures should be available in each laboratory section, including the specimen collection areas. As mentioned in Chapter 5, safety manuals should include fire safety, internal and external disaster plan, radiation safety, exposure control plan, and biological hazard, as well as a hazard communication manual indicating procedures for handling hazardous substance and infection control manuals. The infection control manual usually includes procedures for handling specimens, isolation procedures, handling precautions, disposal policies, decontamination procedures, and hand-washing procedures. It may also include detailed information about accidental percutaneous needlesticks and post-exposure procedures. Since many phlebotomy personnel are decentralized from the clinical laboratory, these policies should be accessible to them at their work stations.

Quality Control (QC) Procedures

QC procedures pertain to maintaining appropriate supplies, reagents, and equipment for laboratory testing. These procedures should be available in each laboratory section, including the specimen collection area. QC records include information about hazards; proper use, storage, and handling; stability; expiration dates; and indications for measuring the precision and accuracy of analytic processes.

Other Procedures Important to Phlebotomists

Other procedures can be useful to phlebotomists based on the type of facility where they work and their specific job responsibilities. There are examples listed below:

- Reporting of critical values (refer to the Clinical Alert on page 158)
- Laboratory test or billing codes
- Inventory procedures for equipment and supplies
- Acceptable symbols, abbreviations, and units of measure (Refer to the Appendices for examples)
- Interdepartmental loans of supplies and equipment
- Use of library resources
- Handling specimens going to or coming from outside organizations
- Instrument and maintenance manuals

BOX 6–3. SAMPLE OF A DRESS CODE POLICY

Happy Hospital strives to present a highly professional and positive image to all patients, customers, and members of the community. Professional dress, good grooming, and personal cleanliness are important aspects of the overall effectiveness and morale of all employees. To establish a standard appearance, the following guidelines will be enforced. Employees who appear inappropriately dressed or groomed will be sent home.

Identification

Name badges will be visibly worn at all times. Stickers, pins, or other types of tokens should not cover the employee or department name.

Daily Hygiene

Having clean teeth, hair, clothes, and body are basic daily requirements. Clean, wrinkle-free clothes, scrubs, or uniforms that are in good condition should be worn.

Hair

Hair should be clean, neat and trimmed. Conservative styles are recommended. Well-groomed, closely trimmed beards, sideburns, and mustaches are allowed. Shoulder length hair should be pulled back and secured.

Nails

Nails should be clean and neatly manicured, conservative in color of nail polish, and not more than 1/4 inch past the fingertip.

Fragrances/Scents

Perfumes and fragrances can be offensive and/or nauseating to patients who are ill. It is recommended that the use of fragrances be minimized or eliminated.

Make-up

Make-up should be conservative and lightly applied. Extreme or excessive make-up is not allowed.

Clothing

Denim clothing of any type or style will not be allowed except on special occasions announced by the hospital administration. Tight-fitting clothing or clothes that are revealing or distracting are not permitted. Shirts should be buttoned up to the second button. Shirttails should be tucked in and tee-shirts with logos or athletic prints will not be allowed. Proper undergarments should be worn at all times. Skirts and dresses should not be shorter than 3 inches above the knee. Shorts are not permitted. Pants/slacks should be worn with a belt if they have belt loops. Tight-fitting leggings are not permitted. It is recommended that male employees who are not involved in patient care wear ties.

Shoes

Shoes should be comfortable, safe in the work environment, clean and polished. Consideration should be made to minimizing noise when walking. Socks and/or proper hosiery should be worn. Sandals or flip-flops are not permitted.

Jewelry

Excessive jewelry is not allowed. When safety is a concern, chains must be worn inside the collar, and long dangling earrings are not acceptable.

Please note that these are minimum guidelines and that individual departments may have more rigid requirements due to safety, infection control, or patient preferences. Consult your supervisor regarding any questions you may have regarding these guidelines.

> **! Clinical Alert**
>
> A **critical laboratory value,** sometimes referred to as a **"panic value,"** is a test result that "represents a pathophysiologic state at such variance with normal as to be life-threatening" unless action is taken by the patient's physician. According to the Clinical Laboratory Improvement Act (CLIA), health care workers are required to report critical values to physicians in a timely manner. This often means paging or telephoning a physician at home and/or during off-hours. While this can be an unwelcomed task, it is important for the patient's welfare and to avoid liability risks. All laboratories should have policies about what should be done when results are within a critical range.[6]

CONTINUING EDUCATION

In addition to procedure manuals, ongoing in-service education programs help increase communication, safety, and efficiency in patient care. With the increasing complexity of patient care services and responsibilities, it is essential for health care workers to attend in-service education sessions within the institution and elsewhere. Certain types of continuing education, such as training about universal standard precautions, fire safety, and radiation safety, are required periodically and are offered by larger organizations. Many of the professional organizations listed in Chapter 1 also provide continuing educational courses that are needed or required for state licensure.

OTHER MODES OF INTRALABORATORY COMMUNICATION

Bulletin boards, posters, checklists, memoranda, newsletters, clipboards, and staff meetings are noncomputerized suggestions for disseminating current information. One person from each work area should be responsible for periodically checking and changing poster information. These methods are useful for reviewing policies, new techniques, and difficult phlebotomy issues.

Computer software and hardware are also available for networking within the laboratory. **E-mail** (electronic mail), voice mail, electronic bulletin boards, product recall notices, and facsimiles (faxes) are all effective ways of communicating. Sometimes off-site laboratory facilities also have a speed-dialing telephone exchanges. All individuals who practice phlebotomy must be familiar with the communications technology in their facilities.

■ EXTRALABORATORY COMMUNICATION NETWORK FOR LABORATORY TESTING

Communication with other health care workers working outside the laboratory can be enhanced by the use of a paper-based or computerized information bulletin or a *floor book* of laboratory services, made available at least in every patient unit, both inpatient and outpatient. This information contains a directory of the laboratory sections with listings of the key staff members, the location of the laboratory, telephone numbers, operating hours, **reference ranges,** instructions, and pertinent standard procedures of the laboratory. The methods used for collection of all specimens, as well as the proper identification, storage, preservation, and transportation mechanisms to be used, are clearly specified. In addition, an alphabetical listing of all laboratory determinations, specimen requirements, special instructions, and tables with reference ranges for each measurement are often included. (Refer to Table 6–1). In some hospitals, this information can be reproduced as a pocket-sized resource or located on a hand palm-sized computer. This is particularly helpful to medical students, residents, fellows, and trainees.

USE OF THE TELEPHONE

The telephone is the most frequently used method of two-way communication in any setting. Health care workers must be aware of the procedures for operating it. These procedures usually include the following:

- Using effective customer service manners.
- Transferring calls.
- Placing the caller on "hold."
- Using the intercom system.
- Modifying and using voice mail messages.
- Organizing conference calls.
- Using the speaker phone.
- Writing legible, complete messages.

Box 6–4 provides suggestions to help the health care worker communicate effectively and politely on the telephone. Additional information on effective communication is presented in Chapter 1.

CONFIDENTIALITY AND PRIVACY

The issues of **confidentiality** and **privacy** will be discussed in more detail in Chapter 17; however, they are mentioned here because they have a profound influence on communication of laboratory test results. Clinical documents such as laboratory and radiology test

Table 6–1.   Sample of a Hospital's *Floor Book* of Laboratory Information

HOSPITAL FLOOR BOOK						
Test No.	Procedure	Specimen	Average Turn Around Time	Laboratory Section	Collected By	Special Instruction
1220	Ionized calcium	SST tube	2 hours	Chemistry	Phlebotomist	—
1221	Serum calcium	SST tube	2 hours	Chemistry	Phlebotomist	—
1558	Complete blood count	EDTA tube	1.5 hours	Hematology	Phlebotomist	Invert tube gently to mix blood and anticoagulant

BOX 6–4.   TELEPHONE TIPS

- Always speak in a polite and professional tone.
- State the department, clinic, or unit name.
- To establish a cooperative relationship, always use phrases such as the following:

    May I help you?

    Pardon me, could you please repeat that.

    Please spell your name.

    I am sorry that I cannot assist you with that matter, let me refer you to someone who can. Thank you.
- If speaking to patients and family members, try to use words that are easy to pronounce, concise, direct, and uncomplicated.
- Articulate words clearly; do not use slang.
- Spelling a term may help you or the receiver understand or recognize what is being said.
- Restate sentences to make sure that you understand the message or instructions.
- Remain neutral in a controversy.
- Reflecting on a response before answering will help clarify your answer; however, pauses that are too long may indicate a lack of interest.
- Ask pertinent questions and have the ability to say that you do not know the answer.

results must be kept confidential and private. Health care workers, including phlebotomists who have access to this information, must be careful not to disclose patient information in a casual, unnecessary fashion. Discussion that does not directly relate to the health care worker's role in caring for the patient should be avoided.

Occasionally a phlebotomist may overhear communication between a physician and the patient. This communication is also considered privileged and must not be shared with others without the consent of the patient. Furthermore, the **Health Insurance Portability and Accountability Act** of 1996 (Public Law 104-191), **HIPAA,** was expanded in December 2000, to protect the security and confidentiality of electronic health information. While primarily designed to apply to insurance plans, the law also applies to all health care providers. The standards detail specific rights for patients regarding protection of their health information; it prohibits disclosure of any health information unless a written consent has been obtained from a patient. Health care providers are required to create "privacy-conscious" practices that include a requirement that only the minimum amount of health information necessary is disclosed. Furthermore, providers and insurance companies must ensure internal protection of medical records, employee privacy training and education, handling privacy complaints, and designation of a privacy officer. A copy of the final rule can be obtained from the Department of Health and Human Services Website at http://aspe.os.dhhs.gov/admnsimp/.[7]

FAX TRANSMISSION OF LABORATORY INFORMATION

As mentioned previously, the new HIPAA laws will affect policies related to electronic transmission of laboratory information. **Fax machines** are widely used because they are efficient, timely, and cost effective, especially when off-site services are offered. Each health care facility or laboratory should have clear policies related to the use of test requisitions or results that are sent or received by facsimile/fax or via computer.

■ COMPUTERIZED COMMUNICATIONS

Personal, hand-held, mini-, mainframe computers and networks have become essential instruments in the clinical laboratory and health care setting; thus, the health care worker needs to become acquainted with computer systems. For example, computer systems carry out functions such as:

- Entering lists of test requisitions for a patient.
- Generating patients' labels, specimen collection lists, and schedules.
- Updating the laboratory specimen accession records.
- Printing lists that identify which test procedures need to be performed on patients' specimens.
- Reporting test results.
- Storing test results.
- Sending laboratory test results to the nursing stations either as individual test reports or cumulative summaries of the patient's laboratory records.
- Sending patient charges to the accounting office.

Computerization of the collection process can significantly decrease errors. Without a computer, collection and specimen information must pass through several people before the sample is actually processed in the laboratory. With a computer, data are continually being checked against the computer files, and authorized individuals can add to and receive information from the accumulated data. With the combined use of hand-held computers and bar code technology, specimens can more easily and accurately be tracked through preanalytic *and* analytic phases of laboratory testing. Computers are also assisting laboratory managers by tracking client calls, generating productivity reports, monitoring courier functions, marketing services, and materials management.

■ REQUISITION FORMS

Laboratory tests are requested by means of the laboratory **requisition form** or a computer-generated order. Therefore the instructions must be explicit, and the design and format of the request forms or computer screens must be carefully considered in order to minimize handwriting, permit convenient handling, generate inexpensive and legible copies, and obtain all necessary information for laboratory testing.

Multiple-part forms, that serve as both laboratory request and report forms, represent one of the most widely used traditional formats for a manual system. These forms are also used when computer failures occur. The forms are usually of a convenient size to be easily attached to 8½ × 11-in. paper as is customarily used for patients' medical records. Also, these forms are easy to transport, handle, sort, and store, and they are cost effective. There are examples in Figure 6–2. The forms are usually manufactured to provide clear copies and easy detachment (perforated edges). Color coding can be used for different request forms for ease of identification, both in the ordering of tests and in the charting of results. The name of the institution is usually included on each request form.

BAR CODES

The use of barcoded labels (Figure 6–2B) for patients' samples to reduce transcription errors and speed up sample processing, is commonplace. **Bar codes** represent a series of

Figure 6–2. A. Multiple-part requisition forms that also serve as report forms can be stamped with Addressograph machines. These forms can be used with a computerized reporting system but are designed to serve as temporary report forms on a manual backup basis. B. If needed, bar-coded labels can be printed with the same information.

(Courtesy of The University of Texas M.D. Anderson Cancer Center, Division of Laboratory Medicine, Houston, TX with permission.)

light and dark bands of varying widths. The configuration of these bands relates to specific alphanumeric symbols (i.e., numbers and letters). In other words, each letter of the alphabet and each number has a specific code (black and white bars of varying widths). When these bands are placed together in a series, they can correspond to a name (patient or test) or a number (identification or test code). When the bar is scanned with a sensitive light or laser scanner, the series of numbers and letters is read into a computer in a precise manner. This technology is very accurate and fast. It saves time, and it keeps personnel from entering or typing information, which reduces clerical errors substantially.

Information that can be converted to bar coded symbology for laboratory uses include the following:[8]

- Patients' names
- Patient identification numbers
- DOB

- Test codes
- Specimen accession or log numbers
- Expiration dates for inventory of supplies and equipment
- Product codes for needles, syringes, specimen collection tubes, etc.
- Billing codes to facilitate accounting
- Sample identification numbers in a particular batch-run on laboratory analyzers

Specimen handling and testing applications for the future may include "two-dimensional" bar code symbologies. There are currently drawbacks to the newer bar codes, including placement of symbols, readability and performance issues, and the cost and availability of equipment. However, the technology has the capability of holding entire databases in the code, thus enabling more options for specimen handling from test orders, logging-in, tracking, testing, and reporting. It uses a technique that stacks multiple linear rows together, which dramatically increases the amount of data that can be encoded compared with the single linear row technology currently used. [9]

Figure 6–3 demonstrates bar codes in a health care facility.

■ TRANSMITTAL OF THE TEST REQUEST TO THE LABORATORY

The test request mechanism formally initiates the cyclic procedure of the laboratory communication network. Two systems are commonly used for this activity. Orders for test requests can be transmitted directly to the clinical laboratory from the requesting authority through an on-line interactive computer system. In many institutions, however, manual requesting systems are still in use, sometimes using bar codes, which are then entered into the computer; other times involving a totally manual system in which the request form also serves as the final report.

On-line computer input of information is the most error-free means of making requests. Because a computer system can perform automatic checks on the input, it does not accept a request for any test that is not in its test-information database. Likewise, it does not accept a sample of plasma or urine for a test restricted to serum. It also allows the person entering the test request to obtain accurate and up-to-date information about specific determinations, such as revised specimen collection requirements, delivery instructions, assay techniques, reference ranges, and fees. Even with hand-held computers that are used for bar code scanning, special comments may be added regarding the patient or sample (e.g., "non-fasting" or "drawn from a CVC line").

In a manual system, the multipart request forms are commonly completed at each patient's unit or clinic by a member of the health care team and delivered to the laboratory. This type of system is more subject to human error, (e.g., lost requisitions, duplicate orders, etc.). These problems can be minimized by instituting a few organizational procedures, such as using a centralized location for all requisition forms, using a sorting system once the requisition slips reach the laboratory, and using a blood collection log. (Refer to Box 6–4.)

Verbal test requests are occasionally used in cases of emergency. The request should be documented on a standardized form in the laboratory prior to the specimen collection (Box 6–5). After the blood is collected, the official laboratory request slip can be filled out and accompany the specimen to the laboratory in the routine manner; or a computerized request can be entered.

Figure 6–3. The use of bar codes can facilitate the following: A. Printing labels and requisition forms. B. Labeling specimens. C. Labeling blood smears. D. Identifying serum aliquot tubes. E. Processing blood samples.

(Courtesy of TimeMed Labeling Systems, Burr Ridge, IL, with permission.)

A

B

C

D

E

BOX 6–4.   DAILY LOG SHEET THAT DOCUMENTS ALL SPECIMENS COLLECTED AND DELIVERED BY SPECIALIZED PHLEBOTOMY PERSONNEL CALLED *LABORATORY LIAISON TECHNICIANS (LLTS)*

DAILY WORK SHEET

UNIT _____   DATE _____   LLT _____

TOTAL PATIENT SERVICES _____   TOTAL STAT SAMPLES _____   7:00–4:00 _____
(# OF VENIPUNCTURES)
TOTAL TIMED SAMPLES _____   3:00–11:00 _____

ROOM #	PATIENT'S NAME	PATIENT #	TESTS TO BE DONE OR SPECIMENS DELIVERED	LOGGED BY	TIME TO BE COLLECTED	TIME COLLECTED	OBTAINED BY	SPECIMEN	COMMENT

(Courtesy of The University of Texas M.D. Anderson Cancer Center, Division of Laboratory Medicine, Houston, TX, with permission.)

■ SPECIMEN LABELS AND BLOOD COLLECTION LISTS

Clear and accurate specimen identification is essential and must begin immediately upon collection, and it must continue through disposal of the specimen. Identification methods vary from manually copying all patient identification information onto the container to using prenumbered bar-coded labels. Manually labeling specimens can be time consuming and prone to transcription errors. These problems can be prevented by using preprinted labels, which are available from many commercial sources. Labeling systems include those that can imprint a patient identification card or electronically print patient identification information onto the specimen label.

Among the most sophisticated, accurate, and efficient labels are those generated by a hospital computer system. Requisition slips for the morning blood collections can be sent to the laboratory on the previous day or entered into the computer at any time. On the basis of the laboratory orders, the computer can generate enough labels containing all the appropriate patient identification criteria for each tube required to be drawn. The labels also list the specific tests requested, the types of specimen collection tubes required for the requested tests, and the unique accession numbers or sample numbers to be used for that particular collection time. Bar codes can be used for any alphanumeric symbols. Smaller transfer labels may also be printed to label special aliquot tubes, collection tubes,

---

BOX 6–5. SAMPLE DOCUMENTATION FORM FOR VERBAL TEST REQUESTS

EMERGENCY REQUESTS FOR LABORATORY TESTS

Nurse:

Requesting Physician:

Location: ICU _____   ER _____   Other _____
             Room: _____

Patient: Patient Id (if available):

Pick up orders on unit:
Tests Ordered: _____
_____
_____
_____

Requested by: _____

Order taken by: _____

Date _____ Time _____ AM _____ PM _____

(Adapted from a form used at The University of Texas M.D. Anderson Cancer Center, Houston, TX, with permission.)

---

cuvettes, and microscope slides. This type of system eliminates the manually written entry log used at smaller facilities for recording the tests and accession number requested for each patient. Additional test requests ordered later in the day are entered into the computer, which assigns a specific time to the tests so that they can be easily separated from those requested in the morning. Labels for later collection can be computer printed or made with an Addressograph machine. Blood-drawing lists are also printed by the computer to provide a list of patients on each floor requiring blood work for the morning draw and the tests ordered, and to identify the assigned sample accession number. The health care worker initials this list after the patient's blood has been drawn, and a copy is left at the nursing unit so that caregivers attending the patient can see which specimens have already been collected. Any additional specimens collected later in the day are documented in the logbook on the floor (see Box 6–4). In this way, the personnel on the health care team has a complete list of the specimen collections taken from each patient throughout the day.

■ SPECIMEN TRANSPORTATION AND DELIVERY

Both the communication network and the quality of laboratory test results depend on the time that specimens are received for processing. Blood and other specimens must be delivered expeditiously.

BASIC HANDLING GUIDELINES

Every health care facility has a specific protocol for specimen transportation and processing. Most laboratories require the use of a leakproof plastic bag for insertion of the specimen container. This bag protects the health care worker from pathogenic (disease-producing) organisms during specimen transportation. Usually, this special transport bag has a pouch on the outside for the laboratory request slip. Thus the potential for contamination of the request slip is eliminated. If possible, the blood in evacuated tubes and microcollection tubes should be maintained in a vertical position to promote complete clot formation, if required, and to reduce the possibility of hemolysis. It is also imperative to handle and transport blood specimens in a gentle manner to prevent hemolyzing the specimens.

Glycolytic action from the blood cells interferes in the analysis of various chemicals (e.g., glucose, calcitonin, aldosterone, phosphorus, enzymes). Because of this, the blood samples should be transported to the clinical laboratory within 45 minutes from the time of collection so that the serum or plasma can be separated from the blood cells. The serum or plasma that is separated from the cells must be handled according to the laboratory procedure. The National Committee for Clinical Laboratory Standards (NCCLS) suggests a maximum time of 2 hours from the time of collection to the separation of sera from plasma. Once separated, sera may remain at room temperature, be refrigerated, be stored in a dark place, or be frozen, depending on the prescribed laboratory method.[10]

For transportation of specimens from remote ambulatory sites, including home health collections, the phlebotomist must still follow the handling guidelines according to Universal Standard Precautions. The phlebotomist should use the same safety equipment he or she would use in a hospital environment (e.g., closed venipuncture system, gloves, disposable laboratory coat, plastic blood collection tubes, and a biohazardous disposal container). In addition, all blood collection equipment and specimens should be transported in an enclosed or lockable container to avoid accidental spills if the automobile is in a collision. The container should have a biohazard warning label on it. Cold packs should be used in the container for transport during hot weather, or the reverse, the vehicle should be heated in cold weather. For home collection, the phlebotomist must be extra careful to dispose of waste properly and to place blood specimens in leakproof plastic bags in an upright position inside a transport container.

CHILLED SPECIMENS

For special types of specimens, chilling is required. If a health care worker is requested to transport an arterial specimen for blood gas analysis, he or she should be aware that the specimen must be transported in an airtight heparinized syringe and placed in a mixture of ice and water. The airtight container and the ice water decrease the loss of gases from the specimen. It is important to use ice water rather than solid chunks of ice; otherwise, parts of the specimen may freeze and hemolysis will result. Speed in specimen transportation is essential to prevent the loss of blood gases. Thus specimens that may require chilling are:

- Blood gases
- Gastrin
- Ammonia
- Lactic acid
- Renin

- Catecholamine[5]
- Parathyroid hormone[11]

PROTECTION OF SPECIMENS FROM LIGHT

Some chemical constituents in blood, such as bilirubin, are **light sensitive** and decompose if exposed to light. Thus, blood collected for light-sensitive chemical analysis should be protected from bright light with an aluminum foil wrapping around the tube. In summary, light-sensitive constituents include the following:

- Bilirubin
- Vitamin B_{12}
- Carotene
- Folate

MICROBIOLOGICAL SPECIMENS

Blood and urine specimens for microbiological culture need to be transported to the laboratory as quickly as possible so that the blood can be transferred to culture media and the urine analyzed. This enhances the likelihood of detecting pathogenic bacteria. Specimens for blood cultures can also be collected directly into culture media, which minimizes possible contamination and speeds the contact with the culture media. (Refer to Chapter 7 for additional information about blood culture collections.)

WARMED SPECIMENS

Specimens that require warming (to body temperature, $37°C$) include those for testing cold agglutinins and cryofibrinogen. These special cases require a heat block for transportation and handling purposes.

SPECIMEN DELIVERY METHODS

In larger facilities the laboratory is most often the department responsible for the delivery of blood specimens to the location where they will be analyzed. However, other types of specimens, e.g., urine, sputum, etc., are commonly delivered by transportation or nursing staff members. In smaller facilities the specimen delivery methods vary widely. Whatever the site, guidelines should be available for safe and efficient delivery of specimens that may include a schedule of pick-ups, how to deliver STAT specimens, where to place specimens, how to "log-in" specimens, etc. Appropriate documentation procedures and open communication among all departments are the keys to successful and efficient specimen delivery.

Hand Delivery

Many specimens are hand-carried and require guidelines for timeliness of delivery to the laboratory. A log sheet for specimens that are hand-delivered to the laboratory is commonly used and is depicted in Box 6–6. For health care workers in a hospital setting, the blood collection trays or carts are typically arranged to hold specimens awaiting delivery to the lab-

BOX 6–6. SAMPLE LOG SHEET TO DOCUMENT DELIVERY OF PATIENT SPECIMENS TO THE LABORATORY

SPECIMEN DELIVERY LOG

Patient Name	Location	Specimens						Date	Time	Escort Name
		CSF	Blood	Urine	Sputum	Other	Test Ordered			

oratory by using test tube racks, a holder for microscopic slides, plastic holders, cups, and/or a leak-proof container for ice water.

Hospital Transportation Department

Typically transportation orderlies or escorts are responsible for moving patients from their nursing units to other service areas such as radiology, physical therapy, etc. However, when they deliver specimens to the laboratory, the following information is required in addition to the test requisitions:

- Type of specimen
- Patient's name and hospital identification number
- Date and time of specimen collection
- Tests ordered
- Time of delivery to the laboratory, i.e., when it was "clocked-in"

Pneumatic Tube Systems

Many hospitals use **pneumatic tube systems** to transport patient records, messages, letters, bills, medications, x-rays, and laboratory test results. Considerations in the use of pneumatic tubes for transporting specimens are mechanical reliability, distance of transport, speed of carrier, control mechanisms, landing mechanism, radius of loops and bends, shock absorbency, sizes of carriers, and laboratory assessment of chemical and cellular components in transported specimens versus hand-carried specimens. It is recommended that blood collection tubes be placed in the pneumatic tube with shock-absorbent inserts padding the sides and with the tubes separated from one another to prevent spillage or breakage. Plastic clear liners are also commercially available so that if leaks do occur, they are visible and are contained to prevent contamination of the tube system, the carrier, and the personnel handling the specimens.

Transportation by Automated Vehicles

Some manufacturers provide transport systems that are automated, motorized, or computerized. Delivery of specimens can be by means of a small container car attached to a network of track that is routed to appropriate sites in the laboratory, nursing stations, or other specimen collection areas. Again, a thorough evaluation of such automated delivery systems needs to include mechanical reliability, transportation distances, speed of the carriers, control mechanisms, soft-landing provisions, radius of loops and bends, shock absorbency, size of carriers, method of cleaning containers, and overall time- and cost-effectiveness. When plans are made to renovate a laboratory area so that it includes this type of transport system, extra space above the ceiling tiles should be considered because the transport vehicles require a sizable right-of-way.

Transportation or Shipping "Infectious Substances"

With the expanded worldwide transport of specimens and the increased attention to security, many air carriers, couriers, customs agents, and federal and state agencies have become more cautious about monitoring transport of hazardous agents. The United Nations Committee of Experts has defined nine hazard classes of dangerous goods as "articles or substances that are capable of posing a significant risk to the health, safety, or to property when transported by air." Infectious substances, defined as substances known to contain, or reasonably expected to contain pathogens (including bacteria, viruses, rickettsia, parasites, fungi, or recombinant microorganisms) are in Class 6 and require specific packaging and handling. Infectious substances include diagnostic specimens, i.e., "any human or animal material such as excreta, secreta, blood and blood components, tissue and tissue fluids, being shipped for diagnostic or investigative purposes." It is the organizations and/or employees' responsibility to comply with the following requirements: [12]

- Provide information and training to all employees who are involved in preparation of specimens for transport
- Properly identify, classify, pack, mark, label and document accordingly
- Make advance arrangements with all carriers of the specimens
- Receive confirmation of prompt delivery
- Notify all carriers of all shipping details

General packing requirements for **infectious substances** being shipped by passenger or cargo aircraft involve the following:

- Packaging must include an inner or primary package, a secondary container, outer package, and the name and telephone number in durable, legible ink of the person responsible for the shipping.
  - The inner packaging must have a watertight primary receptacle (e.g., specimen tubes), a watertight secondary packaging container, and an absorbent material between the primary and secondary containers and must be capable of absorbing all contents of the primary receptacle.
  - For multiple primary receptacles, they should be individually wrapped, separated, and supported to avoid contact among them.

- The secondary packaging must be sufficiently strong, have an overall dimension of at least 100 mm (4 inches), and have an itemized list of contents enclosed between the secondary and outer packaging.
- All outer packages must be marked with "Infectious Substances" labels, the net weight of dry ice (if applicable), the name/address/phone number of the shipper, and a Shippers Declaration indicating that "Inner Packaging Complies with Prescribed Specifications" and "Prior arrangements as required by the IATO Dangerous Goods Regulations 1.3.3.1 have been made."
- Up to 500 mL of blood can be shipped in a primary receptacle and in outer packaging not exceeding 4 liters.
- Substances shipped at ambient or higher temperatures need to be in leakproof primary containers of glass, metal, or plastic.
- When refrigerated or frozen, the refrigerant must be placed outside the secondary packaging with internal support to secure the secondary packaging after the refrigerant has evaporated/dissipated. If dry-ice is used, the pack and outer packaging must allow for the release of CO_2 gas.
- After receiving a specimen from an outside source, it should be immediately identified, logged-in, and checked for sample integrity.

The packing instructions for **diagnostic specimens** are slightly less restrictive but only differ in requirements for the "strength" of the outer packaging material. For infectious substances, the outer packaging must comply with stringent pressure, puncture, vibration, and temperature tests. For diagnostic specimens, the outer packaging should be of sufficient strength for its capacity, weight, and designated use to pass a drop test from a height of not less than 1.2 meters. There are serious fines and legal ramifications for failure to comply with these requirements. [12]

■ REPORTING MECHANISMS

WRITTEN REPORTS

The laboratory report is a feedback mechanism for transmitting vital data from the laboratory to the physician requesting the information. Both the JCAHO and the CAP state that the results should be confirmed, dated, and accompanied by permanent reports that are available in the laboratory, as well as on the patient's medical record via an electronic transmission or a paper-based copy. The CAP also states that each report should contain adequate patient identification, contain the date and hour when the procedures were completed, and be signed and initialed by the laboratory personnel performing the procedure. When electronic reports are used, laboratory documentation on instrument-generated worksheets by personnel performing the procedures is sufficient. The CAP has suggested that health care personnel consider the following when designing a report form.

1. Identification of patient, patient location, and physician.
2. Date and time of specimen collection.
3. Description, source of specimen, and labeled precautions.
4. Compactness and ease of preparing the package for shipment.

5. Consistency in format.
6. Clear understandability of instructions or orders.
7. Logical location in patient's chart for reference laboratory reports.
8. Sequential order of multiple results on single specimens.
9. Listing of reference ranges or normal and abnormal/critical values.
10. Assurance of accuracy of request transcription.
11. Administrative and record-keeping value.

Any unique institutional requirements for an acceptable report should be stated in the laboratory procedure manual and may include criteria such as QC limits, absolute limits, and delta checks.

Results can be documented in one of the following three ways: manual recording of test results, laboratory instrument–printed reports, and electronically generated reports. As previously mentioned, in most manual systems, combination test requisition–report forms are used. These forms may include multiple copies. Most laboratory instruments in use today can generate digital outputs and printed reports. In addition, hospital computer systems can provide patient laboratory trends over a designated period of time.

VERBAL REPORTS

The use of verbal and telephone reports has declined in recent years because computer access to laboratory data is prevalent in most health care environments. If laboratory personnel take an active role in educating clerical, nursing, and physician staff on the acquisition of computerized data, the number of phone requests will decrease.

Verbal reports, although useful for reporting stat results and "panic values or critical" may become a problem in laboratories. The possibility of error is so great that at a minimum, a laboratory should always require proper identification of the patient and the name of the person receiving the report. Documentation of verbally issued reports is recommended and should include the following information: patient name and hospital number, name of person receiving the report, data, information given, and name of person issuing the report (Box 6–7).

COMPUTERIZED REPORTS

Various computer-transmission devices can provide a rapid on-line report system and are, in general, more reliable than verbal reports and faster than waiting for the written report. Most hospitals have terminals located in each patient unit. After the tests have been completed and verified in the laboratory, the results can be immediately displayed in each patient unit. A printer can be attached to each terminal to generate a temporary hard-copy report. Another transmission option transmits fax results. All these methods can provide a written report that is accurate, dependable, and consistent.

Regarding electronic mail (e-mail) reports, the American Medical Informatics Association has issued recommendations for health care professionals, particularly physicians, who use e-mail in patient care. While each health care setting may set policies about the use of e-mail to communicate with patients, the basic recommendations include the following: [13]

- Establish turnaround times for e-mail messages
- Avoid using e-mail for urgent matters
- Inform patients about patient and privacy issues

BOX 6–7. SAMPLE FORM USED BY THE LABORATORY TO ISSUE ORAL RESULTS

TELEPHONE REQUEST FOR RELEASE OF LAB RESULTS

PATIENT NAME: _____

PATIENT ID NUMBER: _____

PHYSICIAN: _____

PERSON REQUESTING INFORMATION: _____

DATE   TEST   RESULTS/INFO GIVEN

TIME OF INQUIRY: _____

DATE OF INQUIRY: _____

REPORTED BY: _____

- Request that patients put their name and patient identification in the body of the message
- Generate automatic replies to acknowledge receipt of a patient's message
- Print a hard copy of all messages, replies, and confirmations of receipt and place them in the patient's paper-based medical record
- Consider obtaining a patient's consent prior to using e-mail for communications
- Never forward the patient's identifying information to a third party without their permission
- Use encryption for all messages
- Do not share professional e-mail accounts with family members for their use
- Use password-protected screen savers for all computers

INTERIM REPORTS AND CUMULATIVE SUMMARIES

Interim laboratory reports are typically used on hospital units at specified times during the day (e.g., 10:00 A.M. and 2:00 P.M.). These reports may include test results completed or in progress. This type of reporting system is often used in facilities that are only partially computerized or as a backup process if the hospital computer system is malfunctioning or down.

Cumulative summaries are a compilation of laboratory reports on one patient over a designated period or after a certain number of tests have been performed on the patient. They are printed at designated times during the week and facilitate the medical record-charting process. They are helpful to nurses and physicians because groups of similar tests are reported together. Trends that reveal laboratory and physiologic changes can be detected more easily than if each laboratory value were reported separately and charted in the medical record at random. With the common use of computerized medical records, it is easier to view cumulative reports.

■ DISTRIBUTION OF RESULTS

The final communication involved in the laboratory communication network is the distribution of test results. Those who receive the laboratory data include nurses, phlebotomists, clerical and medical record personnel (chart attachment); the hospital business officers (patient billing); and laboratory personnel (department record).

CHARTING REPORTS

Manual Methods

So that a chronological type of reporting system is used on the patient's chart, the laboratory reports have traditionally been shingled one upon another. Color coding by the laboratory originating the results aids in coordinating them on a carrier page. The laboratory may also key chronological reports by having a master card prepared in the laboratory for each patient, beginning with the admitting laboratory test results. The results of each day are added to the card, which can be photocopied and sent to the physician.

Computerized Medical Records

As mentioned previously, a health care facility's computer system can easily provide daily laboratory reports and cumulative reports for the patient's computerized medical record. All reports should be available at times convenient for making clinical decisions by the medical staff.

The business office of the health care facility also receives data on-line regarding laboratory procedures. This office must be notified of all laboratory charges, according to data requested and procedural code for patient billing. It is financially advantageous to send reports promptly. Also laboratory copies of test results from previous days, months, or years should be accessible because they are often requested to confirm charges for the hospital stay during insurance or Medicare/Medicaid audits.

SELF STUDY

KEY TERMS

Analytic Phase
Bar Codes
Clinical (or Medical) Record
Confidentiality
Critical Value
Diagnostic Specimens
E-mail
Fax Machines
Health Insurance Portability
    and Accountability Act
    (HIPAA)

Infectious Substances
Light Sensitive
"Panic Value"
Pneumatic Tube Systems
Preanalytical Phases
Privacy
Reference Ranges
Requisition Form
Specimen Collection Manual

STUDY QUESTIONS

The following may have *one* or *more* answers:

1. The key elements common to most medical records are which of the following:

   a. name, DOB, SSN
   b. personal and family medical history
   c. plan of care
   d. discharge summary

2. Medical records serve what purpose?

   a. coordination of care
   b. meet accrediting and licensing
      requirements
   c. provide legal protection
   d. provide research data

3. Guidelines for documentation in health care include which of the following:

   a. accuracy
   b. personal opinions of the situation
   c. completion about each event or procedure
   d. objectivity and timeliness

4. Which of the following data should be considered confidential?

   a. laboratory test results
   b. radiology reports
   c. patient's diagnosis
   d. universal precautions

5. Bar codes can be used for which type(s) of information?

   a. identification of patient names
   b. identification of patient numbers
   c. designation of test to be performed
   d. inventory of supplies

6. What is the most error-free method for requesting a laboratory test?

   a. handwritten requisition
   b. computerized method
   c. verbal method
   d. verbal stat method

7. Sources of preanalytic error can be categorized as follows:

   a. processing variables
   b. specimen variables
   c. physician's attitude
   d. patient variables

8. Telephone responsibilities for health care workers usually include:

   a. using effective customer service manners
   b. using an intercom system
   c. transferring calls
   d. placing people on hold

9. A specimen should be protected from light for which of the following determinations?

   a. bilirubin concentration
   b. hemoglobin level
   c. glucose level
   d. blood cultures

10. A specimen should be chilled for which of the following analyses?

   a. complete blood count (CBC)
   b. bilirubin level
   c. blood gas
   d. glucose level

References

1. Clinical Skillbuilders: *Better Documentation.* Spring House, PA; Spring House Corporation: 1992.
2. Fiesta, J: *20 Legal Pitfalls for Nurses to Avoid.* Allentown, PA; Delmar Publishers: 1994.
3. Krebs, C and Wise, BA: *Medical Assisting, Clinical Competencies.* Albany, NY; Delmar Publishers: 1994.
4. Hamann, LJ: Pre-analytical Variability: A Phlebotomy Perspective. Presented at Current Issues in Phlebotomy. Baltimore, MD: March 6, 1997.
5. College of American Pathologists (CAP): *Laboratory Accreditation Checklists, Proposed Checklist: Laboratory General.* Web page: www.cap.org. Skokie, IL: 2000.
6. Dalton-Beninato, K: Critical Value Notifications are Never Welcome News, *Lab Med* 2000; 31(6) 319–323.
7. QuadraMed: Internet forum on HIPAA Preparedness, Executive Summary. Web page: www.hipaa-iq.com/summary.htm, last updated Jan 30, 2001.
8. Garza, D: Phlebotomy and Bar Coding: Improving Accuracy in Specimen Handling. *Adv Med Lab Professionals* 1999; March 22: 22–27.
9. Allen, M: The Applicability of 2-D Bar Code Symbologies in the Clinical Laboratory, Clinical Note. *Am Clin.* 1999; March: 15–19.
10. National Committee for Clinical Laboratory Standards (NCCLS): *Procedures for Handling and Transport of Diagnostic Specimens and Etiologic Agents.* NCCLS Document H5-A3, Villanova, PA; NCCLS: 1994.
11. National Committee for Clinical Laboratory Standards (NCCLS): *Procedures for the Collection of Diagnostic Blood Specimens by Venipuncture.* NCCLS Document H3-A4, Villanova, PA; NCCLS: June, 1998.
12. Roane, PA: Transporting Infectious Substances, Packaging is Everything! *Adv Med Lab Professionals.* 1999; October 18:7–10.
13. American Medical Informatics Association: Newsline: E-mail Guidelines Introduced, *Health Data Management.* 1998; May: 24.

CASE STUDY

■

Improving Speed and Accuracy in Phlebotomy Practice

The phlebotomists were having an in-service with supervisory technologists to discuss options for improving productivity, accuracy, and for minimizing the number of preanalytical errors occurring in the laboratory. In the previous two years, the specimen collection workload had increased threefold, including the hospital and in-house clinics. Preanalytical errors had also increased and on several occasions they had run out of certain evacuated tubes because they were behind on the inventory counts. One phlebotomist named Billy Bob suggested that bar code technology be considered as a method to improve productivity and accuracy. He had worked at a hospital where they had been in use for several years and thought it could have a positive impact. He began to highlight the benefits of bar code technology and explain how they might be used at the current facility.

QUESTIONS

1. What could Billy Bob say about the benefits and drawbacks of bar code technology?
2. In what ways could bar codes help reduce preanalytical errors?

See Answers in Appendix.

EQUIPMENT AND PROCEDURES

P HLEBOTOMY PRACTICE IS BEST DESCRIBED by what phlebotomists do. Part III answers the following technical questions:

- What tools (supplies and equipment) do I need and how safe are they to use in blood collection?
- How do I prepare myself and the patient?
- How do I perform a venipuncture?
- How do I perform a finger stick?
- What can go wrong, and how can I prevent it from happening?

Building on the knowledge from the first six chapters, Part III highlights technical skills, supplies, and equipment. It is divided into four chapters that describe the supplies, equipment, techniques, and complications associated with phlebotomy practice.

Chapter 7, Blood Collection Equipment, describes and illustrates the latest supplies and equipment necessary for the collection of blood. Emphasis is on anticoagulated and nonadditive blood collection tubes, the importance of color coding, and the use of gloves, syringes, needles, microcollection equipment, specimen collection chairs and trays, and other supplies needed for a safe and effective collection procedure. Safety equipment and safe handling of blood specimens is highlighted.

Chapter 8, Venipuncture Procedures, provides a comprehensive description and illustrations of each step of the blood collection process. It includes a discussion of patient identification, as well as the venipuncture procedure itself. Emphasis is on safe and proper preparation, technique, and collection.

Chapter 9, Skin Puncture Procedures, provides a detailed description and illustration of each step of the skin puncture procedure. Emphasis is on site selection, finger sticks, and blood smear preparation.

Chapter 10, Complications in Blood Collection, describes the complications that occur during the blood collection process and the reasons for their occurrence. Emphasis is on recognition and prevention of these complications, the effects of the patient's physical disposition on the integrity of the specimen, and the interfering effects of drugs and other substances in the blood. Guidelines for specimen rejection are also presented.

SEVEN

■

Blood Collection Equipment

CHAPTER OUTLINE

CHAPTER OBJECTIVES

Upon completion of Chapter 7, the learner is responsible for the following:

1. List the various types of anticoagulants used in blood collection, their mechanisms for preventing blood from clotting, and the vacuum collection tube color codes for these anticoagulants.

2. Describe the latest phlebotomy safety supplies and equipment and evaluate their effectiveness in blood collection.

3. Identify the various supplies that should be carried on a specimen collection tray when a skin puncture specimen must be collected.

4. Identify the types of equipment needed to collect blood by venipuncture.

5. Describe the special precautions that should be taken and the techniques that should be used when various types of specimens must be transported to the clinical laboratory.

■ VACUUM (EVACUATED) TUBE SYSTEMS

Venipuncture with a **vacuum (evacuated) tube** (VACUTAINER [BD VACUTAINER Systems, *Preanalytical Solutions,* Franklin Lakes, NJ]), as shown in Figure 7–1, is the most direct and efficient method for obtaining a blood specimen. The evacuated tube system requires three components: the evacuated sample tube, the double-pointed needle, and a special plastic **holder (adapter)** (Fig. 7–2). One end of the double-pointed needle enters the vein, the other end pierces the top of the tube, and the vacuum aspirates the blood. Vacuum tubes may contain silicon to decrease the possibility of hemolysis and prevent the clot from adhering to the wall of the tube. This convenient system eliminates the need for syringes and consists of disposable needles and tubes. The tubes are available in different sizes and can be purchased in glass or unbreakable plastic. The external tube diameter and length plus the maximum amount of spec-

Figure 7–1.   Vacuum tube (VACUTAINER).

(Courtesy of BD VACUTAINER Systems, *Preanalytical Solutions*, Franklin Lakes, NJ.)

Figure 7–2.   BD Eclipse Blood Collection Needle attached to a holder.

(Courtesy of BD VACUTAINER Systems, *Preanalytical Solutions*, Franklin Lakes, NJ.)

imen to be drawn into the vacuum tube are the two criteria used to describe vacuum tube size (Table 7–1). The smaller sizes (e.g., 2 mL) are useful for pediatric and geriatric collections and can be purchased with different types of anticoagulants, as well as chemically clean or sterile

Table 7–1.   Typical Sizes of Blood Collection Vacuum Tubes

EXTERNAL DIAMETER × LENGTH (MM)	DRAW VOLUMES (ML)
0.25 × 47	2.0
0.25 × 64	3.0
0.25 × 82	4.0
13 × 75	2.0
13 × 75	4.5
13 × 75	5.0
13 × 100	4.5
13 × 100	6.0
13 × 100	7.0
16 × 75	7.0
16 × 100	10.0
16 × 125	15.0

Table 7–2. Specimen Type and Collection Vacuum Tubes

SPECIMEN TYPE	COLLECTION TUBES (STOPPER COLOR/TYPE)	ADDITIVE
Clotted blood/serum	Gray and red	Polymer barrier
	Yellow and red	Polymer barrier
	Gold	Polymer barrier
	Red	None
	Orange	Thrombin
	Yellow and Green	Thrombin
	Brown	Polymergel
Whole blood/plasma	Green and brown	Polymer barrier and lithium heparin
	Green (yellow top)	Polymer barrier and lithium heparin
	Light green	Polymer barrier and lithium heparin
	Light blue	Trisodium citrate
	Lavender (purple)	EDTA (K_3) or EDTA (K_2) or EDTA (Na_2)
	Gray	Sodium fluoride and potassium oxalate
	Green	Lithium heparin
	Green	Sodium heparin or ammonium heparin
	Royal blue	Sodium heparin or EDTA (Na_2)-sterile tube for toxicology and nutritional studies
	Pink	Blood Bank (EDTA)
Clotted blood/serum	Royal blue	No additive; but sterile tube for trace elements, toxicology, and nutritional studies
	Brown	No additive or sodium heparin, but lead-free glass and sterile for lead determinations
Whole blood	Lavender (purple)	EDTA (K_3) or EDTA (K_2) or EDTA (Na_2)
	Green	Lithium heparin, sodium heparin, or ammonium heparin
	Black	Sodium citrate
	Yellow	Sodium polyanetholesulfonate (SPS) or Acid Citrate Dextrose (ACD)

glassware. Each vacuum tube is color coded according to the additive contained within the tube (see Table 7–2 above).

Many tubes are specifically designed to be used directly with chemistry, hematology, or microbiology instrumentation. In these cases, the tube of blood is identified by its bar code and is pierced by the instrument probe, and some sample is aspirated into the instrument for analyses. Use of these *closed systems* minimizes laboratory personnel's risk of exposure to blood. In addition, some tubes have plastic tops or screw-on enclosures around the rubber

As described in Chapter 4, Infection Control, the Federal Needlestick and Prevention Act was enacted in November, 2000. It requires the use of needlestick prevention devices. The holder of the evacuated tube system has a large opening for the blood vacuum tube and a small opening at the other end for needle insertion. Tube holders and blood collection needles are separate devices used in combination to withdraw blood from a patient's vein. Prior to use, the blood collection needle is screwed into the tube holder, which holds the needle and maintains some balance for the vacuum tubes while blood is collected. Various manufacturers have modified the adapter to reduce the risk of accidental needle sticks.

stopper to minimize exposure to blood left on the top of the cap or blood splatters that can occur during cap removal.

Evacuated tubes are also used for transferring blood from a syringe into the tubes. The syringe needle is simply pushed through the top of the tube, and blood is automatically pulled into the tube because of the vacuum. Place the vacuum tube in a rack before pushing the needle into the tube top. A safety syringe shielded transfer device needs to be used to avoid possible exposure to the patient's blood. The plunger must not be pushed down if the tubes are being filled from the syringe because it is extremely hazardous. Also, pushing the plunger may damage cellular components and cause hemolysis because of the forceful expulsion of blood. Specialized tubes and bottles that may fit the adapter are also available for blood culture collection.

The expiration dates of tubes should be monitored continuously. Such monitoring is most easily accomplished with a computerized inventory system; however, routine rotation of stocked supplies and careful checking of phlebotomy trays and carts should also be the responsibility of each phlebotomist.

For instance, BD VACUTAINER Systems, *Preanalytical Solutions* (Franklin Lakes, NJ) developed the Safety-Lok Needle Holder (Fig. 7–3), which has a protective shield so that the blood collector can slide the protective shield over the needle and lock it in place after the needle is withdrawn from the puncture site. This single-use adapter provides immediate containment of a used needle. The BD Eclipse (BD VACUTAINER Systems, *Preanalytical Solutions*, Franklin Lakes, NJ) is a single-use blood collection needle that allows the user to shield the needle after use (see Fig. 7–2). The phlebotomist activates the safety mechanism by closing the shield over the needle until it locks in place.

Another protective holder that provides effective, immediate containment of a used needle is the SIMS Venipuncture Needle-Pro (SIMS Portex Inc., Keene, NH). After removing the needle from the patient's vein, the phlebotomist activates the needle guard by holding the tube holder and pressing the needle guard against a hard surface so that the guard swings over the needle.

Figure 7–3.   Safety-Lok Needle Holder.

(Courtesy of BD VACUTAINER Systems, *Preanalytical Solutions,* Franklin Lakes, NJ.)

Vanishpoint (Retractable Technologies, TX) distributed by Greiner Laborbechnik is a safety blood collection tube holder that provides for the needle to automatically retract into it after blood collection (Fig. 7–4). It can be used for a multitube blood collection with the safety one-step activation to retract the needle after use. It contains no natural rubber latex and thus avoids the possibility of an allergic reaction to the latex.

Another vacuum tube assembly developed to prevent needlestick injuries is the Proguard II (Care Medical Products, Ontario, CA). It is a single-use vacuum tube/needle holder. The used needle is manually retracted into the holder.

Sarstedt, Inc. has the S-Monovette (Sarstedt, Inc., Newton, NC) Blood Collection System (Fig. 7–5), which is a safety device for vacuum collection or a syringe collection technique. It is unique in that the sample collection, transportation, and centrifugation tube is a combined unit.

For any of these blood collection needle and tube holder devices, disposing of the tube holder while it is still attached to the needle ensures that the tube-puncturing needle remains protected during and after disposal. Thus, it significantly reduces the risks of needlestick injuries and blood exposure from the tube-puncturing needle.

■ ANTICOAGULANTS AND BLOOD COLLECTION TUBES

Traditionally, in most clinical laboratories, serum, plasma, or whole blood has been used to perform various assays. More recently, though, heparinized whole blood has become the specimen of choice for the latest clinical laboratory instruments used in stat (immediate)

Figure 7–4. Vanishpoint system.

(Courtesy of Retractable Technologies, Little Elm, TX.)

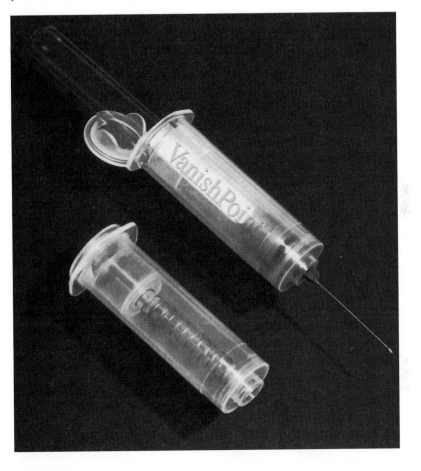

situations. Using whole blood as a specimen decreases the time involved in acquiring the test result because centrifugation is not required prior to laboratory testing.

Many coagulation factors are involved in blood clotting, and coagulation can be prevented by the addition of different types of anticoagulants. These **anticoagulants** often contain preservatives that can extend the metabolism and life span of the red blood cells (RBCs) after blood collection. Anticoagulants and preservatives are used extensively in blood donations to ensure the biochemical balance of certain components of RBCs, such as hemoglobin, pH, adenosine triphosphate (ATP), and glucose. Once transferred, anticoagulants, such as **citrate–phosphate–dextrose (CPD)** and **acid–citrate–dextrose (ACD),** ensure that the RBCs provide the recipient with the means of delivering oxygen (O_2) to the tissues.

Figure 7–5. S-Monovette.

(Courtesy of Sarstedt, Inc., Newton, NC.)

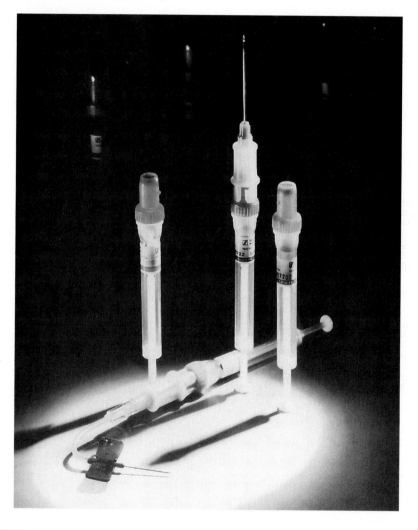

Another major use of anticoagulants and preservatives is in the collection of plasma for laboratory analysis. Specific anticoagulants or preservatives must be used depending on the test procedure ordered. Anticoagulants cannot be substituted for one another. Table 7–3 lists the various laboratory assays along with the types of anticoagulants required and the approximate milliliters of blood that must be collected for each assay.

Coagulation of blood can be prevented by the addition of **oxalates, citrates, ethylene-diamine tetra-acetic acid (EDTA),** or **heparin.** Oxalates, citrates, and EDTA prevent the

Table 7–3. Laboratory Assays and the Required Types of Anticoagulants

TEST NAME	SPECIMEN TUBE (TYPE/COLOR)	WHOLE BLOOD, MINIMUM VOLUME FOR ADULTS (mL)
A$_{1c}$ hemoglobin (see glycosylated hemoglobin)		
ABG (See Blood gases)		
ABO group and type	Whole blood (purple) or serum (red)	5
Acetaminophen (Tylenol)	Serum (red) or plasma (heparin)	1
Acetone	Serum (speckled)	2
Acetylcholine receptor-binding antibodies	Serum (speckled)	3
Acid hemolysis (PNH)	Plasma (light blue)	3
Acid phosphatase, prostatic isoenzyme	Serum (speckled)	2
Acidified serum test (see Hamm's test)		
ACTH (adrenocorticotropic) hormone	Whole blood (purple) (Must be collected in siliconized tube)	1
Activated partial thromboplastin time (see Partial thromboplastin time)		
Activated Protein C Resistance (APCR)	Plasma (blue) (Freeze immediately)	2
Adenovirus antibody	Serum (speckled)	3
Adrenal cortical antibody	Serum (red)	3
Adrenalin (see Catecholamines)		
Albumin	Serum (speckled)	2
Alcohol (ethanol)	Whole blood (gray)	2
Aldolase	Serum (speckled)	2
Aldosterone	Serum (speckled) or plasma (purple or green) *Ice needed for transportation *Patient should be recumbent for at least 30 minutes prior to blood collection	7
Alkaline phosphatase (Alk p'tase)	Serum (speckled)	2
Alkaline phosphatase isoenzymes	Serum (speckled)	2
Alpha$_1$-antitrypsin (AAT)	Serum (speckled)	1
Alpha-fetoprotein (AFP)	Serum (speckled)	3
Alpha$_2$-macroglobulin	Serum (red)	1
Aluminum	Whole blood (royal blue)	7

(continued)

Table 7–3. *(continued)*

TEST NAME	SPECIMEN TUBE (TYPE/COLOR)	WHOLE BLOOD, MINIMUM VOLUME FOR ADULTS (mL)
Amebiasis	Serum (speckled)	3
Amikacin	Serum (speckled)	1
Amino acid	Serum (speckled)	3
Amiodarone	Serum (speckled)	10
Amitriptyline	Serum (red)	3
Ammonia	Plasma (green)	3
Ampicillin	Serum (red)	5
Amylase	Serum (speckled)	2
Amylase Isoenzymes	Serum (speckled)	2
Androstenedione	Serum (speckled) *Deliver immediately	5
Angiotensin-converting enzyme (ACE)	Serum (speckled) *Ice needed for transportation	5
Antibody to hepatitis A virus (anti-HAV)	Serum (speckled)	5
Antibody to hepatitis B core antigen	Serum (red)	3
Antibody to hepatitis BE antigen	Serum (red)	3
Antibody to hepatitis B surface antigen	Serum (red)	3
Antibody identification	Whole blood (red)	7
Antibody screen and blood grouping	Whole blood (red)	5
Antibody titer	Whole blood (red)	5
Anticonvulsants (Dilantin, Mysoline, phenobarbital, carbamazepine, valproic acid)	Serum (speckled)	7
Antidiuretic hormone (ADH, vasopressin)	Whole blood (purple)	3
Anti–DNase B	Serum (speckled)	3
Antinuclear antibodies, fluorescent (ANA)	Whole blood (red)	5
Anti–smooth muscle antibody (ASMA)	Serum (speckled)	3
Antithrombin III	Plasma (light blue)	1
Apolipoprotein A–1	Serum (speckled) Fasting required	2
APTT	Plasma (light blue)	1.8
Arboviruses (St. Louis encephalitis)	Serum (speckled)	3
Arsenic (As)	Whole blood (royal blue)	7

Table 7–3.   *(continued)*

TEST NAME	SPECIMEN TUBE (TYPE/COLOR)	WHOLE BLOOD, MINIMUM VOLUME FOR ADULTS (mL)
Ascorbic acid (see Vitamin C)		
ASO (anti–streptolysin O) titer	Serum (speckled)	3
Aspirin (see Salicylate)		
Autologous blood	Whole blood (red)	5
Bactrim (see Sulfonamides)		
Barbiturates	Serum (speckled)	2
B-cell antigen	Whole blood (red)	3
Benzodiazepines	Serum (speckled)	2
Beta$_2$-microglobulin	Serum (speckled)	3
Bilirubin, total and direct	Serum (speckled) *Protect blood from light	1
Blastomycosis, complement fixation (fungal serology)	Serum (speckled)	4
Bleeding time	Patient	Test performed on patient's arm
Blood cell count, CBC survey (WBC, RBC, Hgb, Hct, MCV, MCH, MCHC)	Whole blood (purple)	3
Blood cell count, differential	Blood smear	Blood smear
Blood cell count, eosinophil	Whole blood (purple)	3
Blood cell count, erythrocyte (RBC)	Whole blood (purple)	3
Blood cell count, leukocyte (WBC)	Whole blood (purple)	3
Blood cell count, platelets	Whole blood (purple)	3
Blood cell count, reticulocyte	Whole blood (purple)	3
Blood gases, arterial (ABG) (pH, pCO$_2$, pO$_2$, HCO$_3^-$, base excess [BE])	Arterial blood (heparinized syringe)	0.6
Blood packed red blood cells	Whole blood (red)	5
Bordetella pertussis antibody (whooping cough)	Serum (red)	3
Borrelia burgdorferi antibody (Lyme disease)	Serum (red)	3
Bromide	Serum (red)	2
Brucella	Serum (speckled)	2
BUN (blood urea nitrogen)	Serum (speckled)	1
Cadmium (Cd)	Whole blood (green, purple) *Use acid-washed syringes	2
Calcitonin	Plasma (green)	3
Calcium	Serum (speckled)	1
Calcium, ionized	Plasma (green)	3
Candida serology, qualitative	Serum (speckled)	3

(continued)

Table 7–3. *(continued)*

TEST NAME	SPECIMEN TUBE (TYPE/COLOR)	WHOLE BLOOD, MINIMUM VOLUME FOR ADULTS (mL)
Carbamazepine (see Tegretol)		
Carbon dioxide (CO_2)	Serum (speckled)	1
Carcinoembryonic antigen (CEA)	Serum (speckled)	3
Cardiac troponins (cTnI, cTnT)	Serum (speckled)	3
Cardiolipin antibodies (anti-cardiolipin antibody IgG and IgM)	Serum (speckled)	3
Carotene	Serum (speckled)	3
Catecholamines (Adrenalin; Epinephrine)	Whole blood (purple) *Ice needed for transportation	20
Ceruloplasmin	Serum (speckled)	3
Chemistry screen (T. protein, Alb, Ca, I phos, Glu, BUN, uric acid, Creat, T. bil, Alk p'tase, LD, ALT)	Serum (speckled)	3
Chickenpox titer	Serum (speckled)	3
Chloramphenicol	Serum (speckled)	4
Chloride	Serum (speckled)	1
Cholesterol	Serum (speckled)	1
Cholinesterase	Serum (speckled)	3
Chromium (Cr)	Serum (royal blue) *Avoid chromium-plated needles; use platinum needles and acid-washed syringes	2
Chromosome analysis	Sterile whole blood (green) (Na heparin)	7
Circulating anticoagulants	Plasma (light blue)	3
Clonazepam	Serum (red) or plasma (purple)	2
CMV, IFA serology	Serum (speckled)	3
Coccidioides immitis (San Joaquin fever)	Serum (speckled)	3
Cold agglutinins	Whole blood (speckled) *Place in warm water and deliver immediately	3
Complement, total	Serum (speckled)	5
Complement—C3	Serum (speckled)	5
Complement—C4	Serum (speckled)	5
Coombs' test, direct (direct antiglobulin test)	Whole blood (red)	3

Table 7–3. *(continued)*

TEST NAME	SPECIMEN TUBE (TYPE/COLOR)	WHOLE BLOOD, MINIMUM VOLUME FOR ADULTS (mL)
Coombs' test, indirect (indirect antiglobulin test)	Whole blood (red)	5
Copper (Cu)	Serum (speckled) or whole blood (royal blue)	3
Cortisol	Plasma (green)	1
Coxsackievirus (Bornholm disease)	Serum (speckled)	3
Coxiella burnetii (Q fever)	Serum (speckled)	3
C-peptide	Serum (speckled)	3
CPK (CK)	Serum (speckled)	1
CPK isoenzymes (CK isoenzymes) (CK-MB)	Serum (speckled)	3
C-reactive protein	Serum (speckled)	2
Creatinine	Serum (speckled)	1
Cross-match	Whole blood (red)	3
Cryofibrinogen	Plasma (green)	1
Cryoglobulin	Serum (speckled) *Immediately place in warm water and transport to lab	4
Cryptococcal antigen	Serum (red)	3
Cyclosporine	Serum (speckled)	3
Cysticercus cellulosae (pork tapeworm)	Serum (red)	3
Cytomegalovirus (CMV), IFA serology	Serum (speckled)	3
D-dimer (D-D$_1$)	Whole blood (blue)	3.5
Dengue virus antibody (breakbone fever)	Serum (speckled)	3
Deoxycorticosteroids	Serum (speckled) or plasma (green)	3
Depakene (see Valproic Acid)		
Desipramine	Serum (speckled) or plasma (green)	5
DHEA	Serum (red) *Immediately place in ice slurry and transport to lab	10
Diazepam (see Valium)		
Digitoxin	Serum (speckled)	2
Digoxin (Lanoxin)	Serum (speckled)	2
Dilantin (phenytoin)	Serum (speckled)	1
Directogen for *Haemophilus influenzae, Streptococcus pneumoniae, Neisseria menigitidis*	Serum (speckled)	3

(continued)

Table 7–3. *(continued)*

TEST NAME	SPECIMEN TUBE (TYPE/COLOR)	WHOLE BLOOD, MINIMUM VOLUME FOR ADULTS (mL)
DNA antibody (anti-DNA)	Serum (speckled)	3
Drug screen	Serum (speckled)	10
EBV–early antigen	Serum (speckled)	3
EBV-IgM	Serum (speckled)	3
EBV-NA	Serum (speckled)	3
EBV-VCA	Serum (speckled)	3
Echinococcus (hydatid disease)	Serum (red)	3
Electrolytes (Na, K, Cl, HCO_3)	Plasma (green) or whole blood (green)	2
Electrophoresis (hemoglobin)	Whole blood (purple)	1
Electrophoresis (immuno)	Serum (speckled)	3
Electrophoresis (SPE)	Serum (speckled)	3
Elution studies	Whole blood (purple)	2
Entamoeba histolytica	Serum (speckled)	3
Eosinophil count	Whole blood (purple)	1
Epinephrine (see Catecholamines)		
E-rosette	Whole blood (purple)	3
E-rosette receptor	Whole blood (purple)	3
Erythrocyte fragility	Whole blood (purple)	1
Erythrocyte osmotic fragility	Whole blood (green)	2
Erythromycin	Serum (speckled)	5
Erythropoietin	Serum (speckled)	5
ESR (sedimentation rate, sed rate)	Whole blood (purple)	3
Estradiol (E_2)	Serum (speckled) or plasma (green)	3
Estriol	Serum (speckled) or plasma (green)	3
Estrogens, total	Serum (speckled)	7
Ethanol (alcohol)	Whole blood (gray)	2
Ethosuximide (Zarontin)	Plasma (green)	3
Euglobulin lysis	Plasma (blue)	4.5
Factor assays	Plasma (blue)	4.5
Fasting blood glucose (FBG)	Plasma (gray)	1
Fatty acids, free	Serum (speckled) *Transport in ice water	10
Febrile agglutinins	Serum (speckled)	7
Ferritin	Serum (speckled)	2
Fetal hemoglobin	Whole blood (purple)	2
Fibrin degradation products (FDP) (FSP)	Plasma (blue)	2
Fibrinogen	Plasma (blue)	1.8

Table 7–3.   *(continued)*

TEST NAME	SPECIMEN TUBE (TYPE/COLOR)	WHOLE BLOOD, MINIMUM VOLUME FOR ADULTS (mL)
Fibrinogen antigen	Plasma (blue)	4.5
Fibrinopeptide A	Whole blood with special tube from hematology	5
Fitzgerald factor	Plasma (blue)	4.5
Flecainide	Serum (red)	3
Fletcher factor (prekallinkrein)	Plasma (blue)	4.5
Fluorescent antinuclear antibody	Serum (speckled)	3
Fluorescent treponemal antibody test (MHA-TP)	Serum (red or speckled)	3
Fluoride	Serum (red)	6
Folate, serum	Serum (speckled)	3
Folate, whole blood (RBC and serum)	Whole blood (purple)	3
Follicle-stimulating hormone (FSH)	Serum (speckled) or plasma (green)	3
Fragility, erythrocyte (RBC)	Whole blood (purple)	2
Francisella tularensis antibody (tularemia)	Serum (speckled)	3
Free, T$_4$ (see Thyroxine, free)		
Free thyroxine index (see Thyroid studies)		
Fungal serology	Serum (speckled)	3
Gamma-glutamyl transpeptidase (GGT) (GT)	Serum (speckled)	3
Gastrin	Serum (speckled)	7
Gentamicin	Serum (speckled)	1
Glucagon	Whole blood (purple)	3
Glucose (FBS and tolerance)	Plasma (gray) or serum (speckled)	1
Glucose-6-phosphate dehydrogenase (G6PD), quantitative	Whole blood (green)	1
Glucose, 2-hour postprandial	Plasma (gray) or serum (speckled)	1
Glycosylated hemoglobin	Whole blood (purple)	1
Gonadotropin HCG-beta (immuno test)	Serum (speckled)	7
Growth hormone (HGH)	Serum (speckled)	1.5
Hamm's test (PNH) confirmation	Plasma (green)	5
Haptoglobin	Serum (speckled)	1

(continued)

Table 7–3. *(continued)*

TEST NAME	SPECIMEN TUBE (TYPE/COLOR)	WHOLE BLOOD, MINIMUM VOLUME FOR ADULTS (mL)
HDL (high-density lipoprotein) cholesterol	Serum (speckled)	5
Heinz body preparation	Whole blood (purple) or (green)	3
Helper T	Whole blood (purple)	2
Hematocrit	Whole blood (purple)	1
Hematology profile (Hct, Hgb, WBC, RBC, MCV, MCH, MCHC)	Whole blood (purple)	1
Hemoglobin	Whole blood (purple)	1
Hemoglobin, plasma	Plasma (purple)	1
Heparin	Plasma (blue)	3
Hepatitis A Ab IgM (Anti-HAV-IgM)	Serum (speckled)	5
Hepatitis B core antibody (HB$_c$Ab) (Anti-HB$_c$)	Serum (speckled)	3
Hepatitis B surface Ab (Anti-HB$_s$)	Serum (speckled)	4
Hepatitis B surface antigen (HB$_s$Ag)	Serum (speckled)	3
Hepatitis C Ab (HCV)	Serum (speckled)	5
HCV RNA	Serum (red)	1
Hepatitis delta antibody and antigen	Serum (speckled)	3
Hepatitis G test	Serum (red)	10
Herpes simplex, virus serology	Serum (speckled)	3
Heterophile antibody (see Monospot)		
Histamine	Serum (speckled)	5
Histoplasmosis	Serum (speckled)	5
HI titer (St. Louis encephalitis)	Serum (speckled)	3
HIV antibody screen	Serum (speckled)	5
HIV antigen	Serum (speckled)	3
HLA typing (microcytotoxicity)	Whole blood (green)	5
Human chorionic gonadotrophin (HCG)	Serum (speckled)	6
Human growth hormone (HGH) (see Growth hormone)		
Human T-cell lymphotropic virus type I (HTLV-1) antibody	Serum (speckled)	2
Hydroxybutyric dehydrogenase (HBD)	Serum (speckled)	5
IgA	Serum (speckled)	1
IgD	Serum (speckled)	1

Table 7–3. *(continued)*

TEST NAME	SPECIMEN TUBE (TYPE/COLOR)	WHOLE BLOOD, MINIMUM VOLUME FOR ADULTS (mL)
IgG	Serum (speckled)	1
IgM	Serum (speckled)	1
Imipramine (Tofranil)	Serum (red)	10
Infectious mononucleosis (see Monospot)		
Inhibitor assay	Plasma (blue)	4.5
Insulin (on ice)	Plasma (purple)	4.5
Intrinsic factor antibody	Serum (speckled)	3
Iron profile (iron, TIBC, and saturation)	Serum (speckled)	3
Kanamycin	Serum (speckled)	5
Lactate dehydrogenase (LD) and LD isoenzymes (LD-1)	Serum (speckled)	3
Lactic acid (on ice)	Plasma (gray)	1
Lanoxin (see Digoxin)		
Latex, IgE, AlaSTAT	Serum (speckled)	0.1
LDL (low-density lipoprotein) cholesterol	Serum (speckled)	10
Lead, blood	Blood (royal blue) or special tube from chemistry	2
LE cell test	Whole blood (green)	3
Legionnaires' serology	Serum (speckled)	3
Leishmania antibody	Serum (speckled)	3
Leptospira agglutination	Serum (speckled)	3
Leucine aminopeptidase (LAP)	Plasma (green)	2
Leukocyte alkaline phosphatase (LAP) stain		Six fresh blood smears
LGV-psittacosis titer	Serum (speckled)	5
LH (see Luteinizing hormone)		
Lidocaine	Serum (speckled)	5
Lipase	Serum (speckled)	2
Lipid profile	Serum (speckled)	10
Lithium	Serum (speckled)	1
Low-density lipoprotein (LDL) cholesterol	Serum (speckled)	5
Lupus anticoagulant (tissue thromboplastin inhibition test)	Plasma (blue) *Deliver immediately	5
Luteinizing hormone (LH)	Serum (speckled)	2
Lyme disease serology	Serum (speckled)	4
Lymphocyte blastogenesis (LBR)	Whole blood (green)	7
Lymphogranuloma venereum	Serum (speckled)	3

(continued)

Table 7–3. *(continued)*

TEST NAME	SPECIMEN TUBE (TYPE/COLOR)	WHOLE BLOOD, MINIMUM VOLUME FOR ADULTS (mL)
Lysozyme, serum	Serum (speckled)	2
Magnesium, serum	Serum (speckled)	1
Malaria antibody	Serum (speckled)	2
Malaria smear		Blood smear
Manganese (Mn)	Whole blood (royal blue) or serum *Use acid-washed syringes	5
Mercury (Hg)	Whole blood (royal blue)	5
Methemalbumin	Serum (speckled)	2
Methemoglobin	Serum (speckled)	3
Methicillin	Serum (speckled)	5
Methotrexate	Serum (red)	2
MHA-TP	Serum (speckled or red)	3
Molecular diagnostic lab tests	Whole blood (purple) *Immediately transport in ice slurry	3×10 mL
Monocyte antigens	Whole blood (purple)	2
Mumps serology	Serum (speckled)	3
Mycoplasma pneumoniae	Serum (speckled)	2
Myelin antibodies	Serum (speckled)	3
NAPA (see Procainamide)		
Nickel (Ni)	Plasma, serum, whole blood *Must prepare collection vials by acid-washing syringes	5
5'-Nucleotidase	Serum (speckled)	2
Nutritional panel	Serum (speckled)	2
Opiates (methadone, codeine, morphine)	Serum (speckled)	3
Osmolality, serum	Serum (speckled)	2
Parathyroid hormone (PTH)	Serum (speckled)	2
Partial thromboplastin time (PTT) (APTT)	Plasma (blue)	1
Penicillin	Serum (red)	5
Pentobarbital	Serum (speckled)	5
pH, blood (see Blood gases)		
Phenobarbital	Serum (speckled)	2
Phenylalanine	Whole blood *Filter paper with low background fluorescence	Droplets used to saturate filter paper (< 0.5)
Phenytoin (Dilantin)	Serum (speckled)	1
Phenytoin (free)	Serum (speckled)	5

Table 7–3. *(continued)*

TEST NAME	SPECIMEN TUBE (TYPE/COLOR)	WHOLE BLOOD, MINIMUM VOLUME FOR ADULTS (mL)
Phosphorus	Serum (speckled)	1
Plasminogen antigen	Whole blood (blue)	5
Platelet function profile	Whole blood (purple)	1
	Whole blood (blue)	7
Pneumocystic serology	Serum (red)	3
Potassium	Plasma (green)	2
Prealbumin	Serum (speckled)	3
Precursor T	Whole blood (purple)	2
Primidone (Mysoline)	Serum (speckled)	2
Procainamide, *N*-acetylprocainamide (NAPA)	Serum (speckled)	2
Progesterone	Clotted whole blood (red)	3
	*Avoid serum separator tube in speckled tube top	
Prolactin	Serum (speckled)	2
Pronestyl (procainamide)	Serum (speckled)	2
Propranolol	Serum (speckled) or plasma (purple)	3
Prostatic acid phosphatase (PAP) (see Acid phosphatase)		
Protein, total	Serum (speckled)	1
Protein, total A/G ratio	Serum (speckled)	1
Proteus OX 19	Serum (speckled)	2
Prothrombin consumption time	Serum (speckled)	3
Protime (International Technidyne Corporation, Edison, NJ) (prothrombin time, PT)	Plasma (blue)	2
PSA (prostatic specific antigen)	Serum (speckled)	1
PTH (see Parathyroid hormone)		
Pyruvate	Whole blood (gray)	5
	*Transport immediately in ice water	
Q fever antibodies	Serum (speckled)	3
Quinidine	Serum (speckled)	1
Rabies virus antibody	Serum (speckled)	3
Renin activity	Plasma (purple)	2
	*Transport immediately in ice water	
Reptilase time	Whole blood (blue)	3.5
Reticulocyte	Whole blood (purple)	5

(continued)

Table 7–3. *(continued)*

TEST NAME	SPECIMEN TUBE (TYPE/COLOR)	WHOLE BLOOD, MINIMUM VOLUME FOR ADULTS (mL)
Rheumatoid factor assay	Serum (speckled)	2
Rickettsial *Proteus* antibodies (*Proteus* OX 19)	Serum (speckled)	3
RPR	Serum (speckled)	2
Rubella	Serum (speckled)	4
Rubeola serology	Serum (speckled)	1
Russell viper venom (RVV) time (Stypven time)	Plasma (blue)	3
Salicylate (aspirin)	Serum (speckled)	2
Salmonella antibody	Serum (speckled)	5
Sedimentation rate (ESR) (erythrocyte sedimentation rate)	Whole blood (purple)	3
Selenium (Se)	Plasma, whole blood, serum (royal blue with heparin or EDTA or no anticoagulant)	3
Serotonin blood (5-hydroxytryptamine)	Whole blood or special tube from chemistry	10
SGOT (AST)	Serum (speckled)	1
SGPT (ALT)	Serum (speckled)	1
Sickling screen	Whole blood (purple)	2
Sjögren's antibody	Serum (red)	7
Sodium, serum	Serum (speckled)	1
SPE (serum protein electrophoresis)	Serum (speckled)	3
Special stains		
Acid phosphatase	Blood smear	
Alkaline phosphatase	Blood smear	
Esterases	Blood smear	
Heinz bodies	Blood smear	
Iron	Blood smear	
Lipid	Blood smear	
PAS for glycogen	Blood smear	
Peroxidase	Blood smear	
Sudan black	Blood smear	
Toluidine blue	Blood smear	
Stypven time (RVV time)	Plasma (blue)	3
Sucrose presumptive (PNH)	Whole blood (blue)	3
Sulfonamides	Serum (speckled)	5
Suppressor	Whole blood (purple)	3
Syphilis (RPR)	Serum (speckled)	2

Table 7–3. *(continued)*

TEST NAME	SPECIMEN TUBE (TYPE/COLOR)	WHOLE BLOOD, MINIMUM VOLUME FOR ADULTS (mL)
T_3 uptake	Serum (speckled)	2
Tegretol (carbamazepine)	Serum (speckled)	2
Teichoic acid antibody	Serum (speckled)	5
Testosterone	Serum (speckled)	7
Theophylline (aminophylline)	Serum (speckled)	2
Thiamine	Whole blood (green)	10
Thiocyanate	Serum (speckled) or plasma (green) or plasma (purple)	8
Thrombin time	Plasma (blue)	3
Thyroglobulin	Serum (speckled)	5
Thyroid antibodies	Serum (speckled)	3
Thyroid studies (T_3, T_4, TSH)	Serum (speckled)	4
Thyroiditis, antithyroglobulin, and antimicrosomal fraction	Serum (speckled)	5
Thyroxine (T_4)	Serum (speckled)	2
Thyroxine (T_4), free	Serum (speckled)	3
Tobramycin	Serum (speckled)	1
Tofranil (see Imipramine)		
TORCH titers	Serum (speckled)	5
Total T_3 (triiodothyronine)	Serum (speckled)	2
Toxoplasmosis serological test, IFA	Serum (speckled)	3
Transaminase (ALT, SGPT)	Serum (speckled)	1
Transaminase (AST, SGOT)	Serum (speckled)	1
Transferrin	Serum (speckled)	2
Trichinella agglutination	Serum (speckled)	3
Tricyclic antidepressants (amitriptyline, nortriptyline)	Serum or plasma (red, green, or purple) [a]Avoid gel separator	3
Triglycerides (fasting)	Serum (speckled)	1
Troponin I (cTnI) troponin T (cTnT)	Serum (speckled)	3
TSH (thyroid-stimulating hormone, or thyrotropin)	Serum (speckled)	2
Tylenol (see Acetominophen)		
Urea nitrogen (BUN)	Serum (speckled)	1
Uric acid	Serum (speckled)	1

(continued)

Table 7–3. *(continued)*

TEST NAME	SPECIMEN TUBE (TYPE/COLOR)	WHOLE BLOOD, MINIMUM VOLUME FOR ADULTS (mL)
Valium (diazepam)	Serum (red)	2
Valproic acid (Depakene)	Serum (speckled)	5
Vancomycin	Serum (speckled)	1
Varicella-zoster immune status	Serum (speckled)	2
Varicella-zoster serology	Serum (speckled)	2
VDRL (RPR) syphilis	Serum (speckled)	2
Vitamin A	Serum (speckled)	3
	*Protect blood from light	
Vitamin B_6	Whole blood (purple)	10
Vitamin B_{12}	Serum (speckled)	2
Vitamin B_{12} binding capacity	Serum (speckled)	3
Vitamin C (ascorbic acid)	Whole blood (green)	5
	*Immediately transport in ice slurry	
Vitamin D (25-OH)	Whole blood (purple)	7
Vitamin E level	Serum (speckled)	5
von Willebrand's factor assay (Rristocetin cofactor)	Whole blood (blue) *Deliver immediately	5
D-Xylose	Serum (red)	3
Zinc	Draw blood with syringe; transfer to special plastic tube from chemistry	5

[a]*Note:* For toxicology and therapeutic drugs, the speckled-topped gel serum separator tube should be evaluated to determine whether the gel serum separator interferes in test results before these tubes are used in drug analysis collections. (See Chapter 12.)

Abbreviations: A/G, albumin/globulin (ratio); Alb, albumin; Alk p'tase, alkaline phosphatase; ALT, alanine aminotransferase; APTT, activated partial thromboplastin time; AST, aspartate aminotransferase; Ca, calcium; CBC, complete blood (count); CMV, cytomegalovirus; CPK, creatine phosphokinase; Creat, creatinine; EBV, Epstein-Barr virus; ESR, erythrocyte sedimentation rate; FBS, fasting blood sugar; Glu, glucose; HB_sAg, hepatitis B surface antigen; HCG, human chorionic gonadotropin; Hct, hematocrit; Hgb, hemoglobin; IFA, indirect fluorescent antibody (test); IgA, immunoglobulin A; IgD, immunoglobulin D; IgG, immunoglobulin G; IgM, immunoglobulin M; I phos, inorganic phosphorus; LD, lactate dehydrogenase; MCH, mean corpuscular hemoglobin; MCHC, mean corpuscular hemoglobin concentration; MCV, mean corpuscular volume; PAS, periodic acid–Schiff; PNH, paroxysmal nocturnal hemoglobinuria; RBC, red blood cell; RPR, rapid plasma reagin; RVV, Russell viper venom (time); SGOT, serum glutamic oxaloacetic transaminase; SGPT, serum glutamic pyruvic transaminase; SPE, serum protein electrophoresis; T. bil, total bilirubin; TIBC, total iron-binding capacity; T. protein, total protein; VDRL, Venereal Disease Research Laboratory; WBC, white blood cell.

coagulation of blood by removing calcium and forming insoluble calcium salts. These three anticoagulants cannot be used in calcium determinations; however, citrates are frequently used in coagulation blood studies. EDTA prevents platelet aggregation and is, therefore, used for platelet counts and platelet function tests. Fresh EDTA-anticoagulated blood allows preparation of blood films with minimal distortion of white blood cells (WBCs). Heparin, a mucopolysaccharide used in assays, such as ammonia and plasma hemoglobin, prevents blood clotting by inactivating the blood-clotting chemicals—thrombin and thromboplastin.

Clinical Alert !

In addition to using the correct anticoagulant for a specific laboratory assay, using the correct amount or dilution of anticoagulant in the blood specimen is important. The blood collection vacuum tubes have been designed for a certain amount of blood to be drawn into the tube by vacuum according to the amount of prefilled anticoagulant in the tube. If an insufficient amount of blood is collected in a tube with anticoagulant, the laboratory test results may be erroneous because of an incorrect blood-to-anticoagulant ratio.

"Partial collection" tubes are available through manufacturers for patient blood collections in which it is anticipated that a "short draw" will be collected. These partial collection tubes will provide accurate laboratory results even though a short draw is collected.

GRAY-TOPPED TUBES

Gray-topped vacuum tubes usually contain (1) potassium oxalate and **sodium fluoride** or (2) **lithium iodoacetate** and heparin. This type of collection tube is primarily used for glycolytic inhibition tests. Thus, sometimes *antiglycolytic agent* is the term for this tube's additive. Because fluoride destroys many enzymes, this additive should not be used in blood collections for enzyme determinations (e.g., creatine kinase [CK], alanine aminotransferase [ALT], aspartate aminotransferase [AST], and alkaline phosphatase [ALP] determinations). Likewise, oxalate distorts cellular morphologic features. Thus, gray-topped tubes should not be used for hematology studies.

GREEN-TOPPED TUBES

The anticoagulants sodium heparin, ammonium heparin, and lithium heparin are found in green-topped vacuum tubes. These tubes are used in various laboratory assays requiring plasma or whole blood, which are mainly chemistry tests. For potassium measurement, heparinized plasma or whole blood, rather than serum, is preferred because sporadic increased potassium levels can occur in serum as a result of potassium released from platelets during blood clotting.[1] Lithium heparin tubes may be used for glucose, blood urea nitrogen (BUN), ionized calcium, creatinine, and electrolyte studies; however, this anticoagulant is not suitable for tests involving the measurement of lithium or folate levels.[2] Similarly, sodium heparin tubes should not be used for assays that measure the sodium concentration. In other cases, a particular procedure will require sodium heparin without lithium or vice versa.

Green-topped vacuum tubes should not be used for collections for blood smears that are to be stained with Wright's stain because the heparin causes the Wright's stain to have a blue background. When used for cytogenetic studies, these tubes must be sterile.

PURPLE-TOPPED AND LIGHT BLUE-TOPPED TUBES

The purple-topped vacuum tubes (containing EDTA) are used for most hematology procedures. Also, this tube is used for molecular diagnostic testing. If a purple-topped tube is underfilled, the patient will have erroneously low blood cell counts and hematocrits, staining alterations, and erroneous morphologic changes to RBCs. Many coagulation procedures, such as PT and APTT, are done on blood collected in light blue–topped vacuum tubes, which contain sodium citrate at a concentration of 3.2 or 3.8 percent. It is becoming preferred to use 3.2 percent since this concentration reduces falsely negative or falsely positive results.[3] If a light blue–topped tube is underfilled, coagulation results will be erroneously prolonged.

RED-TOPPED, ROYAL BLUE-TOPPED, AND BROWN-TOPPED TUBES

The red-topped tubes indicate a tube without anticoagulant for the collection of serum. Thus, the collected blood will clot in this tube. The royal blue–topped tubes are used to collect samples for nutritional studies, therapeutic drug monitoring, and toxicology. The royal blue–topped tube is the trace element tube. The brown-topped tube contains heparin or no additive and is used for blood lead values.

BLACK-TOPPED TUBES

From certain manufacturers, a black-topped tube with buffered sodium citrate is available for blood collections used to determine the erythrocyte sedimentation rate (ESR).

YELLOW-TOPPED TUBES

Sterile blood specimens are also ordered for blood cultures when the patient is suspected of having septicemia (symptoms of sepsis). A major problem with collecting blood for culture is that the patient's sample can become contaminated with microorganisms from the skin. Thus the blood must be collected in a sterile container (vacuum tube, vial or syringe) under aseptic conditions. (See Chapter 12 for blood culture collections.)

As shown in Figure 7–6, blood can be collected directly into vacuum vials that contain culture media. This type of collection minimizes the risk of specimen contamination. The vacuum vials can be purchased with different types of culture media, an unplugged venting unit for aerobic incubation, or a plugged venting unit for anaerobic incubation.

It should be noted that tubes containing ACD (acid citrate dextrose) also use the yellow color code. These tubes are used for specialty blood banking, such as HLA typing.

SERUM SEPARATION TUBES (MOTTLED-TOPPED, SPECKLED-TOPPED, AND GOLD-TOPPED TUBES)

Another collection method is to collect blood in a serum separation tube, such as the VAC-UETTE® serum tube (Fig. 7–7) (Greiner Bio-One, Austria) or BD VACUTAINER Plus SST

Figure 7–6.   BACTEC culture vials.

(Courtesy of BD (Becton-Dickinson and Company), Sparks, MD.)

tube (BD VACUTAINER Systems, *Preanalytical Solutions,* Franklin Lakes, NJ). These tubes contain a polymer barrier that is present in the bottom of the tube. The specific gravity of this material lies between the blood clot and the serum. During centrifugation, the polymer barrier moves upward to the serum-clot interface, where it forms a stable barrier separating the serum from fibrin and cells. Serum may be aspirated directly from the collection tube, eliminating the need for transfer to another container.

PINK-TOPPED TUBES

These tubes have recently received FDA approval for blood bank collections. They contain EDTA.

■ SAFETY SYRINGES

Some patients' veins are too fragile for blood collection with vacuum tubes. Thus safety syringes are generally used for the collection process. Syringes are hazardous and pose an

Figure 7–7. VACUETTE serum tube.

(Courtesy of Grenier Bio-One, Kremsmünster, Austria.)

increased risk of accidental needlesticks. Syringes are sometimes used for collecting blood from central venous catheter (CVC) lines. This procedure is discussed in detail in Chapter 12. A syringe, without the needle, consists of the barrel, the plunger, and the tip. The barrel and the plunger are made to fit together tightly so that when the plunger is in the barrel and drawn back, a vacuum is created. To fit properly, the needle and syringe must be compatible. This vacuum allows blood or other fluids to be aspirated, or sucked, into the

! **Clinical Alert**

To avoid possible needlestick injuries as OSHA requires, use safety syringes, such as the S-Monovette Blood Collection (Sarstedt, Inc., Newton, NC), BD Safety Lok (BD VACU-TAINER Systems, *Preanalytical Solutions,* Franklin Lakes, NJ), Retractable Technologies VanishPoint syringe (Little Elm, TX), SIMS Portex Needle-Pro (Keene, NH), and Bio-Plexus (Tolland, CT) Punctur-Guard needle products. These products are designed to reduce needlesticks by either sliding a cover over the needle after venipuncture or by making the needle "blunt," thereby reducing exposure to a sharp contaminated object.

barrel as the plunger is pulled back. The barrel of the syringe has graduated measurements in milliliter increments. Sizes range from approximately 0.2 to 50.0 mL; however, for specimen collection purposes, 5- to 20-mL syringes are most often used. A needle is usually attached directly on the smooth tip of the syringe. In addition, the health care worker should ensure that the syringe is the correct size for the amount of blood to be collected.

■ NEEDLES

The gauge and length of a needle used on a syringe or a vacuum tube is selected according to the specific task. For example, larger (18-gauge) needles are used for collecting donor units of blood (450 mL or less), whereas smaller (21- and 22-gauge) needles are used for collecting specimens for laboratory assays. When blood is collected from children, a 21- to 23-gauge needle is usually used with a tuberculin, or 3-mL, syringe or with a winged infusion set. The **gauge number** indicates the diameter of the needle; the smaller the gauge number, the larger the needle diameter and higher flow rate. The length of the needle depends on the depth of the vein to be punctured. Needles are usually available as either 1 or 1.5 inch.

Needles are sterilized and packaged by vendors in sealed shields that maintain sterility. These sealed shields are packaged in individual containers that are color coded according to the gauge size of the needles and must be twisted apart before the needles are used in blood collection.[4]

The tip of each needle should be checked for damage. A blunt or bent tip can be harmful to the patient's vein and may result in failure to collect blood.

Different types of needles are used for single- and multiple-sample collections. **Multiple-sample needles** are used with vacuum collection tubes and the holder to allow for multiple tube changes without blood leakage within the plastic holder. The multiple-sample needle has a plastic cover over the tube-top puncturing portion of the needle; this cover creates a leakage barrier. The **single-sample needle** is usually used for collecting blood with a syringe.

It is important to use needles with holders or syringes that are compatible with the needle to avoid the possibility of leaking blood and blood exposure.

THE BUTTERFLY NEEDLE (BLOOD COLLECTION SET)

The butterfly needle, also referred to as a blood collection set or winged infusion set, is the most commonly used intravenous device. It is a stainless steel beveled needle and tube with attached plastic wings on one end and a Luer fitting attached to the other. The most common butterfly needle sizes are 21, 23, and 25 gauge. The butterfly needle is sometimes used in the collection of blood from patients who are difficult to stick by conventional methods (e.g., geriatric patients, cancer patients, pediatric patients).

Clinical Alert ❗

Winged infusion sets, have accounted for the *highest* percentage of needlestick injuries.

Numerous types of *safety* butterfly needles are available and should be used. These safety needles each have a shield that automatically covers the contaminated needle point upon withdrawal from the patient's vein. One example is the Kendall Monoject Angel Wing blood collection set (Fig. 7–8) from the Kendall Co. LP, (Mansfield, MA). It has a stainless steel safety shield that automatically resheaths the needle during withdrawal from the patient. The system includes multisample needle-shielded tube holders and sets for use in drawing blood specimens directly into blood collection tubes and blood culture bottles, as well as multisample needle-shielded transfer tube holders and sets for transferring blood from syringes into collection tubes and blood culture bottles.

BD VACUTAINER Systems *Preanalytical Solutions* has the BD Safety-Lok blood collection set (see Fig. 7–9) that has been designed to shield health care workers from exposed needles. Following venipuncture, a yellow transparent shield is moved over the exposed needle and locked into protective position, creating a barrier between the health care worker and the used needle.

Figure 7–8.   Kendall Monoject Angel Wing blood collection set.

(Courtesy of Kendall Co. LP, Mansfield, MA.)

Figure 7–9. Safety-Lok blood collection device.

(Courtesy of BD VACUTAINER Systems, *Preanalytical Solutions,* Franklin Lakes, NJ.)

Figure 7–10. VACUETTE® safety blood collection set.

(Courtesy of Greiner Bio-One, Kremsmünster, Austria.)

Greiner Bio-One (Kremsmünster, Austria) manufactures the VACUETTE® safety blood collection set (Fig. 7–10). It is a winged needle device with a safety shield. Bio-Plexus (Tolland, CT) produces the PUNCTUR-GUARD winged set for blood collection. The safety device uses an internal hollow blunt built within the sharp outer needle. When the blood samples have been withdrawn, the "internal blunt" is activated *prior* to removing the needle from the vein, thus reducing exposure to a sharp contaminated needle. No matter what type of safety blood collection set is used, it is imperative to use a Luer adapter from the same manufacturer to avoid possible blood leakage and exposure.

Figure 7–11.   Needle disposal systems.

(Courtesy of Datar, Inc., Long Lake, MN.)

NEEDLE DISPOSAL

Needles and syringes must be discarded in rigid plastic containers, which reduces the possibility of needle sticks for the phlebotomist. Each unit is disposable as biohazardous waste. Several sizes of needle-disposal containers (Fig. 7–11) for use at the bedside, on the cart, in isolation, during surgery, on home health care trays, and so on are shown as examples.

■ SAFE ACCESS TO BLOOD SAMPLES

After blood collection, the health care worker must gain access to the blood in the vacuum tube for testing purposes. To protect laboratory personnel against blood exposure during this hazardous step, manufacturers developed several different types of items.

An example is the BD VACUTAINER tube with Hemogard. This device is a vacuum blood collection tube with a plastic shield over the stopper. The shield protects the health care worker from splattering blood when the stopper is removed from the tube. Greiner Labortechnik has blood collection tubes with safety screw caps to minimize aerosol generation.

Tip Tops (Helena Laboratories, Beaumont, Texas) are cone-shaped, flexible polyethylene caps designed to fit 13 and 16 mm blood collection tubes, serum separating columns, and other vials with openings of that size. Each Tip Top has a small opening at the top that allows you to dispense straight from the tube into sample cups and thus provide safety by reducing the risk of accidental spills and exposure to infectious agents. In addition, Helena has the H-Pette, which provides an approach to blood slide preparation that eliminates the hazards of open tubes of blood and transfer pipettes. The H-Pette can be inserted into the stopper of any size blood collection tube for blood transfer to a glass slide.

■ TOURNIQUETS

The tourniquet is a key to successful venipuncture: it provides a barrier to slow down venous flow. Tourniquets are used in specimen collection to apply enough pressure to the arm to slow the return of venous blood to the heart. This slowing of venous return causes pooling of blood in the veins, which makes the veins more visible and easier to feel and find. A tourniquet should *not* restrict arterial blood flowing into the arm. Blood should enter the arm at a normal rate and, with the use of a tourniquet, return to the heart at a slower rate.

Tourniquets that are usually used include the pliable strap, the Velcro type, and the blood pressure cuff. The blood pressure cuff can be used successfully when veins are difficult to find. The most efficient blood barrier provides a resistance that is less than systolic blood pressure but greater than diastolic; or, stated another way, blood flows in but not out. The blood pressure cuff can determine these pressures; consequently, it is a perfect tourniquet.[5]

Another type of tourniquet is the Seraket, which uses a seat-belt design. It allows the phlebotomist to release the venous pressure partially by using a lever that releases some pressure, but not all. Thus, if the phlebotomist needs to tighten the tourniquet again, the lever can be used to adjust the tourniquet. Because errors in laboratory test results can occur from prolonged tourniquet pressure, the Seraket provides a solution to this problem. One drawback of this type of tourniquet, however, is the difficulty in cleaning and decontaminating it if it is soiled with blood.

Velcro-type tourniquets are popular because they are easy to apply and comfortable for the patient. Alternatively, because of major concern for infection control in health care institutions, many facilities now use a disposable natural latex tourniquet strap to help prevent cross-contamination. Many patients are allergic to latex, and thus other types of tourniquets must be available to use to avoid an allergic reaction. Non-latex disposable tourniquets are now available as a good option for the blood collector and patient. If the tourniquets used in the health care facility are not disposable, they must be wiped frequently with 70 percent isopropyl alcohol.

■ BLEEDING-TIME EQUIPMENT

Bleeding time is an assay used to assess the contributions of platelet function and blood vessel integrity to primary blood-clotting abilities.[6] The test is performed by making a minor standardized incision in the forearm or earlobe and recording the length of time required for bleeding to stop. Many procedures have been used to measure bleeding time. Recent advances have led to the development of mechanical devices that are used to create uniform skin incisions for bleeding-time determination. One such device is the Surgicutt (International Technidyne Corporation, Edison, NJ), which provides a uniform surgical incision. The procedure for determining bleeding time is provided in Chapter 12.

■ GLOVES FOR BLOOD COLLECTION

Safety guidelines have been established for health care workers to help them prevent the possibility of acquiring infections, such as hepatitis or those associated with AIDS. These guidelines include the use of gloves during collection of blood from patients. Examples of gloves being used by health care workers include Ultraderm sterile surgeon's gloves (Baxter Travenol Laboratories, Inc., Deerfield, IL), talc-free Eudermic surgical gloves (BD VACUTAINER Systems, *Preanalytical Solutions,* Franklin Lakes, NJ), Medi-Pak latex gloves (General Medical Corp., Richmond, VA), and Lab Safety Supply nonirritating surgical gloves (Lab Safety Supply, Janesville, WI), which are made without talc. It is recommended that phlebotomists not use gloves with talc powder containing calcium because tubes of patients' blood may become contaminated with this powder, and such contamination can result in falsely elevated calcium values. Latex gloves have proved effective in preventing the transmission of infectious diseases to health care workers. However, exposures to latex may result in an allergic reaction in some individuals. Reports of allergic reactions to latex have increased among health care workers in recent years. The National Institute for Occupational Safety and Health (NIOSH) defines latex as "natural rubber latex, the product manufactured from a milky fluid derived from the rubber tree." A **latex allergy** is a reaction to certain proteins in latex rubber. Increasing exposure to latex gloves or the lubricant powder in some gloves also increases the risk of developing allergy symptoms. NIOSH has valuable information on their Web site (www.cdc.gov/niosh/98-113.html) regarding latex allergy prevention, and suggests the following steps to protect oneself from latex exposure:

- Use nonlatex gloves for activities that are not likely to involve contact with infectious materials, e.g., housekeeping, maintenance
- Use powder-free gloves with reduced protein content
- "Hypoallergenic" latex gloves do not reduce the risk of latex allergy, but may reduce reactions to chemical additives in the latex
- When wearing latex gloves, do not use oil-based hand creams, which can cause glove deterioration
- Wash hands with mild soap after using latex gloves
- Clean areas frequently that have been contaminated with latex-containing dust
- Learn the symptoms of latex allergy
- Attend latex allergy educational programs

Researchers have found that latex gloves provide better protection than vinyl gloves.[7] The Safeskin hypoallergenic latex glove (Safeskin Corporation, Coral Gables, FL) outperformed all other brands in the referenced study. Phlebotomists should not, however, use petroleum products or other skin protectants when wearing latex gloves because these substances break down the latex and decrease the active barrier.[8] If a health care worker develops allergenic dermatitis to gloves, she or he should try other brands of gloves or wear cotton gloves under the latex gloves. Erie Scientific (Portsmouth, NH) has UltraFIT glove liners (Fig. 7–12) for individuals who are extrasensitive to latex. These liners are made with 100 percent durable nylon material and can be washed several times for reuse. Another approach suggested by the US Food and Drug Administration (FDA) is to wear latex gloves between two vinyl gloves.[9]

Figure 7–12.   UltraFIT glove liner.

(Courtesy of Erie Scientific, Portsmouth, NH.)

Clinical Alert !

For sensitive individuals, allergic symptoms can begin within minutes of exposure. Mild reactions to latex include skin redness, rash, hives, or itching; severe reactions may involve respiratory symptoms such as runny nose, sneezing, itchy eyes, scratchy throat, and asthma. In rare instances, shock may occur. This can happen to patients and health care workers. In these instances, all latex products should be avoided including latex bandages or tourniquets. Latex-free products are available and include tourniquets, adhesive bandages, arterial blood gas kits, collection tubes, tape, and blood collecting trays. (See PATIENT SAFETY RELATED TO LATEX PRODUCTS in Chapter 5, Safety and First Aid.)

Uarco, Inc. (Barrington, IL) developed adhesive labels that do not stick to gloves. These Glove-Free labels adhere firmly to glass, plastic, and paper, but they do not stick to vinyl or latex gloves. The labels, coated with a special adhesive, aid laboratory safety by eliminating the problem of torn gloves caused by trying to remove an adhering label.

■ ANTISEPTICS, STERILE GAUZE PADS, AND BANDAGES

The health care worker needs **antiseptics, sterile gauze pads,** and bandages for blood collection by either venipuncture or microcollection. Therefore, 70 percent isopropyl alcohol preparation and iodine swab sticks or pads (for blood cultures) are essential items for blood collection.

> ! **Clinical Alert**
>
> In home health care and other ambulatory health care environments where soap and water may not be readily available for the blood collector to wash his or her hands, an antimicrobial safety scrub should be carried with other blood collection items and used before and after blood collection.

■ MICROCOLLECTION EQUIPMENT

Usually, skin puncture blood-collecting techniques are used on infants because venipuncture is excessively hazardous. Skin puncture collection is also indicated for adults and older children when they are severely burned, have veins that are difficult to stick because of their small size or location, must undergo bedside clinical testing, are extremely obese, or must perform home glucose testing.

The volume of plasma or serum that generally can be collected from a premature infant is approximately 100 to 150 μL, and about two times that amount can be taken from a full-term newborn. Larger volumes are obtained from older children and adults.[10]

LANCETS AND TUBES

> ! **Clinical Alert**
>
> A **disposable sterile lancet** should be used to puncture the skin for skin puncture collection. To avoid possible blood-borne pathogen exposure, it is highly recommended to use a "retracting lancet." Surgical blades should not be used for skin puncture due to hazards to the patient and phlebotomist.

For infants, the National Committee for Clinical Laboratory Standards (NCCLS) recommends a penetration depth of no more than 2.0 mm on heelsticks to avoid penetrating bone.[10] The BD Quikheel (BD VACUTAINER Systems, *Preanalytical Solutions,* Franklin Lakes, NJ) lancet (Fig. 7–13) is available for two different incision depths, dependent upon the needs of the infant. The teal-colored Quikheel Infant lancet has a preset incision depth of 1.0 mm and width of 2.5 mm, and the purple-colored Quikheel Preemie lancet has

Figure 7–13.   BD Quickheel lancet.

(Courtesy of BD VACUTAINER Systems, *Preanalytical Solutions,* Franklin Lakes, NJ.)

a preset incision depth of 0.85 mm and width of 1.75 mm. This lancet blade retracts permanently after activation to assure safety to the health care worker.

Also, the BD Genie lancet (Fig. 7–14) is a safety-engineered device for skin puncture blood collection. The Genie lancet is available in an assortment of puncture widths and depths, as well as a needle lancet for glucose testing.

LifeScan, Inc. (Milpitas, CA) produces the Unistik 2 Neonatal, a single-use disposable lancing device that has a penetration depth of only 1.8 mm. It provides protection for infants and for health care workers who have to obtain patient blood samples.

International Technidyne Corporation (Edison, NJ) has produced fully automated, single-use, automatically retracting, disposable devices that provide safety both for the neonate and for the health care worker (Fig. 7–15). Tenderlett jr. for children, Tenderlett for adults, and Tenderlett toddler for infants and toddlers are engineered to incise to the least invasive but most effective depth for optimal blood flow. The Tenderlett incises 1.75-mm deep, Tenderlett jr. incises 1.25-mm deep, and Tenderlett toddler incises only 0.85-mm deep. The retracting blade of each of these devices eliminates potential injury from an exposed blade contaminated with blood.

The Unistik 2 microcollection lancet is also available in 2.4 and 3.0 mm penetration ranges and automatically retracts after incision. The devices are color coded for easy identification of penetration depth.

Figure 7–14. BD Genie lancet.

(Courtesy of BD VACUTAINER Systems, *Preanalytical Solutions,* Franklin Lakes, NJ.)

Figure 7–15. Tenderlett automated skin incision device.

(Courtesy of International Technidyne Corp., Edison, NJ.)

Other devices for microcollection are the Monoject Monoletter Safety Lancets (The Kendall Co. LP, Mansfield, MA) for finger stick collections, the Autolet Lite Clinisafe (Fig. 7–16), both by Owen Mumford Inc., Marietta, GA. The Autolet II Clinisafe is a spring-activated puncture device that allows easy ejection of the lancet and platform, providing safety for both patient

Figure 7–16.   Autolet Lite Clinisafe.

(Courtesy of Owen Mumford, Inc., Marietta, GA.)

and phlebotomist. The Autolet platform can be chosen for the patient's level of comfort and the needed blood volume. These platforms are available in three color-coded depths: white (1.8 mm) for shallow penetration, yellow (2.4 mm) for normal penetration, and orange (3.0 mm) for deeper incisions.

The Autolet Lite Clinisafe features a safety mechanism that inhibits the use of the device unless it is first reloaded with a new lancet and platform. Complying with FDA and Centers for Disease Control and Prevention (CDC) guidelines, both the lancet and the platform can be used only *once* and are simultaneously ejected at the touch of a button.

Superlite lancets have been developed with a slimmer needle and a new bevel to allow for smooth and easy skin penetration, which provides more comfort for the patient.

A laser-based device that is FDA-approved for blood collection is the Lasette (Cell Robotics, Albuquerque, NM). The laser penetrates to a depth of 1 to 2 mm and 250 μm wide. This is a smaller puncture hole than other devices make. Up to 100 μL of blood can be collected.[11]

To collect a reliable small-volume blood sample, it is important to use a properly designed blood collection tube or capillary pipette. In February 1999 the Food and Drug Administration

(FDA), the National Institute of Occupational Safety and Health (NIOSH) of the Centers for Disease Control and Prevention (CDC), and the Occupational Safety and Health Administration (OSHA) issued an advisory on glass capillary tubes. They recommended that capillary tubes be used that are not made of glass and that health care workers use products that include a method of sealing that does NOT require: (1) manually pushing one end of the microhematocrit tube into putty to form a plug; or (2) use products that allow the blood hematocrit to be measured without centrifugation.

The **microcontainers** recommended for use for skin puncture collections are listed in Box 7–1. Usually, microspecimens for blood gas analysis are collected in heparinized Natelson tubes. These tubes may have a color band indicating the presence and type of anticoagulant. The band also identifies the top part of the pipette in reference to sample handling. A red band indicates an ammonium heparin coating in the tube, and a green band indicates a sodium or lithium heparin coating. Because ammonium ions can falsely change the blood pH of the collected blood, sodium or lithium heparin should be used in collections for blood gas analysis. The blood collected in these tubes must be mixed with the heparin by a small metal "flea," or bar, with a magnet (see Chapter 12 for details on capillary blood gas collection). After mixing, the ends are sealed with sealing wax or plastic caps.

AVL Scientific Corporation (Roswell, GA) has developed the AVL microsampler for collection of two 120-µL **arterial blood gas** samples from children or adults. It has a 26-gauge microneedle, which reduces the chances of puncture pain and hematoma formation. The tubes are coated with heparin to prevent clotting, and they automatically fill without bubble formation. This microsampler is used on the radial, brachial, or femoral artery.

Microhematocrit **capillary tubes** are disposable narrow-bore pipettes that are used for packed red cell volume in microcentrifugation. These tubes also have colored bands; a red band indicates a heparin-coated tube, and a blue band indicates no anticoagulant. The Safe-Crit™ (Statspin Inc., Norwood, MA) is a microhematocrit tube made of plastic to avoid the hazard of glass breakage.

Plastic microcollection devices for general laboratory collections (e.g., chemistry, immunology) are usually color coded according to the established protocol for blood collection vacuum tube tops. Thus, purple-topped (lavender-topped) tubes contain EDTA, green-

BOX 7–1.   CONTAINERS FOR BLOOD COLLECTION

- Plastic microcollection devices—various types are needed
  Serum or plasma separator devices
  Different color-coded devices according to additive (i.e., lavender-EDTA, etc.)
- Disposable plastic calibrated microcollection tubes
- Closures for microcollection devices—caps, sealants. Plastic and clay compounds are available for sealing the microcollection devices. However, they pose a hazard because they can become contaminated with blood and even small fragments of capillary glass if the laboratory is still using dangerous glass capillary tubes. Sealants that are in punchcard trays are safer if they are covered between use to avoid hardening of the sealant material.
- Plastic microhematocrit tubes
- Natelson tubes
- Microdilution systems
- Test tubes

topped tubes contain heparin, red- or pink-topped tubes have no additive, and gray-topped tubes have sodium fluoride to inhibit blood enzymes that destroy glucose.

Kendall Co. LP (Mansfield, MA) manufactures the Samplette micro blood collector, which is offered with a full range of anticoagulants and serum and plasma separation gels. One of their collectors is an amber capillary blood separator that provides protection for light-sensitive analytes (e.g., bilirubin).

Electrolytes and general chemistry microspecimens can be collected in the BD Microtainer tube (BD VACUTAINER Systems, *Preanalytical Solutions,* Franklin Lakes, NJ), which has its own capillary blood collector, self-contained serum separator, and Microgard closure, which is safety-engineered to reduce the risk of tube leakage or specimen splatter. Each tube is imprinted with two markings, a minimum 250 μL line and a maximum 500 μL, to assist in collecting appropriate volumes (Fig. 7–17). Alternatively, two or more capillary tubes can be used for electrolyte and general chemistry collection. One advantage of these tubes is that if blood hemolyzes in one capillary tube, another capillary tube containing the patient's sample can be used for the chemical analyses.

The Microvette capillary blood collection system (Sarstedt, Inc., Newton, NC) is another microcollection system that is offered with a full range of anticoagulants and serum separation

Figure 7–17.   Microtainer tube.

(Courtesy of BD VACUTAINER Systems, *Preanalytical Solutions,* Franklin Lakes, NJ.)

Figure 7-18. Safe-T-Fill capillary blood collection device.

(Courtesy of Ram Scientific, Inc., Needham, MA.)

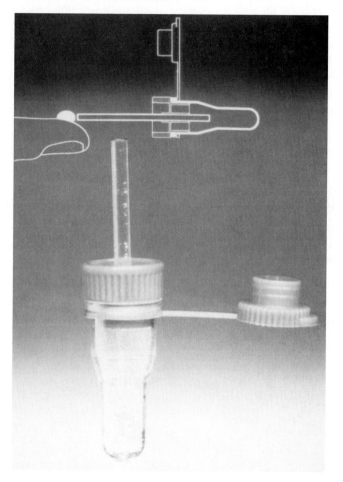

gel. This system can be used to collect, store, and separate samples in the same unbreakable, disposable container.

RAM Scientific Inc. (Needham, MA) has developed an unbreakable plastic capillary-receptacle system called the SAFE-T-FILL capillary blood collection system. The device consists of a plastic capillary inserted into a microtube receptacle (Fig. 7–18). With the attached receptacle, blood flows directly to the bottom of the tube. This system makes the blood drawing safe and clean. The capillary can then be removed, and the tube is closed with the appropriate color-coded cap.

Figure 7–19.   Unopette, a collection and dilution unit for blood samples.

(Courtesy of BD VACUTAINER Systems, *Preanalytical Solutions,* Franklin Lakes, NJ.)

Greiner MiniCollect Capillary tube is a microcollection container made from unbreakable polypropylene with a cap system that eliminates the risk of contamination.

For most chemical assays, lithium and ammonium salts of heparin are the anticoagulants of choice for microcollections. They have rarely been reported to interfere with the determination of electrolytes and most other chemical assays.

Another type of microcollection device is the Unopette (BD VACUTAINER Systems, *Preanalytical Solutions,* Franklin Lakes, NJ), shown in Figure 7–19. This device serves as a collection and dilution unit for blood samples and, thus, increases the speed and simplicity of laboratory procedures. These devices are prefilled with specific amounts of diluents or reagents, or both, for different types of laboratory assays. Some of the more prevalent procedures in which Unopette devices are used include the WBC count, RBC count, platelet count, and RBC fragility.

The standard Unopette test comprises (1) a disposable, self-filling diluting pipette consisting of a straight, thin-walled, uniform-bore, glass capillary tube fitted into a plastic holder and (2) a plastic reservoir containing a premeasured volume of reagent for diluting.

SEALING ITEMS FOR MICROCOLLECTION TUBES

For capillary pipettes and tubes, sealing wax or caps are necessary when the blood is drawn into the tube. Putty-like sealants and plastic closures are available from various manufacturers. The phlebotomist must be sure to follow the instructions with the sealant in order to provide safe sealing during microcentrifugation. A capillary tube device that was developed to reduce the opportunity for blowout of the sealant during microcentrifugation is the

Safe-Cap capillary and Safeplug (Safe-Tec, Inc., Ivyland, PA). SafeCap capillary has a self-sealing plug that was manufactured to permit a more accurate measurement of the packed cell volume and to decrease biohazardous risk to blood splatters and aerosol spray during microcentrifugation.

TRANSPORTING MICROSPECIMENS

Glycolysis in RBCs and WBCs causes a decrease in blood pH that can be detected after a blood gas sample has been stored at room temperature for approximately 20 minutes. Therefore, blood gas microsamples should be immersed in a slurry of ice water from the time of collection until they are delivered to the clinical laboratory. Plastic containers that are small enough to hold these specimens with ice and water should be carried on the specimen collection tray. Ice is usually available on the patient ward. Other items to be carried on a microcollection tray include the following:

1. Seventy percent isopropyl alcohol and Betadine pads.
2. Marking pens for labels.
3. Microcollection blood serum separator tubes.
4. Capillary whole blood cell collectors with 0.23 mg of EDTA (200 μL).
5. Safety lancets for skin puncture.
6. Sterile gauze pads or bandages.
7. Unheparinized plastic microcollection tubes.
8. Heparinized plastic microcollection tubes (250, 400, and 500μL).
9. Heparinized Natelson tubes (75 μL).
10. Unopette devices for collection and dilution procedures.
11. Disposable gloves.
12. Appropriate warming device.
13. Thermometer.
14. Biohazardous waste containers for sharps.
15. Glass microscope slides.
16. Capillary safety tube sealer.
17. Antimicrobial hand gel or foam to wash hands without water and soap.

■ BLOOD-DRAWING CHAIR

! Clinical Alert

In an outpatient clinic that requires blood collections, a **blood-drawing chair** must be available for patients. The chair is designed for maximum safety and comfort of the patient plus easy accessibility to either arm of the patient. The chair should have an armrest for the patient's use during blood drawing. The armrest should lock in place so that the patient cannot fall from the chair if he or she becomes faint. Also, the armrest should adjust in an up-and-down position so that the best venipuncture position for each patient can be achieved.

There are many chair styles and options available for making phlebotomy procedures easier and safer. Options include adjustable armrests, leg extensions, neck pillows or supports, scale mounts, storage cabinets, hydraulic lifts, and foot covers (Custom Comfort, Orlando, FL).

■ INFANT PHLEBOTOMY STATION

As health care services are increasingly being provided at ambulatory sites, including home visits, a safe site is frequently needed for infant blood collections. An infant phlebotomy station (Custom Comfort, Inc., Orlando, FL) provides safety for infant blood collections at off-site locations (Fig. 7–20).

■ SPECIMEN COLLECTION TRAYS

The health care worker needs a specimen tray (Fig. 7–21) to take on blood-collecting rounds. The tray is usually made of plastic and must be amenable to sterilization. The tray should include all necessary collection equipment, and its contents usually differ from one hospital or clinic to another, depending on the patient population. For example, if the phlebotomist works in a children's hospital, he or she needs trays containing microcollection equipment, such as that described earlier. For home health care providers and reference laboratory couriers, the necessary collection supplies, equipment, and collected blood must be carried in an enclosed container with the biohazard symbol shown on the outside. For example, the Loc-Top Lab Tray (Healthmark Industries Co., Detroit, MI), shown in Figure 7–22, is lockable to protect the contents from tampering or accidental contamination. It also has a tight seal to reduce the risk of infection from blood-borne pathogens due to spills or accidents.

Figure 7–20.   Infant phlebotomy station.

(Courtesy of Custom Comfort, Inc., Orlando, FL.)

Figure 7–21. Specimen collection tray.

(Courtesy of BD VACUTAINER Systems, *Preanalytical Solutions,* Franklin Lakes, NJ.)

Figure 7–22. Loc-Top Lab Tray.

(Courtesy of Healthmark Industries, Co., Detroit, MI.)

Health care workers who collect blood from adults usually have the following equipment on their trays or in their safety container:

1. Marking pens or pencils.
2. Vacuum tubes containing the anticoagulants designated in the clinical laboratory blood collection manual.
3. Safety holders for vacuum tubes.
4. Needles for vacuum tubes and syringes.
5. Safety syringes.
6. Tourniquet (Non-latex).
7. Safety blood collection sets (Butterfly needle assembly).
8. Seventy percent isopropyl alcohol, iodine pads or swab sticks.
9. Sterile gauze pads.
10. Bandages.
11. Biohazardous waste containers for used needles and lancets.
12. Safety lancets for skin puncture.
13. Unopette devices for finger stick blood collection.
14. Microcollection blood serum separator tubes.
15. Microcollection capillary whole blood collectors with 0.23 mg of EDTA (200 μL).
16. Disposable gloves.
17. Cloth towel or washcloth.
18. Thermometer.
19. Antimicrobial hand gel or foam to wash hands without water and soap.

■ WEB ADDRESSES FOR SUPPLIERS OF SAFETY BLOOD COLLECTION EQUIPMENT

Baxter Healthcare Corp.
Web site: http://www.baxter.com

Becton Dickinson and Co.
Web site: http://www.bd.com

Bio-Plexus, Inc.
Web site: http://www.bio-plexus.com

Erie Scientific Corp.
Web site: http://www.eriesci.com

Greiner Labortechnik
Web site: http://www.vacuette.com

Healthmark Industries Co.
Web site: http://www.hmark.com

Helena Products
Web site: http://www.helena.com

International Technidyne Corp.
Web site: http://www.itcmed.com

The Kendall Co. LP
Web site: http://www.kendallhq.com

Lab Safety Supply
Web site: http://www.labsafety.com

Lifescan, Inc.
Web site: http://www.lifescan.com

Owen Mumford, Inc.
Web site: http://www.owenmumford.com

RAM Scientific
Web site: http://www.ramscientific.com

Retractable Technologies, Inc.
Web site: http://www.vanishpoint.com

Safe Tec Clinical Products, Inc.
Web site: http://www.safetec.com

Sarstedt, Inc.
Web site: http://www.sarstedt.com

SIMS Portex, Inc.
Web site: http://www.portexusa.com

StatSpin, Inc.
Web site: http://www.statspin.com

SELF STUDY

KEY TERMS

Acid–Citrate–Dextrose (ACD)
Anticoagulants
Antiseptics
Arterial Blood Gas
Blood-Drawing Chair
Capillary Tubes
Citrate–Phosphate–Dextrose
   (CPD)
Citrates
Disposable Sterile Lancet
Ethylenediamine Tetra-acetic
   Acid (EDTA)

Gauge Number
Heparin
Holder (Adapter)
Latex Allergy
Lithium Iodoacetate
Microcontainers
Multiple-Sample Needles
Oxalates
Single-Sample Needle
Sodium Fluoride
Sterile Gauze Pads
Vacuum (Evacuated) Tube

STUDY QUESTIONS

The following may have *one* or *more* answers:

1. Which of the following anticoagulants prevent coagulation of blood by removing calcium through the formation of insoluble calcium salts?

   a. EDTA
   b. ammonium oxalate

   c. sodium citrate
   d. sodium heparin

2. Which of the following anticoagulants is found in a green-topped blood-collection vacuum tube?

   a. EDTA
   b. ammonium oxalate

   c. sodium citrate
   d. sodium heparin

3. For capillary collection from newborns, a lancet of which of the following lengths should be used to avoid penetrating bone?

   a. 1.75 mm
   b. 2.75 mm

   c. 3.00 mm
   d. 3.25 mm

4. Which of the following blood chemical constituents is light sensitive?

   a. glucose
   b. bilirubin

   c. phosphorus
   d. blood gases

5. When blood is collected from a patient, the serum should be separated from the blood cells as quickly as possible to avoid

   a. hemoconcentration
   b. hemolysis
   c. glycolysis
   d. hemostasis

6. The color coding for needles indicates the

   a. length
   b. gauge
   c. manufacturer
   d. anticoagulant

7. From the listed needle gauges, which one has the largest diameter?

   a. 19
   b. 20
   c. 21
   d. 23

8. Which of the following is/are skin puncture equipment?

   a. Tenderlett
   b. Autolet Lite
   c. Samplette
   d. AVL microsampler

9. Which of the following laboratory tests requires that the blood be transported in a slurry of ice water to the laboratory?

   a. bilirubin
   b. CK
   c. blood gas analysis
   d. complete blood cell (CBC) count

References

1. Hyman, D, Kaplan, N: The difference between serum and plasma potassium (letter). *N Engl J Med.* 1985; 313:642.

2. National Committee for Clinical Laboratory Standards (NCCLS): *Evacuated Tubes and Additives for Blood Specimen Collection,* 4th ed. Approved Standard. NCCLS Document H1-A4, Villanova, PA; NCCLS: 1996.

3. Adcock, DM, Kressin, DC, Marlar, RA: Effect of 3.2% vs 3.8% sodium citrate concentration on routine coagulation testing. *Am J Clin Pathol* 1997; 107:105–110.

4. National Committee for Clinical Laboratory Standards (NCCLS): *Procedures for the Collection of Diagnostic Blood Specimens by Venipuncture,* 4th ed. Approved Standard. NCCLS Document H3-A4, Villanova, PA; NCCLS: June, 1998.

5. Scranton, PE: *Practical Techniques in Venipuncture.* Baltimore; Williams & Wilkins: 1977, p. 66.

6. Harker, LA, Slichter, SI: The bleeding time as a screening test for evaluation of platelet function. *N Engl J Med.* 1972; 287:155.

7. Brown, JW, Backwell, H: Putting on gloves in the fight against AIDS. *Med Lab Observ.* 1990; November:47.

8. Personius, CD: Patients, health care workers and latex allergy. *Med Lab Observ.* 1995; March:30–32.

9. Strickland, DA: Latex sensitivity prompts alert. *Med World News.* 1991; April:13.

10. National Committee for Clinical Laboratory Standards (NCCLS): *Procedures for the Collection of Diagnostic Blood Specimens by Skin Puncture.* NCCLS Document H4-A4, Villanova, PA; NCCLS: 1999.

11. News & Views: Lasers to replace lancets? *Lab Med.* 1997; 28:11,689.

EIGHT

■

Venipuncture Procedures

CHAPTER OBJECTIVES

Upon completion of Chapter 8, the learner is responsible for the following:

1. Describe the patient identification process for inpatients, emergency room patients, and ambulatory patients.
2. List essential information for test requisitions.
3. List supplies that would be used in a typical venipuncture procedure.
4. Identify the most common sites for venipuncture, and describe situations when these sites might not be acceptable sites for venipuncture. Identify alternative sites for the venipuncture procedure.
5. Describe the process and the time limits for applying a tourniquet to a patient's arm.
6. Describe the decontamination process and the agents used to decontaminate skin for routine blood tests and blood cultures.
7. Describe the actual venipuncture procedure and the steps that are different using the evacuated tube method, the syringe method, and the butterfly or winged infusion system.
8. Describe the order of draw for collection tubes when using the evacuated tube method, the syringe method, and the butterfly or winged infusion system.
9. List examples and explain reasons for the importance of collecting "timed specimens" at the requested times.
10. Describe the proper method for hand washing.
11. Describe what the terms *fasting* and *STAT* mean when referring to blood tests.

■ BLOOD COLLECTION

In preparing for blood collection, each health care worker generally establishes a routine that is comfortable for him or her. Several essential steps, however, are part of every successful collection procedure. This chapter discusses the following steps in which a health care worker would progress through the blood collection process. These steps were developed from several sources and represent typical scenarios in the blood collection process. Individual facilities may vary the sequence of steps based on the characteristics of their patient populations.[1,2] In some cases, steps may occur simultaneously (e.g., assessing the patient's physical disposition while confirming his or her identity).

1. Preparation of the health care worker.
2. Assessing the patient's physical disposition.
3. Identifying the patient.
4. Approaching the patient.
5. Selecting and preparing equipment and supplies.
6. Finding a puncture site.
7. Preparing the puncture site.
8. Choosing a venipuncture method.
9. Collecting the samples in the appropriate tubes and in the correct order.
10. Labeling the samples.

11. Assessing the patient after withdrawal of the blood specimen.
12. Considering any special circumstances that occurred during the phlebotomy procedure.
13. Assessing criteria for sample recollection or rejection.
14. Prioritizing patients and sample tubes.

■ HEALTH CARE WORKER PREPARATION

Prior to performing any type of specimen collection, the health care worker should have all protective equipment, phlebotomy supplies, test requisitions, writing pen, and appropriate patient information. If patient information is incomplete on test requisitions, the health care worker may not be able to identify the patient correctly or he or she may not know in which tubes to collect the blood. In such cases, assistance from a laboratory supervisor or a nurse is required.

In addition, the health care worker needs a positive and professional disposition prior to beginning the patient encounter. A clear and open mind aids the phlebotomist in a successful dialogue, in listening skills, the venipuncture, and exiting graciously.

■ EXERCISING UNIVERSAL STANDARD PRECAUTIONS

Clinical Alert ❗

All health care workers must be familiar with current recommendations and hospital policies on precautions for handling blood and body fluids. *All specimens should be treated as if they are hazardous and infectious,* according to the universal precautions described in detail in Chapters 4 and 5. Hands should be washed *before* and immediately after specimen collection procedures (Fig. 8–1). A clean pair of gloves should be put on in the presence of the patient as a safety-conscious, reassuring gesture for the patient and the health care worker. A clean, pressed uniform with a laboratory coat also instills a sense of commitment to safety and cleanliness, which is gratifying to patients and promotes a safer work environment for health care workers. Refer to Chapter 6, Box 6–3, to review an example of a Dress Code Policy.

■ ASSESSING, IDENTIFYING, AND APPROACHING THE PATIENT

PHYSICAL DISPOSITION OF THE PATIENT

Factors related to the physical or emotional disposition of the patient often have an impact on the blood collection process or the integrity of the specimen. If the phlebotomist is aware of them, she or he may be able to prepare more adequately for the venipuncture. Sometimes the phlebotomist can get clues about the patient's disposition upon entering a hospital

Figure 8–1. Handwashing technique. A. Handwashing techniques should involve soap lather, friction between hands, and thorough washing between fingers. Foot pedals are preferable for controlling the flow of water. B. Washing should include the wrist areas. C. Lather should be rinsed. Rinsing should continue until all soap is removed. If the water must be turned off by hand, a clean paper towel should be used to grab the faucet.

A

B

C

room. For example, if there is an empty food tray by the patient's bedside, it is likely that the patient has eaten recently. At other times, the cues come after talking to the patient or after the identification process has taken place. It is important that phlebotomists use keen listening skills and professional judgment in asking or confirming issues related to disposition. These factors include:

- **Diet**   Many body substances are affected by the ingestion of foods and beverages. Therefore, it is important to note whether the patient has been fasting or not.
- **Stress**   Excessively anxious or emotional patients may need extra time to calm down prior to, during, or after the procedure. The phlebotomist should be keenly aware of these emotional needs and know how to deal with them. (Refer to Chapter 1 for more details on communication.)
- **Age**   Elderly patients may have more "difficult" or frail veins from which to choose the venipuncture site. (Refer to Chapter 14 for more details about the treatment of elderly patients.)
- **Weight**   Obese patients may require special equipment, such as a large blood pressure cuff for the tourniquet or a longer needle to penetrate the vein.

Effects of these and other factors on blood collection are discussed in more detail in Chapter 10.

PATIENT IDENTIFICATION PROCESS

Clinical Alert

Prior to any specimen collection procedure, the patient must be correctly identified by using a two-step process:

1. The patient should be asked to state his or her first and last names.
2. More important, a confirmatory match should be made among the patient's response, the test requisition, and some type of identification, such as a hospital identification bracelet, a driver's license, or another identification card.

INPATIENT IDENTIFICATION

A hospitalized patient should always wear an identification bracelet indicating his or her first and last names and a designated hospital number (often called a *unit number*). Hospital identification numbers help hospital personnel to distinguish between patients with the same first or last names.

As technology has advanced, so have identification methods. One- and two-dimensional barcode technologies, as previously mentioned in Chapter 6, are evolving to enable more information to be encoded. Barcodes tend to be very accurate and cost-effective for larger organizations, so they are widely used for patient and specimen identification and tracking. There is also wireless technology, such as radio frequency identification (RFID), which uses radio waves to transmit data. The technology has the potential of holding more information than a single linear barcode. Essentially, a "tag" about the size of a penny is created for the patient which will accompany the specimen throughout the laboratory and instantly uploads information as the tag is scanned at various points in the testing process.[3] There is also a wristband available that contains a microchip that stores up to 80 pages of information about a patient. At each step of the preanalytical phase, the information is entered into a palmtop or desktop computer that stores the data in a memory chip. The chip can be removed from the patient's armband to a computer to download information into a database for record keeping. It can also be erased, and reused.[4] Each new identification system must be evaluated for accuracy, usefulness for the end user, cost-effectiveness, training involved, compatibility with existing computer technology, ease of updating records, access and security issues, failure rates, and ability to ensure privacy.

> **! Clinical Alert**
>
> To practice the two-step identification process, the health care worker should, upon entering the room, ask the patient what his or her name is. The health care worker should *not* ask, "Are you Ms. Doe?" because an ill patient on medication may mistakenly utter something, nod, or answer yes. Consequently, the best tactic is to ask, "What is your name?" and let the patient reply. *The patient must be correctly identified by his or her identification bracelet.*

Information on the bracelet may also include the patient's room number, bed assignment, and physician's name (Fig. 8–2). A three-way match should be made with the identification bracelet, the test requisition, and the patient's statement of his or her name. The name card on the bed or door should *never* be used for confirming identity because it is often the last to be changed when patients are discharged and new patients are admitted.

> **! Clinical Alert**
>
> If the patient does not have an identification bracelet, the nurse responsible for the patient must be asked to make the identification. In such cases, the situation and the nurse's name should be documented on the requisition and/or electronically. Specimens should *not* be collected until a positive identification can be made and documented. Drawing blood from the wrong patient can lead to serious consequences, such as incorrect treatment or therapy, and it is a violation for which the health care worker may be counseled or dismissed.

There are cases that usually involve severe burns or patients in isolation, in which the identification may be attached to the patient's bed. These are the *only* circumstances in which a phlebotomist may use a bed-labeled identification tag to confirm identity. This step should be followed up by a nurse's confirmation as well. It should also be documented.

Figure 8–2. Identification bracelet, requisition form, specimen label.

(Adapted from College of American Pathologists: *So You're Going to Collect a Blood Specimen: An Introduction to Phlebotomy,* 6th ed. Northfield, IL, Author, 1999, with permission.)

TEST REQUEST SLIP			
HAPPY HOSPITAL			
Department of Laboratory Medicine			
TEST	RESULT	PERFORMED BY	

DATE REQUESTED __5/22/98__   TIME REQUESTED __7 15/AM__

DATE COLLECTED __5/22/98__   TIME COLLECTED __7 30/AM__

NAME __Peter McLaughlin__

ADDRESS __4129 University Blvd.__
__Houston, Texas__

PATIENT ROOM NO. __1708__   BED NO. __2__

AGE __35__ SEX __M__   HOSPITAL I.D. NO. __601537__

PHYSICIAN __Dr. McGarry__

TODAY ☐   ROUTINE ☐

EMERGENCY ☐   SIGNED *DG*

Sample Requisition Form

Sample Identification Bracelet

Printed information should include the following: patient's name, hospital number, room number, and patient's physician.

Labeled Specimen

Printed information should include the following: patient's name, hospital number, date, time, and phlebotomist's initials.

IDENTIFICATION OF INFANTS AND YOUNG CHILDREN

It is preferable to use the same identification procedures for both children and adults; however, it is not always practical or feasible. This topic will be covered in greater detail in Chapter 11, Pediatric Phlebotomy.

EMERGENCY ROOM PATIENT IDENTIFICATION

Health care workers must also be careful when identifying emergency room patients. Often, when patients come to the emergency room, they are unconscious and/or unidentified. Each hospital has policies and procedures for dealing with these cases that usually involves assigning the patient an identification tag with a hospital or medical record number. This tag may be a multipart form that can be used by health care workers who need some type of temporary identification.

 Clinical Alert

The "emergency identification" tag should be attached to the patient's body by wrist band or other similar device. The temporary identification number will be cross-referenced with the permanent identification number when the patient's identity is confirmed.[1]

AMBULATORY PATIENT IDENTIFICATION

Patient identification for ambulatory patients is usually more difficult to monitor. Most outpatient clinics, however, distribute identification cards to patients before any specimens are collected. If this is the case and the patient has the card available, positive identification can occur in the same manner as with hospitalized patients. These cards can also be used to make an imprinted label for the specimen if an Addressograph machine (Addressograph Company, Chicago, IL) is used. Alternatively, some ambulatory clinics issue identification bracelets to patients. If the patient does not have a patient identification armband or card, it is *strongly recommended* that another form of identification (e.g., driver's license) be checked and documented prior to specimen collection.

Clinical Alert

Some home-bound patients, infants, or children may not have any form of identification available. In this situation, someone else, for example, the nurse or a relative, or the home-bound patient should be asked to confirm the identification by verifying the name, address, and birth date. The phlebotomist should compare this information with the test requests and document the identification process prior to specimen collection. Misidentification of the patient's specimens can result in serious medical consequences, including the patient's death.

Figure 8–3.   Labels and requisition forms.

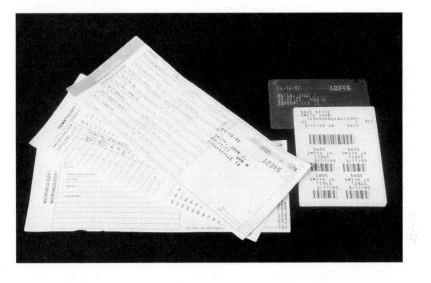

TEST REQUISITIONS

Laboratory tests must be ordered by physicians. The documented requests are usually transmitted in the form of a paper-based requisition or by computer. Computer-generated requests contain the same required information as paper requisitions. In either case, the requisition should contain the following information:

1. Patient's full name.
2. Patient's identification (or medical record) number.
3. Patient's date of birth.
4. Types of tests to be performed.
5. Date of test.
6. Room number and bed.
7. Physician's name and/or code.
8. Test status (timed, **stat,** fasting, etc.).
9. Billing information (optional).
10. Special precautions (potential bleeder, faints easily, etc.).

When requisitions are received in a centralized laboratory department, computer-generated labels that, in some laboratories, also serve as the requisition are often printed as shown above (Fig. 8–3). The numerous types, colors, and styles of labels (e.g., bar-coded labels) and requisitions are discussed further in Chapter 6.

Regardless of whether the requisitions are computer-generated or multipart forms, the health care worker should be familiar with the forms and with the procedures for generating, printing, and using the forms properly. Collection requests should be checked prior to the venipuncture procedure to ensure that there are no discrepancies or duplicates in the test orders.

! Clinical Alert

If the health care worker does not understand the test ordered, a supervisor, a laboratory technologist, or a nurse should be consulted *prior* to the phlebotomy procedure. Knowing which tests are requested helps the health care worker to prepare the patient appropriately and to collect the specimen in the appropriate tubes and in the correct order. Failure to do so results in preanalytical errors, misleading test results, and repeated venipunctures for the patient.

APPROACHING THE PATIENT

In addition to being prepared with the proper equipment and supplies and safety precautions, the health care worker must be emotionally prepared. Such preparation involves adopting a professional appearance and behavior, as well as exercising good communication skills, both as a listener and as a speaker. (Refer to Chapter 1 for more information about professional behavior and communication skills.)

Several professional and courteous behaviors and phrases can help make the patient–health care worker encounter a smooth interaction. The first of these is a polite knock on the patient's door prior to entering the patient's room. The health care worker should introduce him- or herself and state that he or she is from the laboratory and has come to collect a blood sample. As stated previously, making a correct identification is crucial. Once this has occurred, the process may continue. Sometimes, the health care worker may need to explain to the patient that the physician ordered the laboratory test or tests. The health care worker may also need to explain the procedure as supplies are being set up. During setup, the specimen collection tray should *not* be placed on the patient's bed or eating table. As supplies are being readied and the vein is being palpated, the health care worker may try to alleviate some of the patient's fears. It may be reassuring if the phlebotomist shows the patient that the supplies are "new" and "unused." Chapter 1 covers verbal and nonverbal cues for detecting apprehension in patients. Box 8–1 presents a typical scenario of a health care worker–patient interaction.

■ EQUIPMENT SELECTION AND PREPARATION

SUPPLIES FOR VENIPUNCTURE

Supplies for venipuncture differ according to the method used (i.e., **syringe method, evacuated tube system,** or **winged infusion/butterfly system**) and the tests that have been ordered. All methods of venipuncture involve the use of gloves, a **tourniquet,** alcohol pads or disinfectants, cotton balls, bandages or gauze pads, glass microscope slides, needles, syringes or evacuated tube holders, winged infusion sets, plastic capillary tubes, tube sealer, blood collection tubes, laboratory requisitions or labels, marking pens, and discard buckets (Fig. 8–4). Supplies should be readily available and selected just prior to the procedure. Supplies are discussed in more detail in Chapter 7.

BOX 8–1. TYPICAL HEALTH CARE WORKER– PATIENT INTERACTION

Knock on the patient's door.

Health care worker: Good morning. I am Ms. Smith from the laboratory. I have come to collect a blood sample.

Pause to give the patient an opportunity to speak. If the lights are off or dimmed, explain that you need to turn the lights on. Doing so gives the patient a moment to adjust to the idea of bright lights if he or she has been asleep.

Health care worker: What is your name, please? (*In general, it is not wise to ask a patient "How are you?" because most patients in the hospital do not feel well.*)

Patient: I am John Jones.

Health care worker: May I please see your identification (ID) armband?

Check armband against laboratory requisitions and patient's verbal identification. If all three match, proceed.

Health care worker: This will take only a few minutes.

Patient: Will it hurt?

Health care worker: It will hurt a little, but it will be over soon. Please allow me to look at your arm veins.

Proceed with the remainder of the procedure, maintaining a highly professional atmosphere and a respectful attitude.

For certain tests, you may need to ascertain whether the patient has been fasting.

Health care worker: Mr. Jones, when was the last time you ate or drank anything? (*Do not use the term* fast *because some patients may not understand it completely.*)

As supplies are being "readied," the health care worker could demonstrate that s/he is opening a new needle.

Health care worker: Mr. Jones, please notice that I will be using a new needle to collect your blood sample.

At the end of the procedure, say the following:

Health care worker: Thank you, Mr. Jones.

POSITIONING OF THE PATIENT AND VENIPUNCTURE SITE SELECTION

It is important to choose the least hazardous site for blood collection by skin puncture or venipuncture. Several techniques can facilitate the selection of a suitable site. Refer to the Color Plates 6, 7, the front cover sheet and Figures 3–5 and 3–6.

Clinical Alert ❗

Proper positioning is important to both the health care worker and the patient for a successful venipuncture or skin puncture, and efforts to make sure that the patient is comfortable are worthwhile. Patients should *not* stand or sit on high stools during the procedure because of the possibility of fainting. A reclining (supine) position is preferred; however, sitting in a sturdy, comfortable chair with arm supports is also acceptable. Refer to Chapter 7 for more information about blood collection chairs. The health care worker

(continued)

Figure 8–4. Supplies for venipunctures.

! Clinical Alert (*continued*)

can position him- or herself in front of the chair to protect the patient from falling forward in the event of fainting. A slight rotation of the patient's arm or hand may help expose a vein and prevent it from rolling as the needle is inserted. The visibility of veins varies with each individual's skin color, weight, physiologic conditions, gender, and physical features (Fig. 8–5). Therefore, the health care worker must rely on the sense of touch (palpation) to locate the vein. A pillow may be used for arm support of a bedridden patient if the patient is too weak to hold the arm in one position. Equipment should be placed in an accessible spot where it is unlikely to be disturbed by the patient. The phlebotomist can then palpate and trace the path of veins with the index finger.

The most common sites for venipuncture are in the antecubital area of the arm, where the median cubital, cephalic, and basilic veins lie close to the surface of the skin and are most prominent. The median cubital vein is most commonly used; the cephalic vein lies on the outer edge of the arm, and the basilic vein lies on the inside edge. The basilic vein is in close proximity to the median nerve so the other choices are usually preferable. Refer to Color Plate 7, the front cover sheet and Figure 3–5 for exact positions of the veins. Palpating this area usually helps the health care worker get an idea of the size, angle, and depth of the vein. The patient can assist in the process by opening and closing the fist tightly.[2] It is important to remember that veins may also be used for transfusion, infusion, and therapeutic agents. Thus, sometimes veins have restricted use for those purposes.

Figure 8–5. Differences in the visibility of veins. A. Veins are easily visible on a 45-year-old healthy male. B. On a 50-year-old healthy female, the veins are often more difficult to visualize.

A

B

Figure 8–6. Hand and foot veins.

The dorsal side of the hand or wrist, ankle, and foot veins should be used only if arm veins have been determined to be unsuitable (Figs. 8–6 and 8–7).

> **⬢! Clinical Alert**
>
> Reasons for *not* using the patient's arm veins include the following:
>
> • Intravenous (IV) lines in both arms.
> • Burned or scarred areas.
> • Cast(s) on arm(s).
> • Thrombosed veins.
> • Edematous arms.
> • Partial or radical mastectomy on one or both sides.

Hand veins or the veins on the dorsal surface of the wrist are preferred over foot or ankle veins because coagulation and vascular complications tend to be more troublesome in the lower extremities, especially for diabetic patients.

Figure 8–7. Differences in the patterns of hand veins. A. Male. B. Female.

A

B

245

> ⚠ **Clinical Alert**
>
> For hand vein punctures, the posterior surface of the wrist is preferred. *Do not use the anterior side or the palmar venous network* in the wrist, because nerves lie very close to the palmar venous network and can easily be injured by needle probing.

Veins in the wrist or ankle tend to move, or "roll," aside as the needle is inserted; therefore, it may be helpful to have the patient extend the foot or hand into a position that helps hold the vein taut (see Fig. 8–7). Veins of the extremities, however, should be avoided if they are edematous. Some hospitals do not allow health care workers to use the lower extremities for blood-sampling sites. Other hospitals allow sampling from these sites only after permission is granted from the patient's physician. Venipuncture in small veins is facilitated by the use of a 21- to 25-gauge safety butterfly needle. (Fig. 8–8).

Patients who have had mastectomies often have their lymph nodes removed. Without lymph vessels to remove fluid, swelling occurs on the affected side of the body. Thus, blood should not be withdrawn from the mastectomy side if possible. This issue is covered in more detail in Chapter 10.[5]

Figure 8–8. Winged infusion set, or butterfly needle.

(Courtesy of BD VACUTAINER Systems, Franklin Lakes, NJ.)

It is also important to know that arteries do not feel like veins. Arteries pulsate, are more elastic, and have a thick wall. Thrombosed veins lack resilience, feel like a cord, and roll easily.

Clinical Alert !

Nerve damage during a venipuncture is rare but has been known to occur due to excessive needle probing, sudden movements of the patient, etc. (Refer to Chapter 2 for more details.) During the venipuncture, if the patient feels a significant level of pain that appears to be more pronounced than normal, the phlebotomist should discontinue the procedure immediately and ask for assistance from a nurse or supervisor. Only a physician can evaluate whether or not nerve damage has occurred. Nevertheless, the incident should be documented. Color front cover sheet depicts the proximity of nerves in relation to the veins.

WARMING THE PUNCTURE SITE

Warming the puncture site helps facilitate phlebotomy by increasing arterial blood flow to the area and, in some cases, by making the veins more prominent. Although several methods of warming are available commercially, a surgical towel or a washcloth heated to 42°C will not burn the skin. When the towel or cloth is wrapped around the site for 3 to 5 minutes, the skin temperature can increase several degrees. The wrap can be encased in a plastic bag to help retain heat and keep the patient's bed dry. The health care worker may leave the warm wrap on the patient while he or she collects specimens from other patients, and then return to the original patient after several minutes.

TOURNIQUET APPLICATION

A tourniquet or blood pressure cuff may be used to help find a site for venipuncture. The use of a tourniquet makes the veins more prominent and easier to puncture due to venous filling.[2] A soft rubber tourniquet about 1-in. (2.5-cm) wide and about 15- to 18-in. (45-cm) long is most comfortable. To apply it, the health care worker should stretch the ends around the patient's arm about 3 in. (7.6 cm) above the venipuncture area; both ends of the tourniquet can be held in one hand while the other hand tucks in a section next to the skin and makes a partial loop with the tourniquet. The tourniquet should be tight but not painful to the patient (Fig. 8–9). It should not be placed over sores or burned skin, but, depending on the policies of each health care facility, it may be placed over a hospital gown sleeve or a piece of gauze. The partially looped tourniquet should allow for easy release by the health care worker during the venipuncture procedure. During the venipuncture, the health care worker should be able to release the tourniquet with one hand because the other hand will be holding the needle and tubes.

Figure 8–9. Performing a venipuncture procedure. A. The health care worker finished washing hands in the presence of the patient and is greeting him and confirming identification. B. Equipment preparation. C. Site selection. D. Tourniquet application. E. Palpating the site. F. Decontamination with alcohol.

A

B

C

D

E

F

Figure 8–9. (*continued*) G. The venipuncture procedure. H. Removal of tourniquet. I. Tube and needle removal. A safety device may need to be activated, depending on the manufacturer of the equipment. J. Application of pressure. K. Waste disposal. L. Application of bandage.

G

H

I

J

K

L

(*continued*)

Figure 8–9. (*continued*) M. Immediate labeling of tube. N. Adding initials, time, and date. Exiting procedures would include washing hands again, thanking the patient, and carefully storing specimens.

M   N

> ### ⬡ Clinical Alert
>
> The tourniquet should *not* be left on for more than 1 minute because it becomes uncomfortable and causes **hemoconcentration**—that is, increased blood concentration of large molecules, such as proteins, cells, and coagulation factors (see Chapter 10). The patient may be asked to clench and unclench the fist only a *few* times because excessive clenching also results in hemoconcentration. If no vein becomes apparent or "pops up," the patient may be asked to dangle the arm for 1 to 2 minutes to allow blood to fill the veins to capacity, then the tourniquet may be reapplied and the area palpated again. The health care worker should *never* stick a vein unless it can be felt. It is better to defer the patient to someone else who can search for the vein than to take a blind chance.

DECONTAMINATION OF THE PUNCTURE SITE

Once the site is selected, it should be **decontaminated** with a sterile swab or sponge soaked in 70 percent isopropanol (isopropyl alcohol), or with a commercially packaged alcohol pad (see Fig. 8–9 F). This prevents microbiological contamination of either the patient or the specimen. The health care worker should rub the site, working in concentric circles from the inside out. If the skin is particularly dirty, the process should be repeated with a new alcohol pad. The health care worker should also decontaminate his or her own gloved finger if he or she intends to palpate the site again.

Povidone–iodine (Betadine) or iodine preparations are primarily used for drawing blood for blood gas analysis and blood cultures (see Chapter 12, Arterial, Intravenous (IV), and Special Collection Procedures). For some patients, iodine causes skin irritation. Efforts should be made to remove iodine from the skin with sterile gauze after decontamination because excess iodine can interfere with some laboratory tests.

Clinical Alert

The decontaminated area should *never* be touched with any nonsterile object. The alcohol should be allowed to dry (approximately 30 to 60 seconds) or should be wiped off with sterile gauze or cotton after the site is prepared; otherwise, the puncture site will sting, and the alcohol can interfere with test results, such as blood alcohol levels. Blowing on the site to hasten the drying process is not advised because doing so may recontaminate the site.[2]

■ VENIPUNCTURE METHODS

VENIPUNCTURE

Once the puncture site is cleansed, the health care worker may hold the patient's arm below the site, pulling the skin tightly with the thumb. A safety syringe, butterfly, or VACU-TAINER (BD VACUTAINER Systems, *Preanalytical Solutions*, Franklin Lakes, NJ) safety blood collection assembly can be used for venipuncture. (If a safety syringe is used, before the needle is inserted the plunger should be moved back and forth to allow for free movement and to expel all air.) The whole assembly can be held between the thumb and the third or fourth finger. (The index finger may rest on the hub of the needle to guide the needle entry.) The needle should run in the same direction as the vein and should be inserted quickly and smoothly at approximately a 15-degree angle with the skin.[1] To avoid startling the patient, just before inserting the needle, the health care worker should mention to the patient that he or she will "feel a stick." This warning cautions patients and usually alerts them to be still. The health care worker may also need to tell the patient, "Please be very still." Also, there should be no foreign objects (food, chewing gum, a thermometer) in the patient's mouth at the time of the puncture. The needle should be inserted with the *bevel side upward* and directly above a prominent vein or slightly below the palpable vein. The health care worker may need to palpate with one hand after needle insertion if the vein has not been hit. Often, the health care worker can feel a slight "pop" as the needle enters the vein. As the blood begins to flow, the patient may open the fist. The tourniquet can be released immediately or after the blood has been collected, but before needle withdrawal. (While nothing replaces the actual experience, or direct observation of a venipuncture, Figure 8–9 shows photos of various steps in the venipuncture process.)

Box 8–2 describes the specific laboratory procedure used to perform a routine venipuncture.

EVACUATED TUBE SYSTEM

If the evacuated tube (e.g., VACUTAINER) system is used, first the needle should be threaded onto the holder; second, the test tube should be pushed *carefully* into the holder so that the test tube cap is punctured by the inside needle and blood can enter the evacuated tube. If multiple sample tubes are to be collected, each tube should be *gently removed* from the VACUTAINER holder and replaced with another tube. Experienced health care workers

BOX 8–2. SAMPLE PROCEDURE FOR PERFORMANCE OF A ROUTINE VENIPUNCTURE

Performance of a Venipuncture

1. Greet the patient in a friendly, professional manner.

   In an outpatient setting:

   Ask the patient a direct question, "What is your name, sir/madam?" "What is your date of birth?" Compare the name and date of birth stated by the patient with information on the identification card, computer labels, and laboratory request slips. When a blood specimen is required for blood components, an identification bracelet must be worn by the patient. Wash hands in the presence of the patient if possible.

   In a hospital setting (inpatients):

   Knock on the patient's door and enter the room. Compare your request slip or computer labels with the patient's name and hospital number found on the door of the patient's room to make sure you are in the right room. Identify yourself to the patient, stating that you have come to draw blood for some laboratory tests ordered by his or her physician. Compare information on the patient's identification bracelet with that on your computer labels and laboratory request slips. **This information must be identical.** Request a nurse to identify a patient who does not have an identification bracelet. The nurse should also place a bracelet on the patient's wrist except in cases when this is not feasible. Sometimes a patient cannot wear an ID bracelet because his or her wrist is irritated or too edematous for an ID bracelet to fit.

   If this is the case, on the requisition make a note of the nurse who identified the patient. Wash hands in the presence of the patient.

2. Try to gain the patient's confidence and remind the patient that the venipuncture may be slightly painful. Patient's should never be told, "This will not hurt." Exercise Universal Standard Precautions, including use of gloves.

3. Position the patient:

   Procedure for seating the patient (usually outpatients):

   The patient should be seated comfortably in a blood collection chair and should position his or her arm on an armrest, extending the arm so as to form a relatively straight line from the shoulder to the wrist. The arm should be supported firmly by the armrest and should be only slightly bent at the elbow.

   Procedure for having the patient lie down (usually inpatients):

   The patient lies comfortably on his or her back. If additional support is needed, a pillow may be placed under the arm from which the specimen is to be drawn. The patient extends the arm so as to form a relatively straight line from the shoulder to the wrist.

4. Assemble the following supplies for collecting a blood specimen: gloves, blood-collecting tubes, needles, syringe or VACUTAINER holder, tourniquet, 70 percent isopropyl alcohol, and gauze pads or alcohol preparation, pads, iodine and acetone alcohol swab sticks (if blood cultures are to be drawn), and gauze bandage rolls, or paper tape and cotton balls.

5. Select a vein site. Place a tourniquet on the patient's arm. Choose the vein that feels fullest. Look at both arms. Ask the patient to make a fist that makes the veins more prominent and easier to enter. Vigorous hand exercise "pumping" should be avoided because it may affect some test values. Use your index finger to palpate and trace the path of the vein. Thrombosed veins lack resilience, feel cordlike, and roll easily. Feel firmly, but do not tap or rub your finger lightly over the skin because you may feel only small surface veins. Always feel for the median cubital vein first; it is usually bigger and anchored better, and it bruises less. The cephalic vein (depending on size) is the second choice over the basilic vein because it does not roll and bruise as easily. The bend of the elbow is the best place to make a puncture. When this is not possible, other sites include the surface of the forearm, dorsal wrist area above the thumb, volar area of the wrist, knuckle of the thumb or index finger, back of the hand, and back of the lower arm. If a "good" vein cannot be found, try the following:

BOX 8–2. *(continued)*

- Try the other arm unless otherwise instructed.
- Ask the patient to make a fist again.
- Apply the tourniquet, remembering that the tourniquet should never be left on the arm for more than 1 minute.
- Massage the arm from wrist to elbow.
- Tap a few times at the vein site with your index finger.
- Apply heat to the vein site.
- Lower the arm over the bedside or venipuncture chair.

6. Cleanse the venipuncture site. Using an alcohol preparation pad or cotton ball saturated with alcohol, cleanse the area by moving the pad in a circular motion from the center of the vein site outward. The area must be allowed to dry. *Never* touch the skin after the site is cleansed unless you have prepared your gloved finger.

7. Inspect the needle, syringe, or evacuated tube before performing the venipuncture. The appropriate needle is attached to the syringe or the evacuated tube holder and threaded into the holder until it is secure; the needle sheath will lock onto the holder. The cover of the needle must not be removed until you are ready to draw blood so that the needle does not become contaminated. If the needle touches anything but the sterile site, it should be changed. Try to point out to the patient that new supplies are being used, e.g., "I'm opening the clean needle now."

8. Perform the venipuncture:

Evacuated tube method:

Grasp the patient's arm firmly, using your thumb to draw the skin taut. The vein is entered with the bevel of the needle upward. One hand should hold the evacuated tube while the other depresses the tube to the end of the holder.

The tube should be filled until the vacuum is exhausted and the blood flow ceases to ensure a correct ratio of anticoagulant to blood. After each tube is drawn, an additive should be mixed immediately by inverting the tube at least five times. Gentle inversion will prevent hemolysis. *Never* shake a tube of blood after collecting a blood specimen.

Occasionally, a faulty tube will have no vacuum. If a tube is not filling and the needle is inside the vein, another tube should be used. If a tube starts to fill but then stops, the needle should be moved slightly forward or backward. Usually, this adjustment will increase the blood flow. The needle can then be rotated half a turn, and the tourniquet, which may have been applied too tightly, is loosened. Probing is not recommended because it is painful to the patient and may cause nerve damage. If none of these procedures is helpful, the needle should be removed, and an alternate site used.

Syringe method:

A syringe and needle should be used to collect blood from patients with more difficult veins. If the puncture has been made and the blood is not flowing, determine whether you are pulling too hard on the plunger and collapsing the vein. The needle should be drawn back while the plunger is being pulled slightly. Make sure that the bevel is covered by the skin. With the syringe in the right hand, you can use the index finger of the left hand to feel for the vein. After the vein is relocated, keep your finger gently on the vein, and guide the needle to that point. Then, pull gently on the plunger. As soon as the blood starts to flow into the syringe, the needle should not be moved.

Other methods:

A winged infusion set with luer adapters can be used instead of a syringe and needle for very difficult veins. The winged collection set is a closed system. Blood flows from the vein, through the set and directly into a VACUTAINER tube.

If all possibilities have been exhausted, and you have not successfully performed a venipuncture on a patient after two attempts, enlist the aid of a co-worker or a supervisor. Inform the nurse caring for the patient that you have made two unsuccessful attempts to draw blood from the patient. Make a notation of the circumstances on a worksheet.

(continued)

BOX 8–2. *(continued)*

9. The tourniquet is released after the blood is drawn and the patient has opened his or her hand. Releasing the tourniquet allows for normal blood circulation and a reduction in the amount of bleeding at the venipuncture site. After collecting the required sample tubes, withdraw the needle and immediately activate the safety device based on the manufacturer's instructions. Fold a gauze pad or place a cotton ball over the needle, then gently remove the needle. The gauze pad or cotton ball should be held firmly over the venipuncture site.

10. All tubes should be appropriately mixed and labeled at the patient's bedside. Labels must include the patient's first and last names and ID number, the date, the time of collection, and the phlebotomist's initials.

11. Dispose of contaminated materials and supplies in designated containers.

12. Wash hands.

13. Thank the patient.

14. Transport and deliver specimens to the appropriate laboratory.

are able to mix a full tube in one hand while holding the needle apparatus and waiting for another tube to fill. Some health care workers use the dominant hand to change tubes while the other hand keeps the needle apparatus steady. This approach may require the health care worker to switch hands after needle insertion. The position that is the most comfortable for the patient and the health care worker should be used while the needle is simultaneously kept as stable and motionless as possible during tube fillings. (As mentioned previously, remember to release the tourniquet once blood begins to flow into the tubes.) Multiple tubes can be filled in less than 1 minute if the needle remains stable in the vein and the vein does not collapse. So that the proper dilution of blood and additive in the tube is ensured, each tube should be allowed to fill until the blood flow stops. Tubes do not fill completely, so the health care worker must be attentive to when the blood flow ceases. To change tubes, the health care worker should remove the full one from the needle apparatus with a gentle twist-and-pull motion, then replace it with an empty tube, using a gentle push onto the needle apparatus. During the tube exchange, the needle apparatus should be held firmly so that the needle remains in the vein and is not pushed through or pulled out of the vein.

> **! Clinical Alert**
>
> When all tubes have been filled, the needle should be carefully but quickly withdrawn. *Depending on the needle manufacturer,* the safety device should be activated either prior to or immediately upon withdrawal of the needle. (Refer to Chapter 7 for details on equipment safety devices that prevent accidental needlesticks.)

SYRINGE METHOD

If a syringe is used, the same approach to needle insertion should take place as is used for the evacuated tube method. Once the needle is in the vein, the syringe plunger can be drawn back slowly until the required amount of blood is drawn. (It may be helpful to turn the syringe slightly so that the graduated markings are visible.) Care must be taken not to accidentally withdraw the needle while pulling back on the plunger and not to pull hard enough to cause **hemolysis** (e.g., rupture of the cells) or collapse of the vein.

After tourniquet release and collection of the appropriate amount of blood, the entire needle assembly should be withdrawn quickly. Again, the safety device should be activated immediately, depending on the manufacturer's specifications.

WINGED INFUSION SYSTEM OR BUTTERFLY METHOD

A **winged infusion system,** butterfly needle assembly, or scalp needle set can be used for particularly difficult venipunctures (Fig. 8–10). This type of method is useful for the following circumstances:

- Patients with small veins (hand or wrist).
- Pediatric patients.
- Geriatric patients.

Figure 8–10.   Performing a venipuncture procedure with the combination butterfly (double-pointed) needle and evacuated tube system.

A

B

C

D

- Patients having numerous needlesticks (i.e., cancer patients).
- Patients in restrictive positions (i.e., traction, severe arthritis).
- Patients who are severely burned.
- Patients with fragile skin and veins.
- Patients who specifically request it because they feel it is less painful.
- Short-term infusion therapy.

The needles range from ½ to ¾ inch in length and from 21 to 25 gauge in diameter. Attached to the needle is a thin tubing with a luer adapter at the end so that it can be used on a syringe or an evacuated tube system from the same manufacturer. Since the tubing contains air, it will underfill the first evacuated tube by 0.5 mL. This affects the additive-to-blood ratio. Therefore, a red-topped nonadditive tube should be filled prior to any tube with additives. After the first tube, the order of the tube draw should be the same as other methods. When tubes for coagulation are the only ones to be collected, it is suggested that a "dummy" tube be collected and discarded. This fills the tubing with blood so that the correct additive-to-blood ratio is obtained for the coagulation tube. When using the winged infusion system, each tube should be held horizontally or slightly down to avoid transfer of additives from one tube to the next. It is also suggested that small evacuated collection tubes (i.e., 13×75 mm or 4 mL) be used with winged infusion sets to avoid collapsing fragile veins. If using a syringe attached to the luer adapter, a small syringe, such as 5 or 10 mL, should be used for the same reason. Usually a 21- or 23-gauge needle is better than a 25-gauge needle because the small diameter may lead to hemolysis as the specimen is withdrawn. For an infant, however, the 25-gauge needle is the best choice for small veins.

Health care workers should be extra cautious as the needle is removed from the patient because it tends to hang loose on the end of the tubing. Therefore, the safety device that is built into the system should be activated according to the manufacturer's instructions. This may involve a retractable safety enclosure that allows for resheathing or covering the needle once it has been withdrawn (BD VACUTAINER Systems, *Preanalytical Solutions*, Franklin Lakes, NJ) or rotating a device on the needle set that advances a safety blunt prior to withdrawal of the needle from the vein (Puncture Guard Technology, Bio-Plexus, Tolland, CT). (Refer to Chapter 7, Blood Collection Equipment.)

Use of winged infusion or butterfly systems requires training and practice, but they are very popular. Use of this system is, however, more hazardous for health care workers than the use of conventional needles. Failure to activate the safety devices correctly as described by the manufacturers may result in a higher incidence of needlestick injuries.

BANDAGE FOR THE PUNCTURE SITE

A dry, sterile gauze or cotton ball should be applied with pressure to the puncture site for several minutes or until bleeding has ceased. If the patient has a free hand, he or she may be asked to apply the pressure. The patient's arm may be kept straight, slightly bent at the elbow, or elevated above the heart. A bandage should be applied, and the patient should be instructed to leave it on for at least 15 minutes.

If the patient continues to bleed, the phlebotomist should apply pressure her- or himself until the bleeding stops. A gauze bandage can then be applied, and the patient should be instructed to leave it on for at least 15 minutes. If the patient continues to bleed, the unit nurse should be notified.

PROPER DISPOSAL

All disposable or contaminated equipment should be discarded into appropriate containers. Paper and plastic wrappers can be thrown into a wastebasket. Needles and lancets should *not* be thrown into a wastebasket, however, but into a sturdy, puncture-proof, disposable container to be autoclaved or incinerated (see Fig. 8–9 K). Any items that have been contaminated with blood should be disposed of in biohazardous disposal containers as explained in the universal precautions (see Chapter 4, Infection Control. Also refer to Chapter 7, Blood Collection Equipment.)

ORDER OF TUBE COLLECTION

Very often, multiple blood assays are ordered on patients. Whether the health care worker chooses to use a multiple-draw evacuated tube collection system or a plastic syringe, there are certain guidelines for delivery of blood into the proper collection tubes.

The **National Committee for Clinical Laboratory Standards (NCCLS)** and Becton Dickinson, a major manufacturer of blood collection supplies, recommend the following specific order when collecting multiple tubes of blood via the evacuated method or the syringe transfer method:[2,6]

1. Blood culture tubes (yellow top), or blood culture vials or bottles
2. Plain tubes, nonadditive (red top)
3. Coagulation tube (light blue top)
4. Additive tubes:
    a. Gel separator tube
    b. Heparin (green top)
    c. EDTA (purple top)
    d. Oxalate/fluoride (gray top)

For BD VACUTAINER tubes, the order of draw is only slightly different (Fig. 8–11):

1. Blood culture tubes or tubes for sterile samples
2. Plain tubes, nonadditives (red top)
3. Coagulation tube (light blue top)
4. Additive tubes (Heparin, EDTA, potassium oxalate/sodium floride)

BD VACUTAINER SST tubes and BD VACUTAINER PLUS serum tubes are considered additive tubes because they contain silica particles and should be collected after tubes for coagulation studies.[6]

The blood cultures are always drawn first to decrease the possibility of bacterial contamination. The procedure for collection of blood cultures is discussed in Chapter 12 in greater detail. Whenever coagulation studies are ordered for diagnostic purposes (prothrombin time [PT], partial thromboplastin time [PTT]), it is preferable that at least one other tube of blood should be drawn before the coagulation test specimen. This diminishes contamination with tissue fluids, which *may* initiate the clotting sequence. Recent studies, however, suggest that accurate results can be obtained using the *first* tube.[7,8,9] This is particularly important when coagulation studies are the *only* tests ordered. The findings suggest that collecting and discarding the first of two tubes may no longer be necessary in all cases. According to NCCLS recommendations, if *only* a coagulation tube is to be drawn for routine coagulation tests (APTT and PT tests), the first tube drawn may be used for testing. For special coagulation tests (e.g., Factor VIII), the second or third tube should be used.[2] Each health care worker

Figure 8–11.   Example of the order of draw for three tubes. The plain red-topped tube is used first, followed by the light blue-topped tube, the purple-topped tube, and any others that are needed. If two syringes of blood have been withdrawn, the anticoagulated tubes should be filled as soon as possible with the second syringe of blood. Gentle mixing of the anticoagulated tubes should be done as soon as possible after filling.

should use the procedure adopted by his or her own facility. Coagulation tubes should be mixed as soon after collection as possible.

Care should be taken so that the anticoagulant present in the tube does not come into contact with the multisample needle when changing tubes, as some may be carried into the next tube and cause erroneous test results. For example, it is recommended that blood for serum iron be drawn before other specimens with chelating anticoagulants (e.g., EDTA). This will avoid interference in testing the serum iron level. Also, electrolyte determinations include measurement of potassium (K) and sodium (Na). Since the chelating anticoagulant EDTA is usually bound to potassium as EDTA (K_3) or to sodium (Na) as EDTA (Na_2), it is important to collect specimens that require EDTA after a specimen is collected in heparin for electrolytes. The K_3 and Na_2 from the EDTA may falsely elevate the patient's K or Na values. To minimize transfer of anticoagulants from tube to tube, holding the tube horizontally or slightly downward during blood collection is recommended.

Sometimes, when a large volume (more than 20 mL) of blood has been drawn using a syringe, there is a possibility that some of the blood may be clotted. If this occurs, the needle can be *carefully* removed from the hub of the syringe, the top can be removed from the tube, and then the blood can be *carefully* expelled into the tube. Again, it is suggested that the tube be filled by letting the blood run *gently,* not forcefully, down the inside of the tube to avoid hemolysis. If two syringes of blood have been withdrawn, NCCLS recommends taking blood from the second syringe for coagulation studies.[2]

Another factor to be watchful about is the "fill" rate and volume in each tube. This is discussed more fully in Chapter 7. Evacuated tubes with anticoagulants must be filled to the designated level for the proper mix of blood with the anticoagulant. "Partial-fill" tubes are available when it is suspected that the blood specimen will not be adequate.

SPECIMEN IDENTIFICATION AND LABELING

Specimens should be labeled immediately at the patient's bedside or ambulatory setting, and the labels should consistently include the following information[1,2] (see Fig. 8–3):

1. Patient's full name.
2. Patient's identification number.
3. Date of collection.
4. Time of collection.
5. Health care worker's initials.
6. Patient's room number, bed assignment, or outpatient status are optional information.

For hospitalized patients, the tubes should be labeled immediately after the specimen is collected.

Clinical Alert !

Tubes should *not* be prelabeled because they may not be used, then be erroneously picked up and used for another patient. Also, a different health care worker may complete the venipuncture if the initial health care worker is unsuccessful. In that case, the prelabeled tubes may contain the initials of the first health care worker and, therefore, be inaccurate. In addition, if the prelabeled tubes are not used, tearing off the old or unused label may be difficult because of the adhesive; thus, either a new label (from a different patient) would have to be placed on the tube with a partially torn label, *or* the unused tube would have to be discarded. Either option is unsatisfactory, messy, and wasteful.

For the ambulatory care setting, there are mixed opinions about when to label the blood collection tube. The NCCLS suggests that the health care worker "must apply a label to each of the necessary tubes" prior to the actual collection process. Many health care workers (the authors included), however, believe that the same risks exist with prelabeled tubes in the outpatient setting as in the inpatient setting. Therefore, each laboratory procedure manual should contain explicit instructions on labeling requirements, and supervisors should spend ample time not only training new employees in correct identification and labeling practices, but also observing these trainees as they execute such practices.

As mentioned in Chapter 6, for unidentified or unconscious patients who come to a hospital through the emergency room or other unusual circumstances, a temporary identification number can be assigned.

The health care worker should wash hands, then confirm all the information before leaving the patient's hospital room or before drawing blood from another clinic outpatient. The date and time are necessary because requisition forms may indicate the date and time when a laboratory test was *ordered,* rather than the date and time when it was *collected.* The health care worker's initials are necessary to help clarify questions about the specimen if any arise during laboratory processing or testing.

No foolproof method exists for labeling specimens. The health care worker may write directly on the container. Alternatively, commercial collection tubes may have blank affixed labels for this purpose. Similarly, hospitals often use computer-generated labels for collection tubes; however, capillary tubes, microcollection tubes and vials, or other containers without labels must be identified, either by labeling them directly with a permanent felt-tipped pen, wrapping an adhesive label around them, or placing them into a larger labeled test tube for transport. In some cases, small computerized adhesive labels with printed information are available with and detachable from the requisition form.

OTHER CONSIDERATIONS

Because the health care team members (including doctors, medical technologists, clerks, secretaries, and nurses) are all working for the welfare of the patient, they should strive to reduce the total number of daily phlebotomies. To do this, all health care workers involved in patient care duties could follow these suggestions:

- Doctors could write orders on the same line on the chart.
- Orders could be coordinated among all staff physicians working with the patient.
- The laboratory could be notified when multiple timed tests are ordered. For example, if a patient needs a hemoglobin test at 2:00 P.M. and a glucose test at 3:00 P.M., coordinating the times and drawing both specimens during one venipuncture may be possible.
- Therapeutic drug monitoring should be coordinated among laboratory, nursing, and pharmacy personnel.
- Nurses and ward secretaries could organize laboratory orders as much as possible to avoid sending frequent requests minutes apart for multiple venipunctures.
- When orders are transcribed, all of them should be requested at the same time.
- The laboratory should be notified of patient transfers.
- An up-to-date log of room numbers and patients' names should be available on the ward as a resource for laboratory personnel.
- Health care workers should organize requisition forms by patient and floor.
- Any identification discrepancies should be communicated to a nurse.

One hospital has suggested several slogans for their health care personnel regarding phlebotomy:

- A stick in time saves nine.
- We care—several pokes are no joke.
- For their sake, let's stick together.

Table 8–1. Maximum Amounts of Blood to Be Drawn From Patients Younger Than 14 Years

PATIENT'S WEIGHT		MAXIMUM AMOUNT TO BE DRAWN AT ANY ONE TIME (mL)	MAXIMUM AMOUNT OF BLOOD (CUMULATIVE) TO BE DRAWN DURING A GIVEN HOSPITAL STAY (1 MONTH OR LESS) (mL)
lb	kg (approx)		
6–8	2.7–3.6	2.5	23
8–10	3.6–4.5	3.5	30
10–15	4.5–6.8	5	40
16–20	7.3–9.1	10	60
21–25	9.5–11.4	10	70
26–30	11.8–13.6	10	80
31–35	14.1–15.9	10	100
36–40	16.4–18.2	10	130
41–45	18.6–20.5	20	140
46–50	20.9–22.7	20	160
51–55	23.2–25.0	20	180
56–60	25.5–27.3	20	200
61–65	27.7–29.5	25	220
66–70	30.0–31.8	30	240
71–75	32.3–34.1	30	250
76–80	34.5–36.4	30	270
81–85	36.8–38.6	30	290
86–90	39.1–40.9	30	310
91–95	41.4–43.2	30	330
96–100	43.6–45.5	30	350

Adapted from Becan-McBride, K. *Textbook of Clinical Laboratory Supervision.* New York; Appleton-Century-Crofts: 1982.

Other items that should be considered for inclusion in policies and procedures are

1. The number of times that a patient can be punctured by the same health care worker. Generally, a health care worker should not puncture a patient more than twice before calling for a second opinion.
2. The number of times that a patient can be punctured in 1 day. Staff physicians, nurses, and health care workers should coordinate their efforts to minimize the number of patient venipunctures.
3. The total volume of blood that can be drawn daily from a patient, especially a patient in pediatrics or in the nursery (Table 8–1 above).
4. The type of information that a health care worker may provide to the patient about the laboratory tests ordered. In general, the use of good judgment is required. Providing basic information about the tests that have been ordered is acceptable *if* the health care worker is knowledgeable. The health care worker should always emphasize, however, that the patient's physician ordered the tests.
5. The steps to take if a patient refuses to have blood collected. All patients have a right to refuse treatment. In these cases, the health care worker should use good,

sound judgment in explaining to the patient that laboratory results are used to help the physician make an accurate diagnosis, establish proper treatment, and monitor the patient's health status. The health care worker should explain that the patient's cooperation would be greatly appreciated. If the patient continues to refuse, the health care worker must remain professional and acknowledge the right to refuse. The health care worker should indicate to the patient that he or she will make a note of the refusal and notify the patient's physician.

In Chapter 6, Box 6–2 includes examples of what to do in cases when the patient is unavailable, refuses the procedure, or is combative.

ASSESSING THE PATIENT BEFORE LEAVING

Before leaving the patient's side, the health care worker must check the puncture site to make sure that the bleeding stopped. All tubes must be appropriately labeled, and the information on the labels confirmed. Hands should be washed again. All supplies and equipment that were brought in should be removed or discarded appropriately, and the health care worker should thank the patient. An adhesive bandage may be applied. Such bandages, however, are not recommended for infants or young children because of possible irritation and the potential of swallowing or aspirating a bandage.

■ SPECIMEN REJECTION

Each clinical laboratory should establish its own guidelines for specimen rejection. In general, the following factors should be considered:[10,11]

- Discrepancies between requisition forms and labeled tubes (names, dates, times).
- Unlabeled tubes.
- Inadequate volume of blood.
- Hemolyzed specimens (except for tests in which hemolysis does not interfere).
- Specimens in the wrong collection tubes.
- Specimens that were improperly transported (chilled or unchilled).
- Anticoagulated specimens that contain blood clots.
- Use of outdated equipment, supplies, or reagents.
- Contaminated specimens.
- A timed sample is drawn at the wrong time or the time is recorded incorrectly.

When a problem arises, the appropriate investigational channels should be followed. The health care worker who drew the specimen and his or her supervisor should try to solve the problem initially. Errors should be acknowledged and documented with corrective actions. Other personnel may be involved as needed. Communication, honesty, and ethical professional behavior are the keys to an efficient and reliable health care environment. Chapter 10 addresses complications in blood collection.

■ PRIORITIZING PATIENTS

In the course of a day's work at a busy hospital or clinic, a health care worker may have to make decisions about the order in which blood work is obtained. Priorities must be set and adhered to, whether they concern the order in which certain blood tests are drawn on a particular patient or which patients are to be drawn from first among a group. If these distinctions are not made properly, test results can be affected and interpretation of the results may be difficult.

PATIENT PRIORITIES

Timed Specimens

Whenever a test is ordered to be drawn at a particular time, the health care worker is responsible for drawing the blood as near to the requested time as possible. The most common requests for timed specimens are for glucose level determination for which blood should be drawn 2 hours after a meal. The glucose value in the blood is constantly changing, so the blood must not be drawn too early, which yields a falsely elevated result, or too late, which yields a falsely normal result.

Timed specimens are also vital for **therapeutic drug monitoring (TDM).** The laboratory results taken from blood samples for TDM are used in establishing a patient's drug dose. More specifically, TDM is used for the following reasons:[12,13]

- Monitor or confirm overdose.
- Determine the dosage of a medication.
- Establish a baseline measurement after a patient has begun or changed to a new drug therapy.
- Check to see that a drug is not interacting with one the patient is already taking.
- Check to see that if a drug is influenced by the patient's habits, e.g., smokers clear theophylline faster than in nonsmokers, so their serum drug levels will be lower.
- After a change in the patient's kidney, liver or GI functions.
- Within 6 hours after a seizure recurrence (when using antiepileptic drugs).
- When drug toxicity is suspected, i.e., some drugs have a narrow therapeutic window such that the amount needed to benefit the patient is often close to the toxic amount.
- When the patient is noncompliant with the prescribed medications, a physician may need the serum level to confirm that the patient has not taken the drug or has not taken it as prescribed.
- If a patient's condition is not improving after drug therapy, the serum drug level may be subtherapeutic, so a change in dose may be needed.

Usually when a patient is taking a drug orally, blood samples for TDM are drawn right before taking the next dose. This is called the **"trough"** sample because it is usually when the drug is at a low concentration in the patient's serum. **"Peak"** samples are collected for some intravenous (IV) drugs, e.g., antibiotics such as amikacin, gentamicin, and tobramycin, and after IV loading doses of drugs such as phenytoin. "Peak" drug levels represent the highest drug concentration in the patient's blood. Other drugs such as digoxin and lithium take a long time to reach a steady state in the patient's body. Therefore, blood collection should be delayed until the drug reaches the steady state and should be coordinated with the nursing and pharmacy staff to assure proper timing.[12]

In addition to timing, TDM usually requires that the specimen be collected in tubes that do *not* contain gel separators because some gels absorb certain drugs, thus causing falsely lowered results. Other studies indicate that if the samples are processed promptly, some of the effects of gel interference can be minimized; and that acrylic based gels do not exhibit

> ## ! Clinical Alert
>
> Laboratory analyses of drug levels are often used to re-evaluate drug dosages. If blood samples are drawn at inappropriate times, i.e., before the drug has reached equilibrium, or if the "peak" level is erroneously reported as the "trough" level, the wrong dosage will be used to calculate a new dose. It is possible that the patient may then receive an incorrectly calculated dosage. This could be life-threatening. TDM requires careful coordination among all members of the health care team, including the physician and the laboratory, nursing, and pharmacy staff members.
>
> The time of day, e.g., morning versus evening, that blood is collected can have an effect on carbamazepine, cyclosporine, lithium, and theophylline.[12] Again, coordinating the timing with interdisciplinary staff members so as to be consistent from day to day will ensure accurate results.

absorption problems that are linked to silicone or polyester gels. However, it is probably safest to check with the tube manufacturers for specific information on their products.[12,14]

Certain natural hormone levels, such as cortisol, also increase and decrease with the time of day. For instance, a sample of blood taken at 8:00 A.M. shows the highest value for cortisol during the day, whereas a sample taken at 8:00 P.M. usually shows approximately two thirds the value of the morning sample. Therefore, if a health care worker has difficulty obtaining a blood specimen on a patient at 8:00 A.M., someone else should try as soon as possible thereafter, or the test may be canceled until the following day at the discretion of the attending physician. Obtaining a specimen at noon for cortisol level determination may give the physician little information on which to base treatment.

Another hormone, aldosterone, requires another type of timing for blood collection and analysis. The patient must be in a recumbent position for at least 30 minutes prior to blood collection. Serum or plasma can be used in the analyte determination, but heparin or EDTA should be the anticoagulant if plasma is preferred. Because glass interferes in the aldosterone determination, the collecting container should be made of plastic.

To collect blood for a renin-activity test, the health care worker must collect an anticoagulated blood specimen from the patient after a 3-day special diet. In addition, the health care worker must be sure to note whether the patient is in an upright position or **supine** (prone) position when blood is drawn. For this analyte, the blood should be collected from a peripheral vein (e.g., antecubital vein).

Fasting Specimens

When a health care worker works at an institution where inpatients are treated, care should be taken that the patient is not unduly inconvenienced by an order for **fasting blood tests** (i.e., tests performed on blood taken from a patient who has abstained from eating and drinking [except water] for a particular period of time). Fasting levels of glucose, cholesterol, and triglycerides can be important in diagnosing patients and monitoring their progress during the hospital stay. If the health care worker finds that a patient has not been fasting, the health care worker should consult with a physician to determine whether a nonfasting level will be of benefit. The requisition should then indicate that the patient is nonfasting.

Stat Specimens

The term *stat,* which means "immediately," has come to indicate a patient whose medical condition suddenly may become critical and who must be treated or responded to as a medical emergency. When blood work is ordered stat, usually a specimen must be drawn and analyzed *immediately* so that a critically ill patient can be handled properly. Consequently, the health care team should be prepared for immediate response, employ effective technique, and have personnel constantly available for stat blood collections. The health care worker not only should draw the blood quickly and properly but also should ensure its immediate delivery to the laboratory for stat analysis.

SELF STUDY

KEY TERMS

Butterfly System
Decontaminated
Evacuated Tube System
Fasting Blood Tests
Hemoconcentration
Hemolysis
National Committee for Clinical
    Laboratory Standards
    (NCCLS)

"Peak"
Stat
Supine
Syringe Method
Therapeutic Drug Monitoring
    (TDM)
Tourniquet
"Trough"
Winged Infusion System

STUDY QUESTIONS

The following questions may have *one* or *more* answers.

1. A patient may be identified by which of the following means?

   a. patient's chart
   b. nurse

   c. patient's armband
   d. ward clerk

2. Identification procedures for outpatients may include asking for which of the following?

   a. photo identification
   b. birth date

   c. address
   d. identification by a family member

3. The most common sites for venipuncture are in which of the following areas?

   a. the dorsal side of the wrist
   b. the antecubital area of the arm

   c. the middle finger
   d. the middle forearm

4. Palpating the venipuncture site serves what purpose(s)?

   a. provides an indication of the
      size of the vein
   b. distracts the patient from the
      discomfort of the procedure

   c. provides an indication of the depth
      of the vein
   d. helps the phlebotomist determine at what
      angle to insert the needle

5. Using a butterfly needle is beneficial for which of the following?

   a. heel puncture
   b. veins in the wrist or hand

   c. geriatric patients
   d. patients who are burned

6. What effect does warming the site have on venipuncture?

   a. prevents veins from rolling
   b. makes veins stand out
   c. causes hemoconcentration
   d. increases localized blood flow

7. How long should the tourniquet be placed around the patient's arm?

   a. Approximately 4 minutes
   b. Until the needle is removed
   c. Until the entire venipuncture is completed
   d. No more than 1 minute

8. What is the best angle for needle insertion during venipuncture?

   a. 15 degrees
   b. 30 degrees
   c. 45 degrees
   d. 80 degrees

9. What is the suggested order of draw using the evacuated tube system for the following specimens?

   a. blood culture
   b. lavender-topped tube
   c. light blue-topped tube
   d. red-topped tube

10. Containers for the disposal of needles and syringes should have which of the following features?

   a. be puncture resistant
   b. be labeled with a "biohazard" sign
   c. have yellow and black markings
   d. contain antiseptic solution.

References

1. College of American Pathologists (CAP): *So You're Going to Collect a Blood Specimen: An Introduction to Phlebotomy,* 6th ed. Northfield, IL; CAP: 1999.

2. National Committee for Clinical Laboratory Standards (NCCLS): *Procedures for the Collection of Diagnostic Blood Specimens by Venipuncture.* Approved Standard, H3-A4, Villanova, PA; NCCLS: June: 1998.

3. The Observatory: Radio frequency technology in the lab, *Med Lab Observ.* February: 8–9, 2000.

4. Erwin, J: Keeping Track, Patient wristbands hold medical records, *Healthweek;* August 17: 8, 1998.

5. Faber, V, Gingrich, DP: Tips for Drawing Blood from a Mastectomy Arm, *Adv Med Lab Professionals.* June 5: 4, 2000.

6. Becton-Dickinson Systems: Personal communication, Fall, 2000.

7. Gottfried, EL, Adachi, MM: Prothrombin time and activated partial thromboplastin time can be performed on the first tube. *Am J Clin Pathol.* 1997; *107*(6):681–683.

8. Yawn, BP, Loge, C, Dale, J: Prothrombin time: one tube or two. *Am J. Clin Pathol.* 1996; *105*(6):794–797.

9. Adcock, DM, Kressin, DC, Marlar, RA: Are discard tubes necessary in coagulation studies?, *Lab Med* 1997; *28*(8):530–533.

10. Richael, JL, Naples, MF: Creating a workable specimen rejection policy. *Med Lab Observ.* March:37–42, 1995.

11. National Committee for Clinical Laboratory Standards (NCCLS): Procedures for the Handling and Processing of Blood Specimens. Approved Guideline, H18-A2, Villanova, PA: NCCLS: 1994.

12. Warner, AM: Pitfalls in Monitoring Therapeutic Drugs, *Laboratory Medicine*. 1997; *28*(10): 653–663.

13. Sayers, J, Friedman, M: How clinicians use therapeutic drug monitoring. *Lab Med* 1997; *28*(8):524–538.

14. Pruett, S: Tips from the clinical experts: Gel separator tubes for TDM. *Med Lab Observ.* January 1999:14.

NINE

■

Skin Puncture Procedures

CHAPTER OUTLINE

CHAPTER OBJECTIVES

Upon completion of Chapter 9, the learner is responsible for the following:

1. Describe reasons for performing a skin puncture procedure.

2. Identify the proper sites for performing a skin puncture procedure.

3. Explain why controlling the depth of the puncture is necessary.

4. Describe the process of making a blood smear.

5. Explain why blood from a skin puncture procedure is different from blood taken by venipuncture.

■ INDICATIONS FOR SKIN PUNCTURE

Skin punctures are particularly useful for both adult and pediatric patients when small amounts of blood can be obtained and adequately tested. In contrast, venipuncture in children can be hazardous and difficult because of the risk of complications, such as anemia, cardiac arrest, hemorrhage, venous thrombosis, reflex arteriospasm, gangrene of an extremity, danger to surrounding tissues or organs, infections, and injuries from restraining the child during the procedure. It is particularly important to withdraw only the smallest amounts of blood necessary from neonates, infants, and children so that the effects of blood-volume reduction are minimal. A 10-mL blood sample, which could be tolerated by most adults, would represent 5 to 10 percent of the total blood volume in a neonate's body.[1] Sample sizes and procedures for obtaining specimen collections from children are covered in Chapter 11, Pediatric Procedures.

Skin punctures are also useful for the following adult patients:[1]

- Patients with severe burns.
- Obese patients.
- Patients with thrombotic tendencies.
- Oncology patients whose veins are being "saved" for therapy.
- Geriatric patients.
- Those who have fragile veins.
- Patients doing home testing (e.g., blood glucose screening).
- Point of care testing on patients.

Sometimes a skin puncture cannot be used because testing may require larger amounts of blood, interstitial fluids dilute the blood to some extent, and/or a patient has poor peripheral circulation. Specific tests for which skin punctures are not recommended include coagulation studies (because of the interstitial fluid), blood cultures, and erythrocyte sedimentation rate (ESR) determinations.

■ COMPOSITION OF SKIN PUNCTURE BLOOD

The composition of skin puncture blood is significantly different from that of venous blood acquired by venipuncture. It is composed of blood from arterioles, venules, and capillaries, as well as some **tissue (interstitial) fluid,** which is released during the sticking process. The content of arterial blood is greater because the arterial pressure in the capillaries is stronger than the venous pressure. Therefore, skin puncture blood is actually more like arterial blood than venous blood.

■ BASIC TECHNIQUE FOR SKIN PUNCTURE

Many of the steps used for the venipuncture procedure also apply to skin puncture. Basic steps include the following:

1. Preparation for puncture—greeting, identification, handwashing.
2. Choosing supplies and equipment.
3. Positioning the patient.
4. Site selection and warming, if necessary.
5. Cleaning the site.
6. Opening the sterile puncture device within view of the patient.
7. Performing the puncture.
8. Obtaining the specimen.
9. Labeling the specimen.
10. Completing the interaction.

■ PREPARATION FOR SKIN PUNCTURE

Skin puncture procedures involve the same preparation steps as discussed for venipuncture procedures. Such steps include:

- Being emotionally prepared
- Exercising universal standard precautions
- Greeting the patient to put him or her at ease
- Ensuring proper patient identification
- Asking about his or her fasting state
- Asking about latex sensitivity
- Asking about hand preference or dominance
- Labeling procedures appropriately
- Practicing the correct handwashing techniques

For additional discussion of these issues, see Chapter 8.

■ SUPPLIES FOR SKIN PUNCTURE

As mentioned in Chapter 7, Blood Collection Equipment, supplies for skin puncture include the following:

- Disposable gloves
- Lancets or automatic puncture devices
- Micropipettes
- Disinfectant pads
- Cotton balls
- Sterile bandages or gauze pads
- Glass microscope slides
- Diluting fluids
- Microcollection tubes or plastic capillary tubes
- Capillary tube sealer
- Laboratory request slips or labels
- A marking pen
- A biohazard discard bucket

■ SKIN PUNCTURE SITES

Skin puncture in adults most often involves one of the fingers. The fleshy surface of the distal portion of the third (middle) or fourth (ring) fingers of the nondominant hand are the preferred sites for puncture. The fifth (pinky) finger is not recommended because the tissue of this finger is considerably thinner than that of the others; the thumb has a pulse; and the index (pointer) finger may be more sensitive or callused.[1]

For infants or neonates, the following are good sites for skin puncture:[1]

- Lateral or medial plantar surface of the heel
- Plantar surface of a big toe

Refer to Figure 11–3, and to Chapter 11 for further information regarding pediatric phlebotomies.

> **! Clinical Alert**
>
> Skin punctures should not be performed on the following sites:[1]
>
> - Earlobes
> - Central areas of an infant's heel (arch or central curvature)
> - Swollen or previously punctured sites
> - Fingers that are **cyanotic** (bluish in color due to oxygen deficiency), cold, or inflamed
> - Fingers of newborn children
>
> The fingers of infants less than 1 year of age should not be used for skin puncture due to the risk of puncturing the bone and possibly causing **osteochondritis,** inflammation of the bone and its cartilage.[2]

■ WARMING THE SKIN PUNCTURE SITE

Warming the skin puncture site helps facilitate phlebotomy by significantly increasing arterial blood flow to the area. Although several easy-to-use methods of warming are commercially available, a surgical towel or a washcloth heated with warm water to 42°C will not burn the skin. When the towel or cloth is wrapped around the site for 3 to 10 minutes, the skin temperature can increase several degrees.[1]

■ CLEANING THE SKIN PUNCTURE SITE

The skin puncture site should be cleaned with 70 percent aqueous solution of *isopropanol* and thoroughly dried before being punctured because residual alcohol causes rapid hemolysis and may contaminate glucose determinations. Furthermore, alcohol prevents round drops of blood, which are needed for blood smears, from forming. Povidone–iodine (Betadine) preparations are not recommended for use on skin puncture sites because they can falsely elevate potassium, phosphorus, or uric acid determinations.[1]

■ SKIN PUNCTURE PROCEDURE

Microcollection by skin puncture involves many of the same steps used during venipuncture. If the phlebotomist is performing a heel stick, the infant's heel should be held firmly, with the forefinger at the arch of the foot and the thumb below and away from the puncture site (see Chapter 11). If a finger stick is being performed, the patient's finger should be held firmly, with the phlebotomist's thumb away from the puncture site (Box 9–1 and Figs. 9–1 and 9–2). Retractable safety puncture devices are currently available on the market and are widely used in place of the traditional sterile lancet (see Chapter 7).

BOX 9–1.   SAMPLE PROCEDURE FOR PERFORMANCE OF A FINGER PUNCTURE

Procedure for Skin Puncture or Finger Stick

1. Remember the following supplies: gloves, sterile cotton balls or gauze sponges (2 × 2), alcohol swabs, commercial puncture-device, sterile lancets, pipettes, plastic capillary tubes, microcollection tubes, diluting fluids, marking pen or pencil, and bandages. Exercise universal standard precautions, including the use of gloves.

2. Choose a finger that is not cold, cyanotic, or swollen. If possible, the stick should be at the tip of the third or fourth finger of the nondominant hand.

3. *Gently* massage the finger five or six times from base to tip to aid blood flow.

4. With an alcohol swab (70 percent isopropanol), cleanse the ball of the finger. Allow to air dry.

5. Remove the lancet from its protective paper without touching the tip.

6. Hold the patient's finger firmly with one hand and make a swift, deep puncture with the retractable safety puncture device or the lancet halfway between the center of the ball of the finger and its side. The cut should be made across the fingerprints to produce a large, round drop of blood.

7. Wipe the first drop of blood away with clean gauze.

8. *Gently* massage the finger from base to tip to obtain the proper amount of blood for the tests required.

9. Each type of microsample has different collection tube and blood volume requirements. Follow the appropriate manufacturer's instructions. For containers with additives, they should be inverted gently 8–10 times to mix the blood with the additives. Some containers will need to be sealed.

10. Label the specimens and/or outside containers.

11. Remove gloves, dispose of gloves in the proper biohazard container, and wash hands.

Notes

- If the patient's hands are cold, wrap one of them in a warm-to-hot towel 10 to 15 minutes before the puncture is performed. A free-flowing puncture is essential to obtain accurate test results. *Do not use excessive squeezing or massaging to obtain blood.*

- If the sample is not adequate and blood has stopped flowing from the puncture site, a new sterile lancet may be used to repuncture a *different* site.

Clinical Alert

During the opening of the package, if the device accidently touches clothing or brushes against the countertop, it is no longer sterile, and a new device should be opened and used.

Figure 9–1. The finger puncture should involve a quick, deep puncture across the fingerprints, not parallel to them.

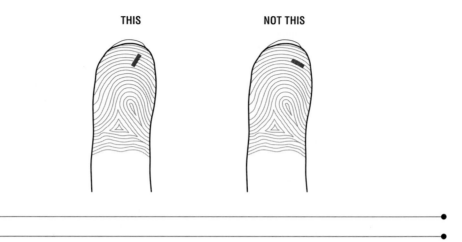

THIS

NOT THIS

Figure 9–2. Skin puncture procedure. A,B. Decontamination of the site. C. A quick puncture is made with a retractable safety puncture device or sterile lancet, and the first drop of blood is wiped off with sterile gauze. D. Blood is collected into a Unopette capillary tube by capillary action.

A

B

C

D

Figure 9–2. (*continued*)   E. Blood is collected into a microcollection tube. F. The patient presses sterile gauze on the finger to stop the bleeding. G. The Unopette capillary tube is inserted into the vial, and the specimen is mixed gently by inverting 8–10 times.

E

F

G

Clinical Alert

If the bone is repeatedly punctured, it can lead to **osteomyelitis,** which is an inflammation of the bone due to bacterial infection.

If a sterile lancet is used, the puncture should be in one sharp continuous movement, almost perpendicular to the site and across the fingerprint. If the puncture is made along the lines of the fingerprint, the blood tends to run down the finger. The average depth of skin puncture should be 2 to 3 mm for adults, and no more than 2.0 mm for small children, to avoid hitting a bone. Special lancets that control the depth of the puncture are available commercially. New laser devices are also now available as skin puncture alternatives. They provide a smaller hole (about 250 μm wide and 1 to 2 mm deep).

Figure 9–3. The blood smear. Blood smears can be made from venous or capillary blood. In both cases, the smears should be made from fresh drops of blood. With the capillary method, the finger puncture should be made in the usual way, and the first drop of blood wiped away. The slide can be touched to the second drop. It should be touched approximately 1/2 to 1 in. (1.3 to 2.5 cm) from the end of the slide. A. A second (spreader) slide should be placed in front of the drop of blood. B. The blood collector should pull the spreader slide into the drop, allowing blood to spread along the width of the slide. When the blood spreads almost to the edges, the spreader slide should be quickly and evenly pushed forward at an angle of approximately 30 degrees. The only downward pressure should be the weight of the spreader slide. The slide should be allowed to air dry. It should *not* be blown on.

If the venous method is being used, the needle should be touched to the slide immediately after it has been withdrawn. A drop about 1 to 2 mm in diameter will suffice. From this point on, the procedure is the same as for capillary blood smears. C. Good smears should have a **feathered edge**, i.e., a visible curved edge that thins out smoothly and resembles the tip of a bird's feather, and should cover approximately half the surface of the glass slide. No ridges, lines, or holes should be visible in the smear. Errors are often the result of too large a drop, too long a delay in making the smear, or using a chipped slide. D. Blood smears should be allowed to air dry after they are labeled.

A

B

C

D

Pressure from the phlebotomist's thumb may be eased and reapplied as the drops of blood appear. The area should not be massaged or milked excessively, however, because doing so causes hemolysis and contamination of the blood specimen with tissue and intracellular fluids. The first drop of blood should be removed with a dry, sterile pad, then capillary tubes (e.g., Unopette tubes [BD VACUTAINER Systems, *Preanalytical Solutions,* Franklin Lakes, NJ]) can be filled, using the second drop and subsequent blood. Blood smears can also be made from subsequent drops of blood. Capillary tubes are filled by **capillary action,** whereby blood flows freely into the tube on contact, without suction. (Refer to Chapter 7, Blood Collection Equipment.) If using a microcollection tube with additives, it is necessary to gently mix the blood in the tube by gentle inversion 8–10 times.

Figures 9–2 and 9–3 above indicate methods for making blood dilutions and blood smears for performing white blood cell **differentials.** (Chapter 7 provides illustrations of different types of microcollection tubes. Also, blood spot testing for newborn screening is covered in Chapter 11.) When filling the capillary tubes, the phlebotomist must not allow air bubbles to enter the tubes because air bubbles can cause erroneous results in many laboratory tests. Blood flow is better and air bubbles are less likely if the puncture site is held downward and gentle pressure is applied. Scooping or scraping up blood from the skin surface is not advised. However, some manufacturers provide devices to "scoop" or catch blood that is free flowing.[1] For a detailed discussion of microcollection devices, refer to Chapter 7.

If multiple specimens are being collected, the "order of draw" should be as follows according to the NCCLS:[1]

- EDTA specimen for hematology tests
- Other tubes with additives
- Nonadditive tubes

Capillary tubes should be carefully and safely sealed with a sealant or with other commercially available devices. They should be properly labelled immediately after collection and mixing.

LANCET DISPOSAL

Used disposable lancets should be placed into a rigid, puncture-resistant biohazard container with a lid.

◼ LABELING THE SPECIMEN AND COMPLETING THE INTERACTION

Hands should be washed after contact with each patient. *Before leaving the patient's side,* the phlebotomist must check the puncture site to make sure that the bleeding stopped. All tubes must be appropriately labeled immediately after collection and mixing, and the information on the labels confirmed. Several tubes may be placed together in a larger labeled container. All supplies and equipment that were brought in should be removed or discarded appropriately, and the phlebotomist should thank the patient. An adhesive bandage may be applied. Such bandages are not recommended for infants or young children, however, because of possible irritation and the potential of swallowing or aspirating a bandage.

SELF STUDY

Capillary Action   **Osteochondritis**
Cyanotic   **Osteomyelitis**
Differentials   **Tissue (Interstitial) Fluid**
Feathered Edge

STUDY QUESTIONS

The following may have *one* or *more* answers.

1. Which of the following are *not* sites for skin puncture?

    a. wrist   c. ankle
    b. vein   d. heel

2. Controlling the depth of lancet insertion during skin puncture prevents which of the following?

    a. puncturing a vein   c. excessive bleeding
    b. bacterial contamination d. osteomyelitis

3. A finger puncture should involve which of the following steps?

    a. puncturing parallel to fingerprint   c. puncturing across the fingerprint
    b. collecting the first drop   d. wiping away the first drop

4. Skin puncture is useful for patients who have which of the following conditions?

    a. obesity   c. fragile veins
    b. burns   d. thrombotic tendencies

5. Which fingers are used most often for skin puncture?

    a. thumb   c. third or fourth finger
    b. second, or index, finger d. fifth, or pinky, finger

6. Test(s) for which skin puncture cannot be used are

    a. routine hematology tests c. coagulation studies
    b. blood cultures   d. erythrocyte sedimentation rate (ESR) determinations

7. Blood from skin puncture is more like arterial blood than venous blood for which of the following reasons?
   - a. the skin has more arterioles
   - b. arterial pressure is stronger in capillaries
   - c. more arterial blood flows in capillaries
   - d. venous pressure is greater in capillaries

8. Capillary or microcollection tubes should be filled with blood in which of the following ways?
   - a. using a syringe to fill the tube
   - b. allowing tube to fill by itself using capillary action
   - c. using suction to pull blood into the tube
   - d. using the tube to scoop droplets off the skin carefully

9. Alcohol should be allowed to dry completely prior to skin puncture
   - a. to prevent stinging
   - b. to prevent dilution of sample
   - c. to prevent lysis of red blood cells
   - d. to allow formation of a round drop of blood

10. The best angle for using two glass slides to make a blood smear is approximately
    - a. 10 degrees
    - b. 15 degrees
    - c. 30 degrees
    - d. 90 degrees

Reference

1. National Committee for Clinical Laboratory Standards (NCCLS): *Procedures and Devices for the Collection of Diagnostic Blood Specimens by Skin Puncture,* Approved Standard, 4th ed. H4-A4. Villanova, PA; NCCLS: September, 1999.
2. Phelan, SE: Fingersticks on children, *Lab Med.* 1999; 30(9): 569–570.

TEN

■

Complications in Blood Collection

CHAPTER OUTLINE

Chapter Objectives
Complications Associated with
Blood Collection
- Fainting (Syncope)
- Failure to Draw Blood
- Hematomas
- Petechiae
- Excessive Bleeding
- Neurologic Complications
- Mastectomy
- Edema
- Obesity
- Intravenous Therapy
- Damaged, Sclerosed, or Occluded
  Veins
- Hemoconcentration
- Hemolysis
- Collapsed Veins
- Allergies
- Thrombosis

- Burned or Scarred Areas
- Infections
- Vomiting
Effects of Physical Disposition on Blood
Collection
- Basal State
- Diet
- Exercise
- Stress
- Diurnal Rhythms and Posture
- Age
- Tourniquet Pressure and Fist
  Pumping
- Other Factors Affecting the Patient
Interference of Drugs and Other
Substances in Blood
Specimen Rejection
Self Study
- Key Terms
- Study Questions

CHAPTER OBJECTIVES

Upon completion of Chapter 10, the learner is responsible for the following:

1. Describe physiologic and other complications related to phlebotomy procedures.
2. Explain how to prevent complications in blood collection and how to handle the complications that do occur.
3. List the effects of physical disposition on blood collection.
4. Discuss the types of substances that can interfere in clinical analysis of blood constituents and the methods used to prevent these occurrences.

Because complications can occur in blood collection, it is extremely important for the health care provider who is collecting the sample to know how to avoid complications if at all possible. If the complications are unavoidable, the health care worker must be knowledgeable of methods that will decrease the negative impact of the complication on the patient, on the quality of the blood sample, or on both.

■ COMPLICATIONS ASSOCIATED WITH BLOOD COLLECTION

FAINTING (SYNCOPE)

Many patients become dizzy and faint at the thought or sight of blood. Also, fasting patients sometimes become faint. Consequently, the health care worker should be aware of the patient's condition throughout the collection procedure. This can be done by asking ambulatory patients if they tend to faint or if they have ever previously fainted during blood collections. If so, they should be moved from a seated position to a lying position. Even for an ambulatory patient without a history of fainting, it is still extremely important to use a blood collection chair with a "locked" arm rest to avoid the possibility of a fall if he or she faints. If a seated patient feels faint, the needle should be removed, the patient's head should be lowered between the legs, and the patient should breathe deeply. If possible, the health care worker should ask for help and move the patient to a lying position. Talking to patients can often reassure them and divert their attention from the collection procedure. Bed-bound patients also experience fainting, or **syncope,** during blood collection, although rarely. In any case, the health care worker should stay with the patient at least 15 minutes until he or she recovers. A wet towel gently applied to the forehead or a glass of juice or water may help the patient feel better.

❗ Clinical Alert

If a patient faints during or after the procedure, the health care worker should try to terminate the venipuncture procedure immediately and make sure that the patient does not fall or become injured. Sometimes, controlling the situation is difficult because of the

Clinical Alert (*continued*) ❗

patient's physical size; however, the health care worker should use common sense about the safest position for a patient. If a patient has fainted and is in a secure position, the health care worker should quickly request assistance from the nursing staff or a physician. A patient who has fainted should recover fully before being allowed to leave and should be instructed not to drive a vehicle for at least 30 minutes. An incident report must be filed with the health care facility regarding the fainting incident and the immediate precautions and instructions provided to the patient to prevent the possibility of long-term complications (e.g., car accident after fainting incident).

FAILURE TO DRAW BLOOD

Several factors may cause the health care worker to "miss the vein." These factors include not inserting the needle deep enough, inserting the needle all the way through the vein, holding the needle bevel against the vein wall, or losing the vacuum in the tube (Fig. 10–1). During needle insertion, the health care worker's index finger can be used to help locate the vein. The needle may need to be moved or withdrawn somewhat, and redirected. In the geriatric patient, the vein may be "tough" during needle entry and may roll; such rolling can cause the needle to slip to the side of the vein instead of properly puncturing it. Thus the health care worker must securely anchor the vein prior to blood collection.

On occasion, a test tube will have no vacuum because of a manufacturer's error or tube leakage after a puncture. Consequently, the health care worker should carry an extra set of tubes in his or her pocket in case this happens during venipuncture. Also, needles for evacuated tube systems have been known to unscrew from the barrel during venipuncture. If this happens, the tourniquet should be released immediately, and the needle removed.

HEMATOMAS

Clinical Alert ❗

When the area around the puncture site starts to swell, usually blood is leaking into the tissues and causing a **hematoma.** This complication can occur when the needle has gone completely through the vein, the bevel opening is partially in the vein, or not enough pressure is applied to the site after puncture. This swelling results in a large bruise after several days (Fig. 10–2). If a hematoma begins to form, the tourniquet and the needle should be *removed immediately,* and pressure should be applied to the area for approximately 2 minutes. If the bleeding continues, a nurse should be notified.

Figure 10–1. Needle positioning and failure to draw blood. A. Correct insertion technique; blood flows freely into needle. B. Bevel on vein upper wall does not allow blood to flow. C. Bevel on vein lower wall does not allow blood to flow. D. Needle inserted too far. E. Needle partially inserted, which causes blood leakage into tissue. F. Collapsed vein.

Figure 10–2. Patient's hematoma several days after a venipuncture.

PETECHIAE

Petechiae, small red spots appearing on a patient's skin, indicate that minute amounts of blood have escaped into skin epithelium. This complication may be a result of a coagulation abnormality, such as platelet defects, and should be a warning to the health care worker that the patient's puncture site may bleed excessively.

EXCESSIVE BLEEDING

A patient usually stops bleeding at the venipuncture site within a few minutes. Patients on anticoagulant therapy, and/or those taking high dosages of arthritis medication or other medication, however, may bleed for a longer period. Thus, anytime a venipuncture is performed, pressure must be applied to the venipuncture site until the bleeding stops. The health care worker *must not* leave the patient until the bleeding stops or a nurse takes over to assess the patient's situation.

NEUROLOGIC COMPLICATIONS

Clinical Alert !

One rare complication that may occur during blood collection is seizures. If a patient begins to have a seizure, the health care worker should immediately release the tourniquet, remove the needle, attempt to hold pressure over the blood collection site, and call for help from the nursing station. No attempt should be made to place anything in the patient's mouth unless the health care worker is authorized to do so.

If the health care worker accidentally inserts the needle all the way through the vein, he or she may hit the nerve below the vein. If this happens, the patient will most likely have a sharp electric tingling sensation that radiates down the nerve. The health care worker should immediately release the tourniquet, remove the needle, and hold pressure over the blood collection site. An incident report on the occurrence should be completed and given to the supervisor.

MASTECTOMY

Clinical Alert !

A woman who has had a **mastectomy** (removal of a breast) may also have **lymphostasis** (no lymph flow) due to lymph node removal adjacent to the breast. Without lymph flow on that particular side of the body, the patient is highly susceptible to infection and some

(continued)

> **!** Clinical Alert (*continued*)
>
> chemical constituents may be altered. Also, the pressure from the tourniquet could lead to injuries in a patient who has had this type of surgery. Thus, venipuncture should never be performed on the same side as that of a mastectomy, unless approved by the physician. If the patient has had a double mastectomy, the back of the hands or finger sticks are alternative methods. However, the physician should be involved in determining suitable sites.

EDEMA

Some patients develop an abnormal accumulation of fluid in the intercellular spaces of the body. This swelling can be localized or diffused over a larger area of the body. The health care worker should avoid collecting blood from these sites because veins in these areas are difficult to palpate or stick, and the specimen may become contaminated with fluid.

OBESITY

Obese patients generally have veins that are difficult to visualize and palpate. If the vein is missed, the health care worker must be careful not to probe excessively with the needle because doing so ruptures red blood cells (RBCs), increases the concentration of intracellular contents, and releases some tissue-clotting factors.

INTRAVENOUS THERAPY

Every time a catheter is used, vein damage occurs. Circulatory blood is rerouted to collateral veins and can result in hemoconcentration. Consequently, patients on intravenous (IV) therapy for extended periods often have veins that are palpable and visible but damaged or occluded (blocked). Whenever a patient has an IV line, the arm with the IV line should not be used for venipuncture because the specimen will be diluted with IV fluid. Instead, the other arm or another site should be considered. Alternatively, sometimes the nurse or the physician can disconnect the IV line and draw blood from the needle that is already inserted. In this situation, the first few milliliters of the specimen should be discarded to remove the IV fluid, and a note should be made on the laboratory requisition form that this step was performed. (Refer to Chapter 12 for more detailed information about blood collection from intravenous lines.)

DAMAGED, SCLEROSED, OR OCCLUDED VEINS

Obstructed, or **occluded, veins** do not allow blood to flow through them; **sclerosed,** or hardened, veins are a result of inflammation and disease of the interstitial substances; and patients' veins that have been repeatedly punctured often become scarred and feel hard when palpated. Because blood is not easily collected from these sites, they should be avoided.

HEMOCONCENTRATION

An increased concentration of larger molecules and formed elements in the blood is called **hemoconcentration.** Several factors can cause this complication, including prolonged (i.e., longer than 1 minute) tourniquet application; massaging, squeezing, or probing a site; long-term IV therapy; and sclerosed or occluded veins.

HEMOLYSIS

When RBCs are lysed, hemoglobin is released and serum, which is normally straw colored, becomes tinged with pink or red. If a specimen is grossly hemolyzed, the serum appears very dark red. **Hemolysis** can be caused by improper phlebotomy techniques, such as using a needle that is too small, pulling a syringe plunger back too fast, expelling the blood vigorously into a tube, shaking or mixing tubes vigorously, or performing blood collection before the alcohol has dried at the collection site. Hemolysis causes falsely increased results for many analytes, including potassium, magnesium, iron, lactate dehydrogenase, phosphorus, ammonia, and total protein.[1] These problems can easily be prevented with appropriate handling. Hemolysis may also be the result of physiological abnormalities. The health care worker should make a note on the requisition form whenever he or she notices that a specimen is hemolyzed.

COLLAPSED VEINS

If a syringe plunger is withdrawn too quickly during venipuncture or the vacuum draw of a tube is too great, the vein may collapse, especially when blood is being collected from smaller veins (see Fig. 10–1F) and veins in geriatric patients. Thus the blood collector should pull slowly on the syringe plunger or use an evacuated tube with a smaller volume during the collection process on patients with smaller veins and geriatric patients. A collapsed vein should *not* be probed with the needle.

ALLERGIES

Clinical Alert

Some patients are allergic to iodine or other solutions used to disinfect a puncture site. If a patient indicates that he or she is allergic to a solution, all efforts should be made to use an alternative method. In addition, some patients are allergic to latex. Several vendors have nonlatex tourniquets, gloves, and bandages for use with patients who have this allergy.

THROMBOSIS

Thrombi are solid masses derived from blood constituents that reside in the blood vessels. A thrombus may partially or fully occlude a vein (or artery), and such occlusion will make venipuncture more difficult.

BURNED OR SCARRED AREAS

 Clinical Alert

Areas that have been burned or scarred should be avoided during phlebotomy. Burned areas are very sensitive and susceptible to infection, whereas veins under scarred areas are difficult to palpate.

INFECTIONS

The health care worker should remember at all times that many patients have transmittable diseases (e.g., hepatitis) and that likewise, he or she can pass an infection to a patient. (For precautionary techniques, refer to Chapter 4, Infection Control, and Chapter 5, Safety and First Aid.)

VOMITING

Sometimes the thought or sight of blood by the patient before or during blood collection leads to vomiting. If this reaction occurs, have the patient take deep breaths and use a cold compress on his or her head. Also, inform the patient's physician of this complication.

■ EFFECTS OF PHYSICAL DISPOSITION ON BLOOD COLLECTION

BASAL STATE

Blood specimens that will be used to determine the concentrations of body constituents, such as glucose, cholesterol, triglycerides, electrolytes, and proteins, should be collected when the patient is in a **basal state**—that is, in the early morning, approximately 12 hours after the last ingestion of food. The results of laboratory tests on basal state specimens are more reliable because normal values are most often determined from specimens collected during this time. Several factors, such as diet, exercise, emotional stress, obesity, menstrual cycle, pregnancy, *diurnal variations,* posture, tourniquet application, and chemical constituents (alcohol or drugs), cause changes in the basal state.

DIET

To ensure that the patient is in the basal state, the physician must require the patient to fast overnight. The term **fasting** refers to abstinence from food and beverages (except water). The required time period necessary for abstaining varies with the test procedures to be performed. Before collecting a specimen, the health care worker should ask the patient if he or she has eaten. Blood composition is significantly altered after meals and consequently is unsuitable for many clinical chemistry tests. If the patient has eaten, and the physician still needs the test, the word *nonfasting* must be written on the requisition form, noted directly on the specimen, or indicated in the organization's computer system.[2]

Inadequate patient instructions are often the cause of mistakes in specimen collection. The health care worker may be asked to explain fasting restrictions to a patient. In such cases, these restrictions must be explained clearly and in detail. Some patients assume that the term *fasting* refers to abstaining from food *and* water. Abstaining from water can result in dehydration, which can alter test results. Thus, the health care worker must ensure that the patient understands what is required of him or her. Written instructions can be given, if available.

Gaining the patient's understanding and cooperation is important and is determined by the professional behavior and the degree of confidence displayed by the health care worker. Casual instructions are apt to be taken lightly by the patient or even forgotten. A health care worker who is organized, attentive, and skilled and who emphasizes important points of the procedure is more likely to get patient cooperation and an accurate test result, and to make the patient more comfortable.

If a procedure involves some discomfort or inconvenience, the patient should be informed. For example, if blood is to be drawn for a timed blood glucose level determination, the patient needs to fast for 8 to 12 hours. Prolonged fasting, however, has been shown to falsely alter blood test results.[2] The health care worker can inform the patient that several specimens will be collected at timed intervals and that he or she may drink water, but that coffee and tea should be avoided because they cause a transitory fluctuation in the blood sugar level.

Normally, serum is clear, light yellow, or straw colored. **Turbid** serum appears cloudy or "milky" and can be a result of bacterial contamination or high lipid levels in the blood. Turbidity is primarily caused by ingestion of fatty substances, such as meat, butter, cream, and cheese, or can occur when an intralipid supplement is included in parenteral nutrition preparations. If a patient has recently eaten fatty substances, he or she may have a temporarily elevated lipid level, and the serum will appear **lipemic,** or cloudy. Because lipemic serum does not represent a basal state and may indicate some chemical abnormalities,[2] a note on the requisition form about the appearance of the serum may be useful to the physician.

EXERCISE

Muscular activity, as a result of moderate or excessive exercise, has a marked effect on laboratory test results, especially when the levels of lactic acid, creatinine, fatty acids, some amino acids, proteins, and some enzymes are being tested. Most of these values, except certain enzyme levels, return to baseline shortly after the exercise stops. The levels of enzymes, such as creatine phosphokinase (CPK), aspartate aminotransferase (AST), and lactate dehydrogenase (LD), can, however, remain elevated as long as 24 hours after a person engages in 1 hour of moderate-to-strenuous exercise.[2]

Research suggests that exercise also has some effects on hemostasis. Some reports indicate that physical exercise activates coagulation, fibrinolysis, and platelet formation. Because different types of exercise were studied, other reports cite conflicting results or no changes in measured hemostatic parameters. Nevertheless, most researchers conclude that some hemostatic changes do occur after strenuous exercise.[3]

STRESS

Patients are often frightened, nervous, and overly anxious, especially prior to blood collection. These emotional stresses can cause a transient elevation in the white blood cell (WBC) count, a transient decrease in serum iron levels, and abnormal hormone (e.g., cortisol, aldosterone, renin, thyroid-stimulating hormone [TSH], prolactin) values.[3,4] Also, mental anxiety can increase blood concentrations of albumin, fibrinogen, glucose, cholesterol, and insulin.[4] Newborns who have been crying violently will have WBC counts that are 140 percent above resting baseline counts. Even mild crying has been shown to increase WBC counts 113 percent. These elevated counts return to baseline values within 1 hour. Consequently, blood samples for WBC counts should be taken approximately 1 hour after a crying episode.[5] Anxiety that results in hyperventilation also causes acid–base imbalances, increased lactate levels, and increased fatty acid levels.[2]

DIURNAL RHYTHMS AND POSTURE

Diurnal rhythms are body fluid fluctuations during the day. Certain hormone levels decrease in the afternoon (e.g., cortisol, adrenocorticotropic hormone [ACTH] TSH, T_4 plasma renin activity, aldosterone, insulin, iron), whereas eosinophil counts increase. Thus, collecting specimens during the designated time periods is important for proper clinical evaluation.

Posture changes are also known to vary laboratory test results of some chemical constituents (e.g., aldosterone and plasma renin activity). This consideration is important when inpatient and outpatient results are being compared. Thus, blood collection should be performed under standardized posture conditions. Changing from a **supine** (or lying) position to a sitting or standing position causes body water to shift from intravascular to interstitial compartments (in tissues). Certain larger molecules cannot filter into the tissue; therefore, they concentrate in the blood. Enzyme, protein, lipid, iron, and calcium levels are significantly increased with changes in position.[6] For example, when the patient's sample is collected while he or she is standing, total cholesterol results will be approximately 10% higher, triglycerides 12% higher, and HDL cholesterol 7% higher than in samples collected when the patient is lying down. The standard position for these blood collections is with the patient sitting.[7] These effects can be more pronounced in patients with congestive heart failure, hepatic disorders, and other, edematous disorders.

AGE

Laboratory test results vary considerably during the stages of life: infancy, childhood (pediatric population), adulthood, and older adulthood (geriatric population). For example, blood cholesterol and triglyceride values increase as a person ages. Various hormone levels, such as estrogen and growth hormone (GH) levels, decrease in geriatric women. GH levels are also decreased in geriatric men.

TOURNIQUET PRESSURE AND FIST PUMPING

Laboratory test results can be falsely elevated or decreased if the tourniquet pressure is too tight or is maintained too long. The pressure from the tourniquet causes biological analytes to leak from the tissue cells into the blood, or vice versa. For example, plasma cholesterol, iron, lipid, protein, and potassium levels will be falsely elevated if the tourniquet pressure is too tight or prolonged. Significant elevations may be seen with as short as a 3-minute application of the tourniquet.[6] In addition, some enzyme levels can be falsely elevated or decreased because of tourniquet pressure that is too tight or prolonged. Also, pumping of the fist before venipuncture should be avoided because it leads to an increase in the plasma potassium, lactate, and phosphate concentrations.

OTHER FACTORS AFFECTING THE PATIENT

Many other factors can affect laboratory test results. Gender and pregnancy have an influence on laboratory testing; thus, reference ranges are often noted according to gender. Geographic factors, such as altitude, temperature, and humidity, also affect normal baseline values. Collecting blood during home health care visits may entail traveling to different regions than the location of the laboratory. Thus, geographic information of this type should be provided on the laboratory requisition slip in order to be considered in the patient's tests results.

Medications may also alter laboratory test results significantly. Consequently, physicians must work closely with pharmacy and laboratory staff to rule out laboratory test results that are altered because the patient is taking medication.

■ INTERFERENCE OF DRUGS AND OTHER SUBSTANCES IN BLOOD

Many prescribed drugs can interfere with clinical laboratory determinations or can physiologically alter the levels of blood constituents measured in the clinical laboratory. The interference of drugs and other substances is so complicated and dependent on the chemical procedures used that only general recommendations are described in this section.

The direct analytic interference of drugs is decreasing with the advent of more specific and sensitive chemical procedures. The physiologically induced abnormalities from various types of drugs, however, are the major causes of interference from medications. Drugs administered to alleviate an illness can induce physiologic abnormalities in one or more of the following systems: hepatic, hematologic, hemostatic, muscular, pancreatic, and renal. The erroneous results may obscure the clinical diagnosis.

Prior to laboratory measurement of chemical constituents, the attending physician should take the necessary precautions in prescribing drugs to the patient. If the patient must be maintained on medication that may cause interferences in laboratory assays, the medication name should be written on the laboratory request form. Unless interference of medications can be avoided by ordering different laboratory assays, medications should be discontinued if possible, and assays should be repeated when false laboratory values are suspected.

Direct analytic interference in laboratory determinations is least likely to occur in blood assays because drug concentrations are usually low. Some drugs or drug metabolites in blood can, however, directly cause falsely decreased or falsely elevated values in laboratory analyses.

A more complete list of such drugs can be found in Young's *Effects of Drugs on Clinical Laboratory Test Results.*[8]

Interference from medications usually causes falsely elevated values rather than falsely decreased values. Some drugs, such as acetaminophen (Tylenol) and erythromycin, can increase serum AST and bilirubin levels and, thus, falsely create a clinical interpretation of hepatic dysfunction without the true presence of hepatic abnormality.[9] Drug-induced elevations of blood constituents can be mistakenly interpreted as falsely increased or normal, when the true values are in the normal range or the subnormal range, respectively.

In addition to prescribed oral medications, intravenous injections of medications and dyes can interfere with laboratory test results. For example, the results of laboratory tests performed after fluorescein angiography may be erroneous owing to interference by the intravenous fluorescein.[10] The results for blood creatinine, cortisol, and digoxin determinations are altered by this dye. Consequently, if the health care worker, nurse, or clinical assistant collects blood in a cardiology section or a specialized health care institution for heart patients, he or she needs to be alert to this potential for laboratory test interference. If he or she is aware of collecting blood from a patient who just had a dye injection, this information must be communicated promptly to the specimen collection supervisor.

Physiologically, drugs can alter blood analytes through various metabolic reactions; the production of blood cells and platelets, as well as their survival times, can be changed. Chemotherapeutic drugs can lead to a decrease in all forms of blood cellular elements and, thus, their metabolic and immunologic processes.

A variety of medications are toxic to the liver (Table 10–1) and, thus, can lead to acute hepatic necrosis.[8] In turn, the hepatic dysfunction leads to an increase in the concentration of blood liver enzymes, such as alanine aminotransferase (ALT), alkaline phosphatase (ALP), and LD. Also, the production of globulins and clotting factors is decreased in patients with drug-induced hepatotoxicity.

Patients receiving medications that may result in renal impairment should be monitored for a possible electrolyte imbalance and elevation of blood urea nitrogen (BUN) levels. Antihypertensive agents given for a long period to lower high blood pressure can lead to kidney damage if the patient is not monitored closely.

Pancreatitis can be caused by corticosteroids, estrogens, and diuretics and causes elevations of serum amylase and lipase values. Aspirin causes **hypobilirubinemia** (a decrease in bilirubin) by expelling bilirubin from the plasma to the surrounding tissue cells.[11]

In addition to medications, other substances such as smoking may affect several laboratory tests' results. Through the action of nicotine from the tobacco, the blood concentrations of glucose, growth hormone, cholesterol and triglyceride increase. Also, alcohol consumption can skew laboratory tests' results, especially hematology results.

Table 10–1. Drugs Toxic to the Liver

Salicylates	Penicillin	Chlorpromazine
Mitomycin	Isoniazid	Methyldopa
Actinomycin	Halothane	Acetohexamide
Thiazides	Chloramphenicol	Chlorpropamide
Trifluoperazine	Sulfamethoxazole	Paramethadione
Sulfachlorpyridazine	Tetracycline	
Phenytoin	Acetaminophen	

Adapted from Sher, PP: Drug interferences with clinical laboratory tests. *Drugs*.1982; 24:24; and Sherlock, S: Progress report: Hepatic reaction to drugs. *Gut*.1979; 20:634.

The health care worker collecting the blood specimen is the link between the clinical laboratory and the patient. Laboratory tests are often ordered without knowledge of the drugs taken or inhaled (i.e., nicotine) or consumed (i.e., alcohol) by a person. Yet, as discussed previously, these drugs will lead to falsely elevated or decreased values. Sometimes during blood collection, a patient will mention that he or she has taken over-the-counter drugs, such as Tylenol, or that he or she has just smoked a cigarette. It is important for the health care worker to communicate the patient's name and the possible drug interference to the clinical laboratory supervisor in charge of specimen collection. The supervisor can then communicate with the attending physician and determine whether the medication or drug will interfere in the laboratory assays. The follow-up communication can lead to better patient care by preventing the presence of interfering substances in laboratory specimens.

■ SPECIMEN REJECTION

Each department or section in the clinical laboratory should establish its own guidelines for specimen rejection. In general, the factors shown in Table 10–2 should be considered.

When a problem arises, the appropriate investigational channels should be followed. The health care provider who drew the specimen and his or her supervisor should try to solve the problem initially. Other personnel may be involved as needed. Communication and honesty are the keys to an efficient and reliable health care environment.

Table 10–2. Complications Leading to Blood Specimen Rejection

Hemolyzed specimen (except for tests in which hemolysis does not interfere)

Nonfasting specimen

Anticoagulated blood containing clots

Improper specimen transportation (e.g., blood gas specimen not transported in slurry of ice water)

Improper blood collection tube

Variation in patient's posture (e.g., aldosterone level changes depending on patient sitting or lying for blood collection)

Lipemic specimen

Insufficient quantity of blood in collection tube

Discrepancies between requisition form and labeled tube (e.g., names, dates, times)

Unlabelled tube

Outdated equipment, supplies, or reagents (i.e., vacuum decreases in old blood collection tube; silicon coating tends to break down with age, etc.)

Contaminated specimen

SELF STUDY

KEY TERMS

Basal State
Diurnal Rhythms
Fasting
Hematoma
Hemoconcentration
Hemolysis
Hypobilirubinemia
Lipemic
Lymphostasis

Mastectomy
Occluded Veins
Petechiae
Sclerosed Veins
Supine
Syncope
Thrombi
Turbid

STUDY QUESTIONS

The following questions may have *one* or *more* answers.

1. Which of the following factors result in failure to draw blood during venipuncture?

   a. losing the vacuum in the tube
   b. tying the tourniquet too tightly

   c. inserting the needle through the vein
   d. puncturing a sclerosed vein

2. Hematomas during venipuncture result from which of the following?

   a. needle bevel is against vein wall
   b. needle bevel is partially inserted in the vein

   c. needle is occluded
   d. patient has coagulation problems

3. Hemoconcentration can be caused by which of the following?

   a. long-term IV therapy
   b. lengthy tourniquet application

   c. excessive needle probing
   d. sclerosed or occluded veins

4. Which of the following is a solid mass derived from blood constituents and can occlude a vein (or an artery)?

   a. hemolyzed RBC
   b. hemolyzed WBC

   c. thrombus
   d. triglyceride

5. If blood is to be drawn for a timed blood glucose level determination, the patient must fast for how long?

   a. 4 to 6 hours
   b. 6 to 8 hours

   c. 8 to 12 hours
   d. 14 to 16 hours

6. Which of the following laboratory test results are affected most if the patient is not fasting?

   a. AST and CPK
   b. triglycerides and glucose
   c. cortisol and testosterone
   d. complete blood cell (CBC) count and prothrombin time

7. An abnormal accumulation of fluid in the intercellular spaces of the body that is localized or diffused is referred to as which of the following?

   a. hemoconcentration
   b. edema
   c. atherosclerosis
   d. hemolysis

8. If a patient is taking high doses of Tylenol, which of the following analyte results is most likely to be affected?

   a. serum bilirubin
   b. CPK
   c. blood glucose
   d. blood cholesterol

9. If the tourniquet is applied for longer than 3 minutes, which of the following analytes will most likely become falsely elevated?

   a. potassium
   b. bilirubin
   c. GGT
   d. parathyroid hormone

10. Emotional stress, such as anxiety or fear, can lead to alterations of which of the following analytes?

    a. serum iron
    b. WBCs
    c. cortisol
    d. RBCs

References

1. Meites, S, ed.: *Pediatric Clinical Chemistry, Reference (Normal) Values,* 3rd ed. Washington, DC; AACC Press: 1989.

2. Statland, BE, Winkel, P: Preparing patients and specimens for laboratory testing. In: Henry, JB, ed.: *Clinical Diagnosis and Management by Laboratory Methods.* Philadelphia; WB Saunders: 1991.

3. Rudmann, SV: The effects of exercise on hemostasis: A review of the literature and implications for research, *Am J Med Technol.* 1987;4(5):215.

4. Guder, WG, Narayanan, S, Wisser, H, et al.: *Samples: From the Patient to the Laboratory.* Germany; Git Verlag Pub: 1996.

5. Becton-Dickinson and Company: *Blood Specimen Collection by Skin Puncture in Infants.* East Rutherford, NJ; Becton-Dickinson and Company: 1982.

6. Statland, BE, Winkle, P, Bokelund, H: Factors contributing to intra-individual variation of serum constituents: Effects of posture and tourniquet application on variation of serum constituents in healthy subjects, *Clin Chem.* 1974;*20*:1513.

7. McNamara, JR: Cardiovascular disease: Laboratory testing adds important information to risk profile, *Clin Lab News.* 2000; *26*(10):12–16.

8. Young, DS: *Effects of Drugs on Clinical Laboratory Tests,* 5th ed. Washington, DC; AACC Press: 2000.

9. Sherlock, S: Progress report: Hepatic reaction to drugs, *Gut.* 1979;20:634.

10. Elin, RJ, Bloom, JN, Herman, DC, et al.: Interference by intravenous fluorescein with laboratory tests, *Clin Chem.* 1989;*35*(6):1159.

11. Routh, J, Paul, W: Assessment of interference by aspirin with some assays commonly done in the clinical laboratory, *Clin Chem.* 1976;22:837.

PHLEBOTOMY CASE STUDY

■

Ambulatory Health Care Collections

Ms. Jeanne Peterson is a health care provider who contracts with two community hospitals to make home health care visits. This morning as she arrived at Lake Mountain Hospital late due to an early winter snowstorm, she noticed she had seven home visits. She quickly threw blood collection equipment in her lockable container and hurried to her first patient, Ms. Verle Ragsdale, an 82-year-old African American woman, who has type II diabetes with myocardial complications. Her physician had requested a complete chemistry profile and protime, in addition to a physical examination. After Ms. Peterson checked Ms. Ragsdale's vital signs, she decided to collect Ms. Ragsdale's blood with a winged infusion blood collection set due to the fragility of her veins. She prepared the site for blood collection and after opening a 25-gauge safety winged infusion needle set, she inserted the needle into the patient's vein in her hand and first collected blood in a light blue–topped tube for the protime, followed by blood collection into a red speckled–topped vacuum tube. After completing the physical exam and blood collection, she labeled the tubes, discarded the biohazardous blood collection items in her biohazardous disposal container, and left Ms. Ragsdale's home with the collected blood and health care equipment, including the blood collection items.

Next, she traveled over the slippery, snow-covered roads to Mr. Ben Sadler's home, a 32-year-old white hemophiliac who had acquired hepatitis C from a blood transfusion. His physician had requested a liver profile. Ms. Peterson introduced herself to Mr. Sadler and prepared her blood collection supplies and equipment for blood collection for Mr. Sadler. As she checked Mr. Sadler's veins, she decided to use a butterfly needle in Mr. Sadler's lower arm due to the sclerosed veins in the antecubital fossa area on both arms. She looked for a blood collection set in her supplies but only found a 23-gauge needle, separate tubing, and a separate luer lok. She put the pieces together and found a needle holder assembly and red-speckled collection tube. After attaching the various pieces, hoping they would work together, she prepared Mr. Sadler's arm for blood collection. She inserted the needle into his vein and as she pushed the tube onto the needle holder assembly, the Luer-Lok became disengaged and splattered blood over Ms. Peterson's laboratory coat and into her face. She immediately pulled the tourniquet off of Mr. Sadler's arm, pulled the needle out of his vein, cleaned the area around him, and ran to his bathroom to wash the blood from her face and eyes.

QUESTIONS

1. Did the health care provider use the proper order of draw for Ms. Ragsdale's laboratory tests? Explain.

2. Was the proper blood collection procedure used for obtaining blood from Ms. Ragsdale? Explain.

3. Was the proper blood collection procedure used for obtaining blood from Mr. Sadler? Explain.

See Answers in Appendix.

PHLEBOTOMY CASE STUDY

■

Venipuncture Site Selection

The medical laboratory technician, Sara Wong, went to collect blood from a 65-year-old hospitalized patient, Mary McDonald. Mrs. McDonald was a diabetic. She had recently undergone a partial mastectomy on her right side. The area around the mastectomy appeared swollen. She had an IV going just below the antecubital area of her left arm. The ordered tests were CBC, differential, and electrolytes. Sara carefully selected a site and was successful on the first attempt to collect the blood samples.

QUESTIONS

1. What would be the preferred site and method of choice for the phlebotomy procedure for this patient?

2. Explain why other sites were eliminated.

3. What special documentation (if any) might be helpful for this phlebotomy procedure?

4. List several techniques that can facilitate the selection of a suitable site.

See Answers in Appendix.

PHLEBOTOMY CASE STUDY

■

Finding the Right Site

A 68-year-old woman, Mrs. Triplet, comes for her annual check up to the oncology clinic. After her visit with her doctor, she is sent to the laboratory to have some "routine" blood specimens collected. The phlebotomist correctly identifies her, prepares the site, supplies, and equipment and inquires about which arm Mrs. Triplet prefers to have the puncture performed on. Mrs. Triplet says, "Well, it doesn't really matter to me but I had my mastectomy done 5 years ago on this side and they usually stick me over here," as she points to her left arm.

QUESTIONS

1. How should the phlebotomist proceed?
2. Why would a mastectomy make any difference in site selection?
3. Does the length of time after a mastectomy make any difference?

See Answers in Appendix.

SPECIAL PROCEDURES AND POINT-OF-CARE TESTING

THE PRACTICE OF PHLEBOTOMY INVOLVES specialized duties and functions in certain circumstances. Part IV describes the special procedures and work settings that are becoming part of the expanding role of health care workers. Each new activity can be learned alone or along with other, more routine duties. For some phlebotomists, a procedure that was previously "special" and off limits is now routine. For others, phlebotomy may require special training in pediatrics, geriatrics, or IV therapy.

Chapter 11, Pediatric Procedures, focuses on the special attention and technical skills necessary for dealing with infants and children. The chapter describes effective communication with children and parents; different procedures for blood collection, including heel sticks, neonatal screening procedures, and the dorsal hand vein technique; and special concerns regarding diagnostic testing for children.

Chapter 12, Arterial, Intravenous (IV), and Special Collection Procedures, covers site selection and puncture procedures for blood collection for arterial blood gas determinations; the Allen test; bleeding-time tests; blood cultures; glucose and lactose tolerance tests; and therapeutic drug monitoring (TDM) tests. Also discussed are blood collections through intravenous lines, central venous catheters, blood donor room collections, and emergency room blood collections.

Chapter 13, Elderly, Home, and Long-term Care Collections, highlights procedures that are becoming more routine in the care and monitoring of patients in these settings. Emphasis is on point-of-care testing, such as glucose monitoring, blood gas and electrolyte analysis, and cholesterol screening.

Chapter 14, Urinalysis and Body Fluid Collections, describes the various alternative procedures for urine and other body fluid collections, including cerebrospinal fluid, seminal fluid, amniotic fluid, and specimens for microbiological cultures. Emphasis is on proper collection and safe handling of the specimens.

Chapter 15, Specimen Collection for Forensic Toxicology, Workplace Testing, Sports Medicine, and Related Areas, describes specimen collections related to drug testing in forensic toxicology and workplace testing. Emphasis is on the role of the health care worker in appropriate sample collection, handling various types of samples, detecting altered specimens, securing the chain of custody, and transporting the specimen.

ELEVEN

■

Pediatric Procedures

CHAPTER OUTLINE

Chapter Objectives
Age-Specific Care Considerations
Preparing Child and Parent
- Psychological Response to Needles and Pain
- Room Location
- Equipment Preparation for a Friendlier Environment
- Positions for Restraining a Child
- Combative Patients
- Interventions to Alleviate Pain
- Sucrose Nipple or Pacifier
Prevention of Disease Transmission
- Precautions to Protect the Child
- Latex Allergy or Alert

Pediatric Phlebotomy Procedures
- Microcapillary Skin Puncture
- Heel Stick
- Neonatal Screening
- Finger Stick
- Venipuncture
- Collecting Blood from IV Lines
Self Study
- Key Terms
- Study Questions

CHAPTER OBJECTIVES

Upon completion of Chapter 11, the learner is responsible for the following:

1. Describe fears or concerns that children in different developmental stages might have toward the blood collection process.

2. List suggestions that might be appropriate for parental behavior during a venipuncture or skin puncture.

3. Identify puncture sites for a heel stick on an infant and describe the procedure.

4. Describe the venipuncture sites for infants and young children.

5. Discuss the types of equipment and supplies that must be used during microcollection and venipuncture of infants and children.

6. Describe the procedure for screening neonates for phenylketonuria (PKU).

Drawing blood from a pediatric patient requires much expertise and knowledge. Not all **pediatric phlebotomies** are finger sticks, so the novice health care worker must study anatomy and physiology, be familiar with special types of equipment that are available, observe the various techniques as they are performed by an experienced health care worker, and practice the techniques to develop the necessary skills.

Performing venipunctures on young patients is technically and emotionally challenging for the health care worker because of these patients' small size and because children are less emotionally and psychologically prepared to cope with pain. Therefore, a successful outcome requires the use of good interpersonal skills in dealing with children and their concerned, apprehensive parents.[1]

With proper training in technique and an understanding of pediatric psychological development, the delicate task of drawing blood from a frightened child need not strike fear or dread in the heart of the health care worker. Skills should be perfected on older children first, then, when confidence is attained, venipunctures can be attempted on younger children. When learning the techniques, the health care worker should remember to ask for help if needed and to allow adequate time to develop the necessary skills.

■ AGE-SPECIFIC CARE CONSIDERATIONS

Age-specific care considerations are shown in Table 11–1. It describes not only the fears and concerns of the pediatric patient at various ages, but also suggests parental involvement at each stage, and provides competencies and tips for the phlebotomist.

■ PREPARING CHILD AND PARENT

Preparing the child and the parent for the blood collection procedure involves the following steps:

1. Introduce yourself. Be warm, friendly, establish eye contact, and show that you are concerned about the child's health and comfort. When you interact with a pediatric patient and his or her parent, you should instill a sense of trust and confidence in the parent and the child. A calm, confident approach is the first step in limiting their anxiety and obtaining their cooperation.

2. Correctly identify the patient. A hospitalized infant usually has an identification bracelet on his or her ankle. Newborns who are not yet named are usually referred to by their last names (e.g., Baby Boy Smith, Baby Girl Jones) and are identified by a unique identification number. If the mother is still in the hospital after delivery, the baby may wear a bracelet that is cross-referenced to the mother for breastfeeding times and so forth. Keeping identifications straight is always crucial, but especially so when specimens from twin babies must be collected and labeled.

Table 11-1. Age-specific Care Considerations and Competencies for Phlebotomists

AGE	FEARS AND CONCERNS	COMMUNICATION	COMFORT	SAFETY	PARENT BEHAVIOR
0–6 months	• Totally dependent on and trusts parents and other adults	• Introduce yourself to caregiver • Explain procedures	• Keep patient warm • Warm site of puncture if needed • Parent may hold child • Use very gentle approach • Use of a distraction, such as light pen, key ring, or bell, may minimize fear	• Keep side rails up during procedure • Do not leave any supplies or discarded items on bed • Encourage parent to hold or cuddle infant after procedure • Use appropriate microcollection supplies and equipment	• Parent may hold child as an aid to the phlebotomist and to provide comfort
6–12 months	• Fear of strangers • Fear of separation from parent • Limited language use	• Introduce yourself to caregiver • Talk slowly to infant • Try to make eye contact with infant	• Keep patient warm • Warm site of puncture if needed • Allow familiar health care worker to perform procedure • Allow parent to be in close proximity • Allow child to use pacifier, hold teddy, blanket, or other comforting items	• Do not separate from caregiver unless absolutely necessary • Keep side rails up • Do not leave any supplies or discarded items on bed • Encourage parent to hold or cuddle infant after procedure • Use appropriate microcollection supplies and equipment	• Parent may assist by holding, explaining to, and comforting the child • Parent may help identify comforting toy

(continued)

309

Table 11-1. (continued)

AGE	FEARS AND CONCERNS	COMMUNICATION	COMFORT	SAFETY	PARENT BEHAVIOR
1–3 years	• Self-centered • Fear of injury • Fear of long separation from parent	• Introduce yourself to both child and caregiver • Child will understand simple commands and may choose to cooperate • Take it slowly, do not rush patient, he or she needs time to think about your requests • Allow child to touch supplies but dispose if they become contaminated • Ask parent to also explain procedure in familiar terms	• Keep patient warm • Warm site of puncture if needed • Allow familiar health care worker to perform procedure • Allow parent to be in close proximity • Allow child to use pacifier, hold teddy, blanket, or other comforting items	• Try not to separate from parent unless absolutely necessary. If needed, reinforce that it is only for a short period of time • Keep side rails up • Do not leave supplies or discarded items on bed • Use appropriate microcollection supplies and equipment	• Parent may assist by holding, explaining to, and comforting the child • Parent may help identify comforting toy • Encourage parent to praise child after procedure
3–5 years	• Self-centered • Fear of injury • Enjoys pretending and role playing	• Introduce yourself • Talk to child in simple terms • Allow child to touch equipment • Try using familiar cartoon characters (Disney, Sesame Street) in the explanation • Perhaps use toys to demonstrate procedure • Child may pretend he or she is the doctor and will "help" with the procedure • Provide tokens for bravery	• Allow child to have familiar things or people near by • Give child time to verbalize his or her fears	• May tolerate separation from parent • Able to recognize danger and obey simple commands • Needs close supervision • Keep side rails up • Do not leave supplies or discarded items on bed • Use appropriate microcollection supplies and equipment	• Parent may be present to provide emotional support and to assist in obtaining the child's cooperation • Encourage praise for bravery

Table 11-1. (continued)

AGE	FEARS AND CONCERNS	COMMUNICATION	COMFORT	SAFETY	PARENT BEHAVIOR
6–12 years	• Less dependent on parents • Fear losing self-control • More willing to participate • Tries to be independent • Curious	• Introduce yourself • Child may be interested in health concepts, "why" and "how" • Explain "why" the blood is needed • Involve child in the procedure	• Try not to embarrass the child but offer them a comforting toy or familiar object • May want parent to hold child's hand • Take it slowly, allow time for repeat questions • Allow child some input on decisions (e.g., color of bandage, etc.)	• Side rails should be left up after procedure • Do not leave supplies or discarded items on bed • Use appropriate microcollection supplies and equipment	• Child may ask parent to leave room
13–17 years	• Actively involved in anything concerning the body • More independent • Embarrassed to show fear • Needs privacy • May act hostile to mask fear	• Introduce yourself • Use adult vocabulary, do not "talk down" • Explain procedure thoroughly • Ask if he or she would like to help with the procedure • Ask what might make them more comfortable • Allow time for questions or to handle supplies	• Maintain privacy • Take extra time for explanations and or preparation • Offer them the opportunity to have parent close by • Give them time to recover after the procedure if they have cried	• Use same strategies as adult • Use appropriate collection supplies and equipment depending on the size of the individual and the physical and emotional tolerance to procedure	• Child may not want parent to be present
Children with special problems or mental disabilities	• Fears are similar to the behaviors of the developmental level • Need relaxed, gentle approach	• Use strategies that are appropriate for the developmental stage	• Use strategies that are appropriate for the developmental stage	• Use strategies that are appropriate for the developmental stage	• Use strategies that are appropriate for the developmental stage

3. Find out about the child's past experience with blood collections. This can be accomplished easily by asking whether the child has ever had blood collected. The child and the parent can then tell about their experiences with past procedures and provide you with valuable information about the approaches that worked effectively for them and those that were not as successful.

4. Develop a plan. Asking the parent how cooperative his or her child will be is a simple and accurate means of predicting the level of the child's distress. Usually, the younger child with poor venous access will experience more distress. A successful plan involves not only the parent's ability to make educated choices about what will be most helpful but also one's knowledge of pediatric phlebotomy techniques. If possible, allow the child to have some control by asking him or her from which arm or finger he or she prefers blood to be taken. After assessing the experiences, anxiety, and fears of the parent and the child, tailor the procedure for optimal success.

5. Explain and demonstrate the procedure at their eye level. When explaining what you will be doing, use words appropriate for the child's age. Children interpret words literally, so be careful of your choice of words. Use of a doll, puppet, or stuffed animal in the demonstration can help you relate to the child in a nonthreatening manner. If the child has a favorite doll, blanket, or toy, he or she should be encouraged to hug it for comfort and support.

6. Establish guidelines. Tell the child and the parent that the procedure will most likely be successful on the first attempt, but if not, it will be attempted only once more. Then another health care worker will be called in to complete the procedure.

7. Be honest with the child who asks whether the puncture will hurt. Some children cannot separate pain from fear. Instructing the child to say when he or she feels pain will help the child to make this distinction. The child should be told that saying "ouch" or making faces is acceptable, but that he or she must make an effort to keep the arm absolutely still. Also tell the child that if the procedure hurts too much, it can be momentarily stopped; but that the quicker the procedure is performed the less painful it will be. Tell the child it is okay to cry if it does hurt and remind him or her that it will only be for a short time. Reassure the child that the blood will be collected as quickly as possible so that the pain will be brief.[2]

8. Encourage parent involvement. Most recent research demonstrates that **parental involvement**—the parent's presence and support—has the most beneficial effect on the child's anxiety.[3] Some parents, however, may be reluctant to be present because they do not understand how they can assist or because they do not want to be a part of a procedure that will cause their children pain. Each parent's ability to assist must be assessed, and if after discussing his or her role, the parent is still reluctant to participate, his or her wishes should be respected.

Studies have shown that parental behavior influences the child's behavior during the procedure. The following parental behaviors and examples will have a positive effect on relieving the child's distress.[3,4]

Behaviors:	*Examples:*
Distraction	"Look at Mommy"; "Tell the nurse about your doll"
Emotional support	Hugging, stroking hair, patting, and saying soothing words
Explanation	"We need to take a tiny bit of blood from your finger"; "Mommy will help you hold your arm so that we can finish quickly"

PSYCHOLOGICAL RESPONSE TO NEEDLES AND PAIN

Children especially fear needles, and an emotionally distraught child has difficulty separating fear from actual pain. Many children perceive that a "shot," or needle, hurts more than anything else that has ever happened to them. Children's drawings of hospital procedures often depict huge needles that go entirely through the limb.[2] Nevertheless, with proper preparation, the child and the parent can develop coping skills to help alleviate the fear and thereby diminish the "hurt."

ROOM LOCATION

For psychological reasons, the best room location for a painful procedure is a treatment room away from the child's bed or playroom. For a hospitalized child, the bed should be a safe, secure place to rest and sleep, not a place associated with pain. If the child shares a room with another child, performing the procedure at the bedside can upset the roommate as well. If the child cannot be moved to a treatment room, privacy should be maintained by drawing a curtain between the beds and speaking in a calm, quiet manner.

EQUIPMENT PREPARATION FOR A FRIENDLIER ENVIRONMENT

Just the sight of needles, syringes, and a person in a white laboratory coat can be frightening to a child. Nurses and other health care providers working with children frequently wear bright, colorfully printed uniforms or smocks to create a friendlier environment. Equipment, too, can be modified to appear less threatening. As an example, prepare the phlebotomy equipment and supplies prior to entering the room in which the child is located so that the child does not become even more anxious in the health care environment. Use shorter needles if possible, and keep threatening-looking supplies (e.g., needles) covered and out of sight. If the hospital policy requires goggles or face shields for blood-exposure precautions, put this equipment on after greeting the child. At the completion of the procedure, reward the child with praise, a special Band-Aid with cartoon characters, a sticker, an age-appropriate toy, or, with parental permission, a lollipop. If no parent is present to assist in relieving the child's anxiety, you or the nurse in charge may cuddle and offer a pacifier to an infant or gently stroke or talk softly to sooth a small child.

POSITIONS FOR RESTRAINING A CHILD

To ensure that a child does not move the limb during venous access, physical restraint may be required. A supportive parent can assist with restraining while providing comfort to the child.

Two preferred methods of restraining a child to immobilize the arm are the vertical position and the horizontal, or supine, position.[2,5] In both cases, the mother's face is in close proximity to the child's, thereby providing a comforting and secure feeling. The vertical technique, which works well for toddlers, requires the parent to hold the child on the lap. As the parent hugs and holds the child's body and the arm not being used, the health care worker can firmly hold the other arm to perform the procedure (Fig. 11–1).

In the horizontal position, the child lies supine, with the health care worker on one side of the bed and the parent on the opposite side. The parent gently but firmly leans over the child, restraining the near arm and the body while holding the opposite extended arm securely for the health care worker (Fig. 11–2).

Figure 11–1. Vertical position for restraining a child to perform a phlebotomy.

Figure 11–2. Horizontal, or supine, position for restraining a child to perform a phlebotomy.

Neonates and infants younger than 3 months usually do not require restraint. Consequently, they can be managed by the health care worker alone.

COMBATIVE PATIENTS

At times, a child will become uncooperative even after the proper steps have been followed to elicit cooperation. Children may become combative—kicking and thrashing—if force is used. Because sharps are involved in blood collection, the health care worker must be certain that the procedure can be performed safely. Using force to the point of potential physical injury is unethical and unprofessional. Therefore, if the risk of injury to the health care worker or the child is likely, the blood collection attempt should be discontinued, and the nurse or the physician notified.[6] In such instances, alternative coping measures or pharmacological intervention may be necessary prior to the next attempt.

INTERVENTIONS TO ALLEVIATE PAIN

Depending on the anticipated duration of the procedure, the severity of the child's illness, and the anxiety of the child, pharmacological intervention may be used to alleviate pain and anxiety. A topical anesthetic, **EMLA (eutectic mixture of local anesthetics),** which is an emulsion of lidocaine and prilocaine, can be applied to intact skin. This local anesthetic is ideal for use on children prior to venipuncture or starting intravenous (IV) therapy because it does not require a needle. EMLA penetrates both the epidermal and dermal layers, anesthetizing to a depth of 5 mm. It is applied to the skin as a patch or a cream that is then covered with a transparent occlusive dressing. Optimal anesthesia occurs after 60 minutes and may last as long as 2 to 3 hours. Drawbacks to the use of EMLA are cost, the need to apply it 60 minutes prior to the procedure, and having to know in advance the location of the vein to be used. Two separate locations may be anesthetized if the child has difficult venous access. EMLA has minimal side effects but may cause pallor at the application site or erythema due to the adhesive covering; however, EMLA should not be used if the child is allergic to local anesthetics.[2,7] Recent product information from Astra Pharmaceuticals indicates that EMLA can be used on neonates (minimum of 37 weeks gestation) and children weighing less than 20 kg. However, the area and duration of application should be limited.

SUCROSE NIPPLE OR PACIFIER

Giving an infant a **sucrose nipple or pacifier** to suck during and immediately after phlebotomy offers some degree of comfort, although it does not alleviate the pain. Once the infant is crying vigorously and the heart and respiratory rates have increased, a pacifier has no significant effect on changing the rates. Infants given pacifiers or sucrose nipples have, however, been shown to be more alert following the procedure and to be less fussy and to cry for a shorter duration.[8]

■ PREVENTION OF DISEASE TRANSMISSION

If a child is in isolation, a sign posted on the door will describe the type of isolation and the personal protective equipment (PPE) to be worn. Isolation categories are based on the mode of transmission (see Chapter 4, Infection Control).[9] All necessary supplies—a gown, gloves, and a mask—should be available at the room. Hands should be washed according to policy before and after gloving. Usually, an anteroom is available before the isolation room, where you may wash and put on the protective equipment.

Universal standard precautions should be followed throughout pediatric phlebotomy procedures. All children should be treated as if they could be potentially infectious. To prevent transmission of blood-borne pathogens, standard precautions should always be used in addition to transmission category isolation precautions.[9] (See Chapter 4, Infection Control, and Chapter 5, Safety and First Aid.)

PRECAUTIONS TO PROTECT THE CHILD

Premature babies, newborns, infants, and children who are chronically ill, immunocompromised, or have extensive burns are more likely to be susceptible to environmental microorganisms. To protect these children, some hospitals may require PPE, gowns, gloves, and masks to be worn as indicated before entering the room. Remove the PPE according to policy and dispose of them in the appropriately marked container. Hands should be washed and a clean gown and gloves put on before attending to the next child or infant.

LATEX ALLERGY OR ALERT

Some children and health care workers may be allergic to latex. Usually, a sign posted on the door will note the child's allergy, or the child may wear a bracelet indicating a **latex allergy** or a latex alert. Several brands of nonlatex gloves should be available for use with children who have this allergy. Children with spina bifida and those with congenital urinary tract abnormalities or neurogenic bladders are particularly sensitive to latex. [10,11]

■ PEDIATRIC PHLEBOTOMY PROCEDURES

Two methods are used to obtain blood from infants and children: microcapillary skin puncture and venipuncture. The previously described steps for preparing the child and the parent should be taken before the procedure is performed.

MICROCAPILLARY SKIN PUNCTURE

Skin punctures are useful for pediatric phlebotomy when only small amounts of blood need to be obtained and can be adequately tested. It is particularly important to collect only the smallest amounts of blood necessary from neonates, infants, and children so that the effects of **blood volume** reduction are minimal.

> **! Clinical Alert**
>
> Small infants can become anemic if too much blood is taken in the course of a day.

A 10-mL sample taken from a premature or newborn infant is equivalent to 5 to 10 percent of the infant's total blood volume. Calculation of blood volume is based on weight. It can be calculated for any size person if the weight (in kilograms) of the individual is known. The total blood volume of a person is calculated by multiplying weight (kg) by the following blood volumes:

115 mL/kg	Premature infants
80–110 mL/kg	Newborns
75–100 mL/kg	Infants and children
70 mL/kg	Adults

Clinical Alert ⬣!

A 3-kg infant (approximately 6.6 pounds) will have a total blood volume between 225 to 300 mL. It is important to monitor how much of this is withdrawn each day.[12] Table 8–1 provides the maximum amounts of blood to be drawn from infants and children.

When performing skin punctures, the hematology specimens are collected first to minimize platelet clumping, then chemistry and blood bank specimens. Each laboratory has approved procedures for phlebotomy including the volume of blood that is required for each test; these procedures should always be followed.

Sites

The heel of the infant or neonate is the most desirable site for skin puncture to obtain capillary blood. The most medial or lateral section of the plantar, or bottom, surface of the heel should be used (Fig. 11–3). For children older than 1 year, the palmar surface of the tip of the third or fourth finger may be used instead (see Chapter 9, Skin Puncture Procedures). The plantar surface of the great toe is rarely used and only in children older than 1 year.

Equipment for Microcapillary Sampling

(See Chapter 7, Blood Collection Equipment, for additional information.) The following equipment is necessary for pediatric skin puncture procedures:

1. Sterile automatic disposable pediatric safety lancet devices (in different incision depths for neonates, larger infants, and children).
2. Seventy percent isopropyl alcohol swabs in sterile packages.
3. Sterile cotton balls or gauze sponges.
4. Plastic capillary collection tubes and sealer.
5. Microcollection containers and BD Unopettes.
6. Glass slides for smears.
7. Puncture-resistant sharps container.
8. Disposable gloves (nonlatex if child is allergic).

Figure 11–3.   Recommended sites for infant heel sticks. Shaded areas (in red) are the preferred site for puncture.

9. Compress (towel or washcloth) to warm heel if necessary.
10. Marking pen.
11. Laboratory request slips or labels.

Special Equipment for Capillary Blood Gas Collection

See Chapter 12, Arterial Intravenous (IV), and Special Collection Procedures, for details on capillary blood gas collection. The following supplies are needed for this procedure:

1. Heparinized plastic capillary tube and caps or sealer.
2. Metal filing and magnet.
3. Container of ice water.
4. Warm compress (towel or washcloth).
5. Clean, dry towel.
6. Sterile gauze sponge.

HEEL STICK

⚠ Clinical Alert

Microsamples from the heel are preferred for routine laboratory, platelet count, blood chemistry, and drug level determinations for **neonates** and infants who have not begun to stand. If an infant has compromised circulation to the extremity, is in shock, or has edema or infection at the heel, another site should be used. Avoid **heel stick** in an area that has many previous puncture sites because such a stick could cause an infection.

The safety lancet should be of proper pediatric size, making an incision that is less than 2.0-mm deep (see Fig. 11–4). Major blood vessels lie 0.3 to 1.6 mm beneath the skin at the dermal–subcutaneous junction in newborns. If an incision goes deeper, the **calcaneus** or heel bone may be hit and may lead to **osteomyelitis.**

Clinical Alert ❗

Commercially available safety heel-incision devices are designed specifically for use on infants and premature babies. As an example, the Tenderfoot (International Technidyne Corp., Edison, NJ) heel incision device (Fig. 11–4) can be obtained in different calibrations for heel sticks on infants, premature infants, and toddlers. The standard size makes an incision 1.0 mm in depth. The size of incision for premature infants is 40 percent smaller to ensure safety for these infants.

Figure 11–4. Tenderfoot heel incision device.

(International Technidyne Corporation, Edison, NJ.)

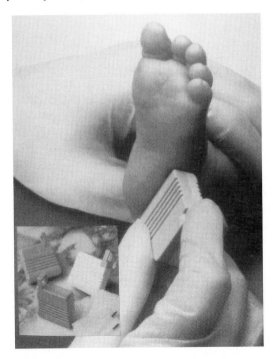

Specific guidelines for performing a heel stick include the following:

- Do not puncture the anteromedial aspect or the posterior curve of the heel because a puncture at either site could injure the underlying calcaneus. Figure 11–3 shows the proper sites for a heel puncture.
- When holding the infant's foot, be firm but gentle. A **premature infant**, in particular, has delicate tissue that may bruise easily. Holding the foot too tightly also restricts blood flow.
- Avoid excessive milking or squeezing, which causes **hemolysis** and dilutes the blood with interstitial and intracellular fluid.
- Avoid covering puncture sites with adhesive bandages because newborn skin is fragile and may macerate under the bandage.

Heel Warming

The amount of blood that can be obtained from a single heel stick is limited, so to obtain an adequate sample, prewarming the heel may be indicated. Prewarming the heel increases blood flow dramatically and arterializes the specimen. This step is essential for drawing specimens for capillary blood gas analysis.

There are several methods of warming the heel; however, a surgical towel or a washcloth heated with warm water to 39 to 42°C works well. If the temperature of the towel exceeds 44°C, it may burn the infant. Wrap the warm, wet towel around the infant's foot, and encase the wrap in a plastic bag to help retain heat and to keep the patient's bed dry. Prewarming the site for 3 to 5 minutes is effective in raising the skin temperature several degrees. Chemical heel-warming packs are also available commercially for this purpose. Caution should be used if the towel is heated in a microwave oven because heating is uneven, and the towel may have hot spots. Depending on the institution's policy, the nurse may be called in advance to prewarm the infant's heel, or one may apply the warm wrap, attend to another patient, then return in a few minutes to perform the heel stick.[13]

Procedure

Hands should be washed and then gloves put on. Also, if required, the health care worker may don a gown and a mask. The infant must be identified properly. If the infant is not wearing an identification bracelet, the floor nurse must identify the infant. The heel area should be inspected and assessed for proper warmth. If it is cool or a blood gas specimen is to be collected, prewarm the foot with a warm, wet towel or a chemical heel-warming pack, according to policy. When the heel has been warmed and dried, the side of the heel should be disinfected with the alcohol swab, using firm circular motions, starting at the center of the area and working outward. Allow the alcohol to dry. Blowing on the area to hasten drying is not advised because doing so will contaminate the area. To ensure that the site is dry and free of alcohol, it should be wiped with a sterile cotton ball or gauze sponge.

The nondominant hand should hold the infant's ankle "tennis racket" style: forefinger across the arch and thumb supporting the heel. The infant's foot should be gripped firmly but carefully to prevent bruising or injury and to avoid restricting blood flow. Using the dominant hand, the pediatric lancing device should be held perpendicular to the heel. As mentioned previously, an automatic safety lancing device will control the incision depth, which should not exceed 2.0 mm. The skin should be pierced with the lancet. The first drop of blood should be wiped away with the sterile gauze sponge because this drop of blood contains excess tissue fluid. As the drops form, blood is drawn into the capillary tubes and the microcollection containers, both of which should be held at a downward angle, not horizontally. Intermittent, gentle pressure with the forefinger may facilitate the blood flow. Massaging or milking the area is not advisable, however, because doing so causes hemolysis or dilution of the blood with tissue fluids.

Clinical Alert !

If the blood flow is inadequate for collection of all required specimens, a second puncture may be needed at another heel site. In such cases, the skin is prepared as before. A puncture device should *never* be reused, and no more than two punctures should be attempted. Box 11–1 provides a sample nursery procedure for performing a heel stick on an infant.

Care of the Heel After Collection

When collection is complete, the heel should be evaluated, a sterile gauze sponge placed over the puncture site, and pressure applied until the bleeding stops. An adhesive strip should not be used because, as mentioned before, infants have delicate skin that may macerate under the Band-Aid or may be damaged when the strip is removed.

Clean Up

Used lancing devices are disposed of in a sharps container. The infant's bed is checked for any equipment or trash left behind. Used gauze sponges, gloves, and gowns should be disposed in a biohazardous waste container. Hands should be washed after removing the gloves.

Complications From Heel Stick

Clinical Alert !

Some complications associated with neonatal heel sticks include cellulitis, osteomyelitis of the calcaneus, abscess formation, tissue loss, scarring of the heel, and calcified nodules. Calcified nodules occur most commonly in infants who, as preemies (premature babies) or neonates, received multiple heel sticks. In neonates, these nodules appear as small depressions, which progress to firm nodular lesions that appear 4 to 12 months later, migrate to the skin surface, and disappear by 18 to 20 months.[14]

BOX 11–1. SAMPLE NURSERY PROCEDURE FOR PERFORMING A HEEL STICK ON AN INFANT

Principle:

To obtain blood specimens from infants with the least amount of trauma while maintaining good isolation techniques.

Procedure:

1. Locate the entrance to the nurseries (intensive care, intermediate care, and low risk).
2. Place blood collection tray on the table near the scrub sinks outside the nurseries.
3. Remove rings, watch, and laboratory coat.
4. Wash hands with regular soap. Control the water with foot pedals.
5. Put on a gown with ties in the back.
6. Wear sterile gloves.
7. Pick up tray with two clean paper towels and enter nursery area.
8. Find the small metal cart and place tray on a clean diaper on the cart.
9. Discard paper towels.
10. Identify the baby by making sure that the information on the request slip is identical to that on the baby's armband.
11. After ensuring that the skin is warm, perform a heel puncture on appropriate sites to obtain specimens for all the tests requested.
12. Hold clean cotton gauze over the puncture site until bleeding stops. Do not put adhesive strips on the baby's feet.
13. Remove all collection equipment from the crib to avoid harming the baby.
14. Before collecting blood from the next baby, wash hands at the sink inside the nursery proper and change gloves.
15. Initial the log book for all work completed.
16. Remove gown and gloves and discard in proper receptacle.
17. Wash hands.
18. When moving from one nursery area to the other, repeat the complete procedure and put on a clean gown and gloves.

Notes:

1. The baby's heel may be punctured a maximum of two times. Do not stick a baby more than twice to obtain a specimen at any given time. If a particular baby must always be punctured the maximum number of times, notify the phlebotomy supervisor and the baby's primary nurse.
2. Do not puncture a foot if bruises, abrasions, or sloughing skin is present. Call the situation to the attention of the baby's nurse.
3. To help obtain a free-flowing puncture from a baby who does not bleed freely, have a nurse wrap the baby's heel in a warm towel 10 to 15 minutes before the puncture is made. Prewarming the site is also necessary for collection of all specimens for capillary blood gas analysis.
4. Use only a gentle massage when obtaining blood. Excessive massaging dilutes the blood with tissue fluids and may cause hemolysis. It is sufficient to massage with your thumb and forefinger.
5. Never repuncture old puncture wounds.
6. Never remove a baby from its crib or change its position in any way without the approval of a nurse.

NEONATAL SCREENING

In the United States, **neonatal screening** for **phenylketonuria (PKU)** and **hypothyroidism** is mandatory by law. These diseases can result in severe abnormalities, including mental retardation, if not discovered and treated early. Blood spot testing for these and other diseases is performed before the newborn is 72 hours old. If blood is collected before the newborn is 24 hours of age, the screening must be repeated before the infant is 14 days old.[5]

Recently the National Newborn Screening Task Force recommended more education and standardization among states for newborn screening procedures and policies. Less than half of the states screen for congenital adrenal hyperplasia, a disorder as common as PKU. All but three states currently screen for galactosemia, and all but eight states screen for sickle cell disease. Only six states screen for cystic fibrosis, and only New York state currently screens for HIV. The following Web sites should be reviewed for more specific information: Maternal and Child Health Bureau (MCHB) of the Health Resources and Services Administration (HRSA) at www.mchb.hrsa.gov and the American Academy of Pediatrics (AAP) at www.aap.org.[15]

The heel is the most frequently used site for collection of blood for screening. Appropriate collection cards are kept in the hospital laboratory or the nursery. Circles are printed on the filter paper portion of the card; one blood drop is to be placed in each circle. It is important not to touch or contaminate the circle areas with substances other than the newborn's blood. Wash hands and put on gloves. Then, positively identify the newborn and prepare the infant in the same manner as for a heel stick. Once the puncture is made and the blood drop appears, the circle area is touched on the filter paper with the blood until the circle is filled. If the circle does not fill entirely, the heel is wiped and another, larger drop is expressed to a different circle. Do not add a second drop of blood to a previously used circle. Only one side of the filter paper should be used. Allow the paper to air dry thoroughly in the horizontal position. Direct application of blood from the heel to the card is the technique of choice; however, blood from a heparinized capillary tube may be applied if care is taken not to scratch or dent the filter paper. Make sure all the information on the screening card is completed correctly so that follow up can be done if the results are abnormal. The screening card should be placed in an appropriate envelope and sent to the laboratory within 24 hours (Box 11–2).

FINGER STICK

Clinical Alert !

A finger stick to obtain blood for routine laboratory analysis is usually preferred for children older than 1 year. Also, a finger stick may be necessary if a child has damaged veins from repeated venipuncture or if the veins are covered with bandages or casts. Do not perform a finger stick if the extremity has compromised circulation, is edematous, or is infected.

BOX 11–2.   PKU COLLECTION PROCEDURE

Principle:

It is a state requirement that a PKU screening be performed on all newborn patients. The test determines the level of phenylketonuria in the blood.

Procedure:

1. Pick up completed PKU slips at nursing unit or PKU health department forms in a physician's office.
2. Properly identify patient, and explain the procedure to the parent(s).
3. Place patient's foot (limb) in dependent position.
4. Sterilize skin with alcohol; allow to *dry* and puncture with disposable safety lancet.
5. Allow drops to form and apply *directly* to filter paper. Apply blood to only one side of the paper while viewing from the other side to ensure *complete saturation* of entire circle. All five circles *must* be completely filled.
6. Allow card to dry thoroughly in a horizontal position (minimum of 3 hours). *Do not* stack wet samples.
7. Reference laboratory personnel will mail the newborn screen in an envelope provided by the State Health Department within 24 hours to the State Health Department. In a physician's office, the health care worker may be responsible for placing the card in a mailer to the Health Department.

Notes:

Specimens may be considered unsatisfactory if

1. All circles are not completely filled.
2. All filled circles are not thoroughly saturated.
3. Uneven saturation is present because of multiple-sample application or the use of capillaries.
4. The specimens appear to be contaminated.
5. Clotted or caked blood is present on the filter paper.
6. Elution of blood from the filter paper is incomplete.
7. The filter paper is separated from the form.
8. The specimen is received more than 5 days following the date of collection.

(Courtesy of Hermann Hospital Clinical Laboratories, Houston, TX, with permission.)

Precautions

Use a proper-sized pediatric safety lancet designed for the age and size of the child. An automatic lancet controls the puncture depth, which should not exceed 2.0 mm in small children. The distance from the skin surface to bone or cartilage in the middle, or third, finger is between 1.5 and 2.4 mm. Automatic incision devices are available in sizes that incise to depths of 1.75 mm, 1.25 mm, and 0.85 mm for toddlers. For a detailed description of the blood collection procedure and supplies, refer to Chapter 9, Skin Puncture Procedures, and Chapter 7, Blood Collection Equipment.

VENIPUNCTURE

Venipuncture in children is used when larger quantities of blood are needed for sampling. The veins of the antecubital fossa or the forearm are most accessible and are chosen for most toddlers and children. Dorsal hand veins are preferred sites for venous access in neonates and well newborns. Other sites for venipuncture are the medial wrist, the dorsum of the foot, the scalp, and the medial ankle. If the **neonate** or child is receiving fluid or medication intravenously, the distal veins should be avoided for phlebotomy and preserved for IV therapy. Venipuncture is indicated for blood sampling for routine laboratory tests, sedimentation rate, blood cultures, cross-matching, coagulation studies, and drug and ammonia levels. Do not use veins in an extremity or area if there is edema or infection or if an IV line is present. Avoid deep veins in a child with hemophilia or other bleeding disorders.

Precautions

Remove the tourniquet before withdrawing the needle. Do not use alcohol preparation pads to apply pressure because they sting and prevent hemostasis. Instead, apply pressure with the gauze sponge or a cotton ball for 3 minutes to prevent a hematoma. For neonates, use small, winged safety (butterfly) needles. If feasible, use winged safety needles for small children as well.

Equipment for Venipuncture

The equipment necessary for a pediatric venipuncture includes the following:

1. Winged safety infusion needle (23 or 25 gauge) or transparent hub needle (21 gauge × 1 in. or 23 gauge × ¾ in.).
2. Syringes slightly larger than the volume of blood needed.
3. Large-bore or 19-gauge needle.
4. Seventy percent isopropyl alcohol swab in a sterile package.
5. Cotton balls or gauze sponges.
6. Appropriate specimen containers.
7. Tourniquet (nonlatex if child is allergic).
8. Sterile disposable gloves (nonlatex if child is allergic).
9. Blood culture:
   a. bottles, aerobic and anaerobic.
   b. iodine swabs.
10. Paper tape and adhesive strip (only for use with older children).
11. Marking pens.
12. Biohazardous waste container.

Dorsal Hand Vein Technique

The dorsal hand vein technique is appropriate for neonates and infants who are younger than 2 years old. Although the neonate will not need restraint, an older infant can be wrapped snuggly in a receiving blanket or restrained by an assistant to minimize movement. As for all procedures, the infant should be positively identified before beginning. Select the hand that has easily visible veins (Fig. 11–5). No tourniquet is necessary. The phlebotomist's middle finger and forefinger should encircle the wrist and are used to apply pressure to distend the dorsal veins (Fig. 11–6). Placing one's thumb against the infant's fingers, the infant's wrist can be flexed downward as the dorsum of the infant's hand is examined. Be careful not to bend the wrist too much or the vein may collapse. Lightly brushing a finger across the back

Figure 11–5. The hand that is selected should have veins that are easily visible.

Figure 11–6. Positioning of health care worker's fingers for dorsal hand vein technique.

of the infant's hand as it is palpated helps select the best vein and determine its direction. Never attempt the venipuncture if one cannot see or feel the vein. Once the optimal vein has been chosen, the finger tourniquet should be released to allow blood to recirculate. Disinfect the back of the infant's hand with the alcohol swab. Take time and allow the area to air dry, then wipe with sterile gauze. Select the appropriate needle according to the size of the vein. Next, the phlebotomist should reposition fingers on the infant's wrist as a tourniquet and flex the infant's hand with his or her thumb. The transparent hubbed needle should be bevel up, parallel to the vein. The needle should be angled about 15 degrees to the skin. The skin should be pierced 3 to 5 mm distal to the vein, then advanced slowly and carefully until the vein is punctured. As soon as blood appears in the hub, the needle should stop advancing. The blood may flow slowly as the venous pressure is very low. A few seconds should pass, then if no blood appears, it may be necessary to reposition the needle gently. The needle need not be held because the surrounding skin will hold it in place.

As soon as the blood begins to flow, the microcollection tubes should be filled *directly from the hub*. Caution is advised to avoid bumping the hub and pushing the needle through the vein. The finger tourniquet should be released intermittently to allow the vein to refill. If the blood flow slows or stops, gently rotating the needle without advancing it may reestablish the flow. Once the necessary tubes are filled, a dry gauze sponge should be placed over the puncture site, while applying pressure as the needle is quickly withdrawn. Pressure should be maintained for 2 to 3 minutes or until the bleeding stops. An adhesive strip may be used to cover the puncture site on well babies and older infants. Tape should not be used on ill neonates because their skin is fragile. The infant may be comforted by offering a sucrose nipple, if permitted. All used supplies should be discarded in the appropriate biohazardous containers. Gloves and the gown should be discarded, and hands washed.

Dorsal hand vein venipuncture has several advantages over skin puncture: it is less stressful for the infant and the health care worker, there is less dilution of the specimen with tissue fluids and less hemolysis, and fewer punctures are required.[13,16,17] However, a major disadvantage is collecting blood using a needle without a safety device.

Venipuncture at Other Sites

The procedure for performing venipuncture on children is similar to that for adults (see Chapter 8). The differences include the necessary preparation of the child and the parent, assistance in restraining the child, and the use of special pediatric-sized needles or safety winged infusion sets. After the child is securely positioned, place the tourniquet proximal to the selected vein to distend it. If necessary, the limb may be lowered, rubbed-gently, or even warmed to promote dilation of the vein. Disinfect the site thoroughly. Allow the alcohol to dry completely. Then, hold the two wings of the infusion set together in the dominant hand as the other hand pulls the skin below the puncture site taut. When inserting the needle in children, it is best to insert 3 to 5 mm below the vein. When blood appears in the tubing, release the wings of the infusion set. The skin will hold the needle in place, or paper tape can be used to secure it. Gently aspirate the syringe until the required amount of blood is withdrawn. Release the tourniquet and apply pressure over the puncture site with a gauze pad as the infusion set is quickly removed. Ask the parent or the nurse to hold pressure on the site until the bleeding stops, then apply the adhesive strip. Remove the syringe from the infusion set, attach the large-bore needle, and insert it into the collecting tubes to be filled.

Scalp Vein Venipuncture

Scalp veins may be used on infants when access to other veins is difficult or undesirable. Figure 11–7 shows the scalp veins used for peripheral vascular access.

Additional equipment required for this procedure includes a disposable razor and a large, flat rubber band. A 23- or 25-gauge safety winged infusion set (butterfly needle) is used for the venipuncture. The appropriate procedures should be followed: hand washing and gloving, preparing the infant, and positioning with an assistant to provide restraint. If the scalp veins are not readily visible through the hair, a disposable razor may be used to shave the hair carefully in the frontal or parietal scalp area. A prominent vein may be occluded proximally with a finger as in the dorsal hand vein technique. Feel for a pulse to prevent hitting an artery. If a vein cannot be distended with the finger, a large, flat rubber band may be placed around the upper head as a tourniquet.[5] (Placing a gauze pad under an area of the band helps in removing it after the procedure.) Disinfect the scalp with a povidone–iodine (Betadine) preparation or with alcohol, allow the scalp to dry, and then wipe it with sterile gauze. After the scalp is inspected for the desired vein, release the tourniquet to permit refilling of the veins. Reapply finger pressure or the rubber band. Hold the skin taut with the nondominant hand distal to the site to be punctured. Hold the infusion set with the two wings folded together and the bevel of the needle up. Position the needle at a 15-degree angle over the vein in the direction of the blood flow. Puncture the skin, and slowly advance the needle until blood begins to flow into the tubing of the needle set. Attach the syringe. Gently and slowly aspirate the blood to prevent hemolysis or occlusion by the vein wall. When sufficient blood

Figure 11–7.   Scalp veins frequently used for peripheral vascular access in infants.

(From Ball, J, Bindler, R.: *Pediatric Nursing: Caring for Children.* Norwalk, CT; Appleton & Lange: 1995, p 823, with permission.)

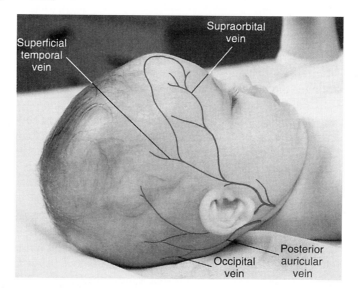

is collected, release the finger tourniquet or rubber band. Place the sterile gauze pad over the puncture site, and apply pressure before quickly removing the needle. Apply additional pressure for several minutes to ensure that the bleeding has stopped. Fill the collecting tubes in the usual fashion. Comfort the infant by stroking him or her softly, or by offering a pacifier if permitted. Be sure all used supplies are removed from the bed area.

COLLECTING BLOOD FROM IV LINES

Hospitalized children who are undergoing IV therapy, whether for total parenteral nutrition (TPN), administration of an antibiotic, or chemotherapy, often have poor veins. They may have a heparin or saline lock or a central venous catheter when long-term access is required. Some blood tests can be performed with blood drawn from these lines; however, one must check with the nurse in charge or the doctor and verify the policy because some hospitals limit the number of times that a line can be accessed. Also, confirm the amount of blood that can be drawn on the basis of the child's weight (see Table 8–1).

Equipment

The equipment required for blood withdrawal from IV lines includes the following:

1. Syringe filled with 5 mL of normal saline.
2. Syringe filled with 5 mL of heparinized flush solution (1 mL for heparin lock).
3. Five-mL syringe for discard.
4. Syringe for blood specimen.
5. Small blood collection tubes.
6. Large-bore needle for transferring blood to tubes.
7. Nineteen- to 25-gauge needles for gaining access to heparin lock.
8. Isopropyl alcohol or povidone-iodine (Betadine) swabs.
9. Double stopcock for central line.
10. Luer-Lok (Becton-Dickinson, Franklin Lakes, NJ) catheter cap.
11. Sterile 4 × 4 in. gauze sponge.
12. Mask.
13. Gloves (nonlatex if child is allergic).

Procedure for Heparin or Saline Lock

When collecting blood from a heparin or saline lock, disinfect the catheter cap with an alcohol or a povidone–iodine (Betadine) swab. Check patency of the line by flushing with a small amount of normal saline. Attach a needle to the discard syringe, and insert it into the cap of the lock. Gently withdraw approximately 2 to 3 mL of fluid and blood, remove the syringe and needle, and discard in a sharps container. Insert another needle and syringe to collect the blood sample. When a sufficient amount of blood has been obtained, withdraw the needle and fill the collection tubes. Clean the cap of the heparin lock, then insert the syringe with the heparinized flush solution, slowly injecting the solution.

Procedure for Central Venous Catheter

Wash hands, put on a mask and gloves, open a sterile 4 × 4 in. gauze sponge, and place it under the catheter port to serve as a sterile field. Open the sterile stopcock and attach the discard syringe to the access port closest to the child. Attach the blood-collecting syringe to the next port and the normal saline–filled syringe to the distal port, all with sterile technique. Clean the connection site with alcohol swabs. Two or three swabs must be used to clean the site for 2 minutes. Then, allow the connection to dry. Clamp the catheter, then remove the catheter cap. Connect the preassembled stopcock setup, ensuring a tight seal. Unclamp the catheter, open the stopcock to the discard syringe, and withdraw 3 to 5 mL of fluid. Close that port, then open the stopcock port to the collection syringe and aspirate the required amount of blood. Close that port, and remove the syringe. An assistant can attach the large-gauge needle and fill the collection tubes. Attach the syringe with the heparinized solution to that port. Open the distal port. Gently aspirate to clear the stopcock of air, holding the syringe vertically to allow bubbles to rise. Tap the syringe to free any bubbles sticking to its side. Flush the catheter with 5 mL of saline, close that port, and then open the port to the heparinized solution and flush with 5 mL. Reclamp the catheter and remove the stopcocks. Clean the connection site of the catheter with a new alcohol preparation pad, then attach a new Luer-Lok cap.[5] Discard used items in the appropriate containers. Remove gloves and mask and wash hands.

SELF STUDY

KEY TERMS

Age-Specific Care
    Considerations
Blood Volume
Calcaneus
Eutectic Mixture of Local
    Anesthetics (EMLA)
Heel Stick
Hemolysis
Hypothyroidism

Latex Allergy
Neonatal Screening
Neonates
Osteomyelitis
Parental Involvement
Pediatric Phlebotomies
Phenylketonuria (PKU)
Premature Infant
Sucrose Nipple or Pacifier

STUDY QUESTIONS

The following questions may have *one* or *more* answers.

1. Performing a phlebotomy on a child is challenging because of which facts?

    a. a child is less emotionally mature
        than an adult
    b. a child is small

    c. smaller equipment must be used
    d. a child's blood clots more quickly

2. Which of the following describes the behavior of an adolescent undergoing a painful procedure?

    a. fears separation from parent
    b. embarrassed to show fear

    c. fears injury to body
    d. may not want parent present in room

3. Which of the following are important steps in preparing the child and the parent for a pediatric phlebotomy?

    a. assess their past experience
        with blood drawing
    b. perform the phlebotomy as
        quickly as possible

    c. ask the parent to leave the room
    d. use a doll or a puppet to demonstrate the
        procedure

4. Which is the *best* location for performing a phlebotomy on a hospitalized child?

    a. bedside in a chair
    b. playroom

    c. treatment room
    d. in his or her bed

5. The preferred technique(s) for restraining a child is/are which of the following?

   a. vertical—child sitting in parent's lap   c. mechanical restraint
   b. total sedation   d. supine with parent leaning over child

6. Which of the following are acceptable interventions to alleviate pain?

   a. xylocaine injection   c. ice pack
   b. sucrose nipple   d. EMLA cream

7. Which is the preferred site for a heel stick?

   a. anteromedial aspect   c. posterior curve
   b. medial or lateral aspect d. a previous puncture site

8. Warming the heel provides which of the following benefits?

   a. arterializes blood   c. prevents hemolysis
   b. dramatically increases blood flow   d. hastens hemostasis

9. Complications of heel sticks may include which of the following?

   a. osteomyelitis   c. paralysis of the foot
   b. abscess formation   d. calcified nodules

10. What is the optimal depth of a finger stick in a child?

    a. greater than 3.0 mm   c. less than 2.4 mm
    b. less than 0.5 mm

11. What is/are the preferred technique(s) for obtaining blood in neonates?

    a. finger stick   c. dorsal head vein technique
    b. heel stick   d. antecubital fossa venipuncture

12. Neonatal blood screening is used to identify which disease(s)?

    a. syphilis   c. cystic fibrosis
    b. hypothyroidism   d. PKU (phenylketonuria)

References

1. Mehne, C: Cultivating a tender touch. *Mt Today.* September:12–16, 1992.
2. Colaizzo, D, Tesler, M: Children's pain: 4, *Nurseweek.* 1994; March:14–15.
3. Jacobson, PB, Manne, S, Gorfinkle, K, et al.: Analysis of child and parent behavior during painful medical procedures. *Health Psychol.* 1990; 9(5):559–576.
4. Manne, S, Bakeman, R: Adult–child interaction during invasive medical procedures, *Health Psychol.* 1992;11(4):241–249.
5. Ball, J, Bindler, R: *Pediatric Nursing: Caring for Children.* Norwalk, CT; Appleton & Lange: 1995.
6. Kelly, S: Pediatric blood collection made easy. *Lab Med.* 1993; 24(4):247–248.
7. Robieux, I, Eliopoulos, C, Hwang, P, et al.: Pain perception and effectiveness of the eutectic mixture of local anesthetics in children undergoing venipuncture. *Pediatr Res.* 1992;32(5):520–523.
8. Marshall, RE: Neonatal pain associated with caregiving procedures. *Pediatr Clin North Am.* 1989;36(4):885–903.

9. National Committee for Clinical Laboratory Standards (NCCLS): *Protection of Laboratory Workers from Instrument Biohazards and Infectious Disease Transmitted by Blood, Body Fluids, and Tissue; Approved Guideline.* M29–A. Villanova, PA; NCCLS: December 1997.

10. Centers for Disease Control and Prevention: Anaphylactic reactions during general anesthesia among pediatric patients. *MMWR.* 1991; *40*(28):437–443.

11. Food and Drug Administration (FDA): Allergic reactions to latex-containing medical devices. *FDA Med Alert.* Mar 29, 1991.

12. National Committee for Clinical Laboratory Standards (NCCLS): *Procedures and Devices for the Collection of Diagnostic Blood Specimens by Skin Puncture.* 4–A4, Villanova, PA; NCCLS: September 1999.

13. Clagg, ME, Jamieson, B: *Pediatric Phlebotomy.* American Society of Clinical Pathologists (ASCP) Fall Teleconference Series, No 9434, Chicago: ASCP; Sept 6, 1990.

14. Sell, EJ, Hansen, MD, Struck-Pierce, S: Calcified nodules on the heel: A complication of neonatal intensive care. *J Pediatr.* 1980; *96*(3).

15. American Academy of Pediatrics (AAP) Task Force on Newborn Screening: Newborn Screening: A Blueprint for the Future—A call for a National Agenda on State Newborn Screening Programs. *Pediatrics*, 8/2000; 389–422, Vol. 106, No. 2.

16. Clagg, ME: Venous sample collection from neonates using dorsal hand veins. *Lab Med.* 1989;*20*(4): 248–250.

17. Johnston, V: News and Views: venipuncture better for newborns? *Lab Med.*1998; *29*(6):329.

TWELVE

∎

Arterial, Intravenous (IV), and Special Collection Procedures

CHAPTER OUTLINE

CHAPTER OBJECTIVES

Upon completion of Chapter 12, the learner is responsible for the following:

1. Explain the special precautions and types of equipment needed to collect capillary or arterial blood gases.

2. Describe the equipment that is used to perform the bleeding-time test.

3. Discuss the requirements for the glucose and lactose tolerance tests.

4. Differentiate cannulas from fistulas.

5. List the steps and equipment in blood culture collections.

6. List the special requirements for collecting blood through intravenous (IV) catheters.

7. Differentiate therapeutic phlebotomy from autologous transfusion.

8. Describe the special precautions needed to collect blood in therapeutic drug monitoring (TDM) procedures.

9. List the types of patient specimens that are needed for trace metal analyses.

Depending on the specific needs of individual clinical settings, health care workers may be required to perform a variety of special tests or procedures in addition to routine skin punctures and venipunctures. This chapter presents the basic techniques and precautions for various special tests. Extensive training sessions and supervision should accompany the student in these procedures because they can harm the patient if performed incorrectly.

■ ARTERIAL BLOOD GASES

Arterial blood gases (ABGs) provide useful information about the respiratory status and the acid–base balance of patients with pulmonary (lung) disease or disorders. In addition, critically ill patients with other diseases, such as diabetes mellitus, benefit from ABG measurement, which is used to help manage their electrolyte and acid–base balance. Arterial blood is used rather than venous blood because arterial blood has the same composition throughout the body tissues, whereas venous blood has various compositions relative to metabolic activities in body tissues.

Arterial puncture to obtain arterial blood for blood gas evaluation requires skill and knowledge of technique. A health care provider must undergo extensive training on arterial punctures, including demonstration of the procedure, observation, and, under the supervision of a qualified instructor, several performances on patients.

RADIAL ARTERY PUNCTURE SITE

When an ABG analysis is ordered, the experienced health care worker, nurse, medical technologist, or physician should palpate the areas of the forearm where the artery is typically close to the surface. The **radial artery**, located on the thumb side of the wrist (Fig. 12–1), is the artery most frequently used for blood collection for ABG analysis.[1] This artery has widespread collateral flow, which means that the hand area is supplied with blood from more than one artery. Arterial blood flows into the hand from both the radial and the ulnar arteries. In addition, the radial artery lies over ligaments and bones of the wrist and can be easily compressed to lessen the chance of a hematoma during the procedure. A drawback to using the radial artery is its small size.

To use the radial artery for blood collection for ABG analysis, the health care provider must first perform the **Allen test** to make certain that the ulnar and radial arteries are providing collateral circulation. The Allen test is performed as follows: (1) The health care provider compresses both arteries with the index and middle fingers, and the patient is asked to tightly clench his or her fist repetitively in order to squeeze the blood out of the hand (Fig. 12–2A). (2) The patient is then asked to open his or her hand (Fig. 12–2B), and

Figure 12–1.   Technique of radial artery puncture.

(From Saunders, CE, Ho, MT, eds.: *Current Emergency Diagnosis and Treatment.* Norwalk, CT; Appleton & Lange: 1992: p 922, with permission.)

the health care provider releases the pressure on the ulnar artery. (3) The hand should fill with blood within 5 to 10 seconds (Fig. 12–1C); if so, the Allen test is positive. If color returns to the hand after 5 to 10 seconds, the Allen test is negative. A negative Allen test indicates the inability of the ulnar artery to supply blood to the hand adequately and shows a lack of collateral circulation. Thus, the radial artery should not be used in a negative Allen test since this artery might be accidentally damaged during puncture, resulting in total lack of blood flow to the hand.

BRACHIAL AND FEMORAL ARTERY PUNCTURE SITES

The **brachial artery** is an alternative site for blood collection for ABG analysis. The brachial artery is in the cubital fossa of the arm, as shown in Figure 12–3. Another choice,

Figure 12–2.   Allen test. A. Using the index and middle fingers, the health care worker compresses the patient's ulnar and radial arteries. The patient tightly clenches his or her fist repetitively. B. The patient opens the hand, and the health care worker releases the pressure. C. If the patient's hand refills with blood (i.e., color returns) within 5 to 10 seconds, the test is positive; if not, the test is negative.

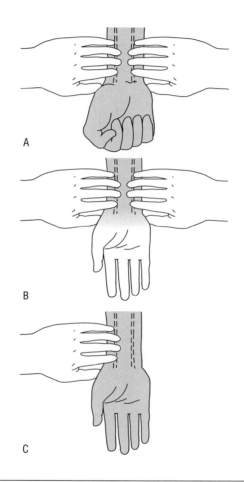

the **femoral artery**, is the largest artery used in ABG collections. It is located in the groin area of the leg, lateral to the femur bone, as shown in Figure 12–4. Even though the brachial and femoral arteries are larger than the radial artery, they are used less frequently because they lack collateral circulation. The brachial artery lies close to the median nerve, which can be accidentally punctured. However, a recent four-year study on blood collections from the brachial artery has demonstrated that brachial artery puncture is an acceptably safe procedure and a very reasonable alternative to radial artery puncture.[2] The femoral artery is a site sometimes used on patients with cardiovascular disorders. The possibility of releasing plaque from the inner wall of the artery in geriatric patients, however, is a definite

Figure 12–3. Arteries in the arm.

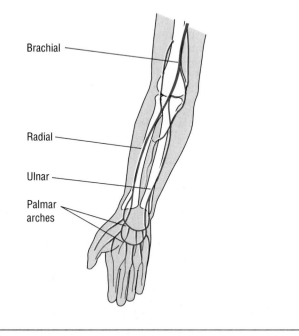

Brachial

Radial

Ulnar

Palmar
arches

disadvantage of using the femoral artery as a puncture site. Usually, the femoral artery is the last choice for an arterial puncture site, and the health care provider must have expertise in obtaining blood from this artery.

PREPARATION OF SUPPLIES AND PATIENT

The necessary equipment and supplies, as listed in Table 12–1, should be gathered and organized for a successful arterial puncture. The patient must be properly identified and informed of the arterial puncture procedure. It should be determined that the patient has been in a stable state for at least the previous 30 minutes (i.e., no respirator changes). The health care provider should attempt to calm the patient before drawing the specimen if the patient appears anxious. The anxiety can lead to hyperventilation, which will falsely alter the ABG levels. Before proceeding, the health care provider must also determine whether the patient is on anticoagulant therapy or is allergic to iodine or lidocaine, and the patient's temperature, oxygen concentration from the respirator (if applicable), and respiratory rate must be recorded.

RADIAL ABG PROCEDURE

When an ABG analysis is ordered, the experienced phlebotomist, nurse, or physician should wash his or her hands, put on gloves, a facial mask, and a protective laboratory coat, and palpate the radial artery in the radial sulcus of the forearm. The radial artery in the patient's

Figure 12–4. Arteries in the leg.

nondominant hand is usually the best choice. With the forefinger or first two fingers, the health care worker should press at these sites to find the artery. The thumb should never be used for palpating because there is a pulse in the thumb that may be confused with the patient's pulse. Any site that has a hematoma or that was previously used for an arterial puncture should be avoided. The patient's arm should be positioned with the wrist slightly extended and rotated. Check for adequate collateral circulation using the Allen test.

The safety syringe should be quickly covered, mixed with the anticoagulant, labeled, and placed in ice water immediately in an effort to prevent the blood gases from escaping into the atmosphere. Ideally, the specimen should be analyzed within 10 minutes of collection. Therefore, the specimen should immediately be labeled and transported to the laboratory.

Table 12–1. Equipment and Supplies for an Arterial Puncture

Tincture of iodine solution or chlorhexidine

One-half to 1 percent lidocaine to numb site

Prefilled heparinized safety syringe, 1 to 5 mL (especially designed plastic syringe for collections for ABG analysis)

Cover for syringe

Needles (20 to 22 gauge, for collections for ABG analysis)

Needles (25 to 26 gauge, for lidocaine administration)

Safety syringe for lidocaine administration (1- or 2-mL plastic syringe)

Gauze squares to be held on site after puncture

Plastic bag or cup with crushed ice and water

Patient identification label

Laboratory requisition slip

Waterproof ink pen

Alcohol pad

Adhesive bandage strip

Oxygen-measuring device to record on laboratory requisition slip the oxygen concentration on patient receiving oxygen

Thermometer to record patient's temperature on laboratory requisition slip

Mask

Gloves (nonlatex if patient is allergic)

Protective laboratory coat or smock

Biohazardous waste containers for sharps

Clinical Alert ❗

Once the radial artery site is chosen, the area should be cleaned well with tincture of iodine solution. No tourniquet is required because the artery has its own strong blood pressure. As in venipuncture, a safety syringe with a needle can be used to withdraw the sample. The safety syringe, however, should be small (1 or 5 mL). The addition of liquid lithium heparin to coat the syringe barrel will anticoagulate the blood. Using too much liquid heparin is probably the most common preanalytic error in blood gas measurements.[3] Therefore, the amount of anticoagulant should be 0.05 mL of liquid heparin (1000 IU/mL) for each milliliter of blood. The health care worker should pull the skin taut and pierce the pulsating artery at a high angle, usually no less than 45 degrees. Little or no suction is needed because the blood pulsates and flows quickly into the syringe under its own pressure. When enough sample has been drawn (usually about 1 mL), the health care worker withdraws the needle carefully to avoid introducing bubbles into the syringe and applies gauze and direct manual pressure on the site for at least 5 minutes. Before leaving the patient, the health care worker should clean the puncture site with an alcohol pad to remove the excess iodine solution, and a pressure bandage should be left on. If bleeding from the site persists, the health care worker should apply more manual

(continued)

Arterial blood results for some analytes (e.g., ammonia, glucose, lactic acid, alcohol) may differ from venous blood results because of metabolic activities. Therefore, arterial blood samples should be collected for the blood gas measurements only when specifically requested by the attending physician. In such situations, the request slip must indicate that arterial blood was collected for the analytes.

■ CAPILLARY BLOOD GASES

Arterial blood is the specimen of choice for testing the pH, oxygen (O_2) content, and carbon dioxide (CO_2) content of the blood. Skin puncture blood is less desirable as a specimen source because it contains blood from capillaries, venules, arterioles, and fluids from the surrounding tissue. In addition, common collection methods for capillary blood gas specimens employ an open collection system in which the specimen is temporarily exposed to room air, theoretically allowing for a brief exchange of gases (both O_2 and CO_2) before sealing the specimen from the air.

Blood for **capillary blood gas analysis** is often collected from small children and babies for whom arterial punctures can be too dangerous. They are collected from the same areas of the body as other capillary samples, such as the lateral posterior area of the heel, or the ball of the finger. (See Chapter 11, Pediatric Procedures.)

When a capillary blood gas analysis is ordered, the health care worker should choose a site and prewarm the area to ensure that good blood flow is obtained and that blood can be quickly collected, anticoagulated, and sealed from contact with room air. To prewarm the site, the health care worker must wrap a cloth or towel that is saturated with warm water around the foot or hand for 3 to 10 minutes. Care should be taken that the warming cloth is not too hot; if the warmed cloth can be held comfortably in the hand, it is not too warm for the patient. When the health care worker is prepared to collect the blood gas specimen, the towel should be removed and the area dried. The puncture site should be cleaned and entered in the usual manner for skin punctures (as discussed in Chapter 9). A heparinized capillary tube (Fig. 12–5) with a volume of at least 100 μL should be used to collect the specimen. A metal filing may be inserted into the tube before collecting to help mix the specimen while it is entering the tube. It is extremely important that the specimen be collected with *no air bubbles,* which can distort the values obtained from the specimen. When the tube is full, the ends should be sealed with plastic caps or clay (according to individual laboratory protocol), and a magnet should be used to draw the metal filing back and forth across the length of the tube to mix the specimen completely. The tube should then be labeled and submerged in a slurry of ice water for transfer to the laboratory. The sample should be analyzed

Figure 12–5.   Capillary blood gas tube.

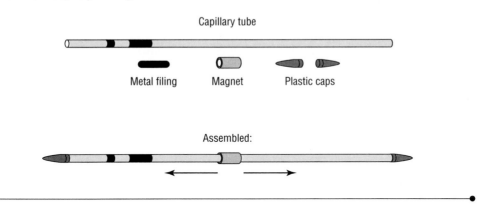

immediately in the laboratory; however, if the specimen is stored horizontally, capped, and in the slurry of ice water, it can be kept as long as 2 hours without serious degradation. The skin puncture site should be pressed with a clean gauze sponge until the bleeding stops.

■ BLEEDING-TIME TEST

The **bleeding-time test** is a useful tool for testing platelet plug formation in the capillaries. It is generally used along with other coagulation tests for diagnosing coagulopathies or problems in hemostasis, such as thrombocytopenia, qualitative platelet defects, vascular abnormalities, and von Willebrand's disease. This diagnostic tool is most frequently used as a preoperative screening test.

The test is performed by making a minor standardized incision in either the earlobe or the forearm and recording the length of time required for bleeding to cease. The duration of bleeding from a punctured capillary depends on the quantity and quality of platelets and the ability of the blood vessel wall to constrict.

Many methods have been used to measure bleeding time, the oldest dating to 1910 when Duke originally described a method in which a lancet was used to make a puncture wound in the earlobe. This test was difficult to standardize, did not allow space for repeat testing, and often caused undue apprehension in the patient. Ivy improved the bleeding-time test in 1941 by using a lancet to make puncture wounds on the forearm while maintaining a constant venous pressure with a blood pressure cuff. Both methods are difficult to reproduce because of several variables (e.g., depth of puncture, length of puncture).

Clinical research has led to the development of automated incision-making instruments for bleeding-time tests. One is called Surgicutt.[4] It is a sterile, standardized, easy-to-use, disposable instrument that makes a uniform, surgical incision. This instrument is a spring-activated surgical steel blade housed in a self-containing plastic unit from which the blade protracts and retracts automatically, eliminating the variable of blade incision. The following steps provide the procedure for the Surgicutt Bleeding Time Test.[5]

1. Prior to beginning the procedure, patients should be advised that there is an occasional scarring problem inherent in the bleeding time test. Butterfly-type bandages can reduce the potential scarring by applying one to the incision area for a 24-hour period. If there is ooze from the incision, as may be encountered in severe primary hemostatic disorders, then a pressure-type dressing should be used in conjunction with the butterfly-type bandage. If the puncture site is still bleeding beyond 15 minutes, the test should be discontinued by applying pressure to the area. A physician should be notified. The patient can also be asked if he or she has taken aspirin or other salicylates within the previous 2 weeks; these drugs interfere with the test.

2. Materials and supplies should be prepared before beginning the procedure. The following items are needed:

   - Surgicutt instrument. Each self-containing unit is sufficient for a single bleeding time determination. If package has been broken, do not use.
   - Gloves.
   - Antiseptic swab.
   - Blood pressure cuff (sphygmomanometer).
   - Filter paper disk (one to two Whatman's no. 1 filter paper disks per bleeding time test).
   - Butterfly-type bandage.

3. Place the patient's arm on a steady support with the volar surface exposed. The incision is best performed over the lateral aspect, volar surface of the forearm, approximately 5 cm below the antecubital crease. Avoid surface veins, scars, bruises, and edematous areas. Lightly shave the area if body hair will interfere with the test.

4. Place the blood pressure cuff on the upper arm. Inflate the cuff to 40 mm Hg. The time between inflation of the cuff and the incision should be 30 to 60 seconds. Hold at this exact pressure for the duration of the test.

5. Cleanse the area with an antiseptic swab and allow to air dry. Remove the Surgicutt device from the package, being careful not to contaminate the instrument by touching or resting the blade-slot end on any unsterile surface.

6. Remove the safety clip. (Safety clip may be replaced if the test is momentarily delayed; however, prolonged exposure of Surgicutt to uncontrolled environmental conditions prior to use may affect its sterility.) Once safety clip is removed, DO NOT push the trigger or touch the blade slot.

7. Hold the device securely between the thumb and the middle finger. Gently rest it on the patient's forearm and apply minimal pressure so that both ends of the instrument are lightly touching the skin. A horizontal incision parallel to the antecubital crease is the most sensitive technique for the bleeding time.

8. Gently push the trigger, starting the stopwatch simultaneously. The blade will make an incision 5 mm long by 1 mm deep. Remove the device from the patient's forearm immediately after triggering. After 30 seconds, wick the flow of blood with filter paper. Bring the filter paper close to the incision, but DO NOT touch the paper directly to the incision, so as not to disturb the formation of a platelet plug.

9. Wick the blood every 30 seconds thereafter until blood no longer stains the paper. Stop the timer. Bleeding time is determined to the nearest 30 seconds. Reference

ranges vary from one health care facility to another. Most, however, are in the approximate range of 2.0 to 8.0 minutes.

10. Remove the blood pressure cuff and cleanse the incision site with an antiseptic swab. Apply the nonallergenic butterfly-type bandage for 24 hours.

The Simplate R (Retractable) and Simplate II R are sterile, disposable devices (Fig. 12–6) used to make uniform incisions for the bleeding-time test. The spring-loaded blades are contained in a plastic housing. When triggered on the forearm, Simplate R and Simplate II R provide one and two incisions, respectively, 5-mm long by 1-mm deep. Simplate II R is used for duplicate determinations. These devices standardize bleeding-time testing by producing uniform incisions that provide reliable and reproducible results.

POSSIBLE INTERFERING FACTORS

The bleeding-time test is only a screening test, so the results of this test alone are insufficient to diagnose a specific condition. A prolonged bleeding time may indicate the need for further testing (e.g., platelet count). In addition, the following items should be considered:

- The ingestion of aspirin-containing products up to 7 to 10 days prior to testing may affect results.
- Other drugs (e.g., dextran, streptokinase, streptodornase, ethyl alcohol, mithramycin) may cause a prolonged bleeding time.

Figure 12–6.   Simplate R (retractable) bleeding device.

(Courtesy of Organon Teknika Corp., Durham, NC.)

There are other variations of this same procedure using different devices. For reproducible results, it is important to follow the manufacturer's instructions and to teach all health care workers in the same manner.

■ BLOOD CULTURES

Blood cultures are often collected from patients who have **fevers of unknown origin (FUO).** Sometimes during the course of a bacterial infection in one location of the body, **bacteremia** or **septicemia** (presence of bacteria or toxins in the blood) may result and become the dominant clinical feature. Blood cultures aid in identifying the specific bacterial organism causing the infections, and when combined with antibiotic sensitivity tests can provide information to the physician about which antibiotic works best against that particular species of bacteria. In the case of a patient who experiences fever spikes, it is generally recommended that blood cultures be drawn before and after the spike, when bacteria may be most likely present in the peripheral circulation. It is best to collect one set (two bottles) of aerobic and anaerobic cultures at the time the order is given. Thirty minutes later, a second set of anaerobic and aerobic cultures should be obtained. A request for "second site" blood cultures that are obtained concurrently on opposite arms is useful when the physician suspects bacteremia due to a local internal infection. A "second site" culture, however, is *not* a very effective tool for *routine* blood culture orders and provides relatively little information that properly spaced, timed blood cultures cannot provide.[6]

Prior to beginning the procedure, the health care provider should briefly explain the test to the patient. Then, the following steps should be taken for blood culture collection:

1. The necessary equipment and supplies should be gathered and prepared next to the patient as listed in Table 12–2.
2. After donning gloves (nonlatex if patient has latex allergy), locate the vein, loosen the tourniquet, scrub the site of the venipuncture with alcohol for 60 seconds to rid the site

---

Table 12–2.   Equipment and Supplies for Blood Culture Collections

Gloves (recommended sterile gloves for aseptic technique)

Three alcohol/acetone or alcohol preps

Two iodine tincture scrub swabsticks

Two blood culture vials (one for anaerobic microorganisms and one for aerobic microorganisms)
   or
SPS evacuated tubes

Needles (22 or 20 gauge) or blood collection set

Safety syringe or evacuated safety tube assembly

Sterile gauze pads

Nonlatex bandages

Nonlatex tourniquet

Patient identification labels

Laboratory requisition slip and pen

Biohazard waste container

of excess dirt, and then scrub with the iodine tincture for at least 45 seconds. Next, clean the site again with a second iodine tincture ampule, moving outward in circles. The phlebotomist's gloved forefinger should also be cleaned in the same manner. If the patient is known to be hypersensitive to iodine, omit the iodine scrub and clean the site twice with alcohol. A blood culture preparation kit is available commercially from Medi-Flex Hospital Products, Inc. (Overland Park, KS) (Fig. 12–7). This kit, the Blood Culture Prep Kit II, provides another method for preparing to collect blood culture specimens. It is a two-step prep system without pads or swab sticks. Through a recent study, it was shown the blood culture collection sites prepared using iodine tincture instead of iodophor (e.g., povidone) were superior in combating contamination sites where cultures were collected by "non-phlebotomy" personnel.[7]

3. Clean the area of the venipuncture with the second iodine tincture swab stick by beginning in the center and rubbing the swab outward in concentric circles covering an area approximately 4 inches in diameter. Do not go back over any area that has been prepped (Figs. 12–8 and 12–9). Allow the area to dry for 1 minute in order for the antiseptic to be effective against skin bacteria.

As the venipuncture site dries, prep the tops of the blood culture vials or SPS evacuated tubes with a new iodine tincture swab stick, then wipe the tops of the vials with a new alcohol prep. This wipes the iodine away and decreases the likelihood of iodine entering with the blood into the vial. For some manufacturers of

Figure 12–7.   Blood culture prep kits.

(Courtesy of Medi-Flex Hospital Products, Inc., Overland Park, KS.)

Figure 12–8. Arm preparation for collection of blood culture specimens.

Puncture Site

Figure 12–9. Scrubbing a blood culture venipuncture site with the providone–iodine prep system. (Courtesy of Medi-Flex Hospital Products, Inc., Overland Park, KS.)

blood culture vials, it is recommended to clean the vial top with *only* alcohol after removing the cap from the vial. *The prepping of the vials should occur IMMEDIATELY prior to the blood collection.*
Removal of the entire metal ring on some manufacturer's bottles introduces air into the vials and can cause contamination. *Read* the manufacturer's directions on blood culture vials before using them because they may vary as to size of blood sample needed and preparation requirements.

4. The venipuncture procedure can be performed three different ways. These include:
   - Using a safety syringe and then transferring the blood from the syringe into the blood culture vials. It is important to use a safety syringe with a cylindrical needle shield that locks in place over the needle. Thus, the tube end of the culture vial can be inserted into the shield during blood injection, which will reduce needlestick risk and reduce risk of blood splatter from dislodged tube covers. If the blood culture specimen from an adult is collected with a syringe, it is commonly recommended to have a 20-mL collection and transfer the first 10 mL to the anaerobic vial and then 10 mL to the aerobic vial. If the blood collector can only collect 3 mL or less, the entire amount should be placed in the aerobic vial. For pediatric patients younger than 10 years old, it is recommended to collect 1 mL of blood for each year of life for the blood culture workup.[8]
   - Using a safety butterfly assembly (safety blood collection set) and transferring the blood via a direct draw adapter that fits directly over the blood culture vial (Fig. 12–10) for a safe method to collect blood. Using this method, blood is transferred to the aerobic vial first since the assembly tubing contains air.

Figure 12–10. BACTEC direct draw adapter.

(Courtesy of BD-Becton-Dickinson and Company, Sparks, MD.)

- Using a safety holder/needle apparatus to collect blood in the yellow-topped evacuated tubes containing **sodium polyanethole sulfonate (SPS)**, or in bottles, such as the BACTEC culture collection kit (BD-Becton-Dickinson and Company, Sparks, MD), that are shaped to fit into the barrel apparatus just as an evacuated tube would, thereby eliminating one step (see Fig. 7–6).

POSSIBLE INTERFERING FACTORS

> ### Clinical Alert
>
> For any of these blood culture collection procedures, the venipuncture site MUST NOT be repalpated after the venipuncture site is prepared for blood collection. Relocating the vein by repalpation after sterilization recontaminates the site. Thus, make a mental note of the vein's location in relation to skin features such as a mole, crease, freckles, etc. Exceptions: It can be repalpated if
>
> 1. The health care worker is wearing sterile gloves and has not contaminated the finger used for palpating the site.
> 2. The health care worker has cleaned the gloved palpating finger with the iodine scrub.

If blood culture collections are ordered with other laboratory tests, blood culture specimens *must* be collected *first*. If an evacuated blood collection tube is used prior to the blood culture vials or SPS evacuated tubes, the needle can become contaminated.

When entering the needle into the venipuncture site, do not scrape the needle across the skin since this can contaminate the needle, and thus, blood cultures.

Also, the anaerobic blood culture vial *must* be inoculated first in all procedures except the butterfly assembly method because injection of air into the anaerobic bottle can cause the death of some anaerobic microorganisms and result in a false-negative culture.

Some culture vials contain resin beads that neutralize antibiotics in the patient's blood specimen. If not neutralized, the antibiotics can inhibit bacterial growth and cause false-negative results.

The blood should always be delivered gently to the vials and/or the tubes to prevent hemolysis of the cells. This is performed by directing the flow from the needle or the syringe hub along the side of the tube without foaming or extra pressure on the plunger. Evacuated tubes fill themselves, and therefore, the blood does *not* need to be forcefully ejected from the syringe. Then, invert the vials and/or tubes gently. After collecting the blood, remove the iodine from the patient's skin with an alcohol prep. The health care provider must initial the patient identification labels, indicate the time of collection on the labels, and attach a label to each vial or tube. Indicate on the request form and on the vials which culture (number) was collected if a series of blood cultures have been ordered.

Two studies have shown that the practice of changing needles after collecting blood for culture and inoculating the blood specimen into culture vials has little if any effect on the contamination of blood collected for culture.[9,10,11] In addition, changing needles after collecting blood for culture can lead to a needlestick injury to the phlebotomist. Careful skin cleansing was shown to be a more important factor in minimizing the specimen contamination rate than is the common practice of replacing the needle used for venipuncture with a fresh, sterile needle before inoculating the blood into culture media.

Clinical Alert !

Blood collected for culture must **not** be obtained through **intravenous (IV) catheter** lines if it cannot be obtained by venipuncture. Contamination rates may increase if the indwelling catheter is used to obtain culture specimens.[12] The only exception is if blood culture specimens are collected to determine if bacterial contamination is in the line. In this case, blood culture specimens need to be collected both from the IV line and by venipuncture for determination of the bacterial source. If using a syringe, a 20-mL size is the largest syringe that should be used with an IV line because larger sizes may collapse the catheter wall. Also, if possible, blood should be collected below an existing intravenous line because blood above the line will be diluted with the IV fluid. Another source of error may involve failure to follow the sterile procedure, which results in contamination of the blood culture and misinformation for the clinician. For instance, palpating the venipuncture site after the site has been prepared without first cleaning the gloved finger can result in contamination of the culture. Likewise, failure to wipe the iodine from the tops of the vials with alcohol or using too little blood for the culture can result in a false-negative culture.

The Isostat system (Isolator microbial tubes) manufactured by Wampole Laboratories (Cranbury, NJ) is a special blood culture tube system (Figs. 12–11 and 12–12). The Isolator microbial tube has (1) a stopper that fits standard blood collection vacuum holders, (2) lysing and anticoagulating agents, (3) reagents in the tube that inactivate human immunodeficiency virus (HIV) within the normal 60-minute transport and processing time, and (4) containment adapters that help protect health care workers and laboratorians against infection due to aerosol spray or breakage during centrifugation. Using this tube affords the advantage of faster microbial test results. It also helps safeguard the laboratorian since the reagents in the Isolator tube inactivate HIV within the normal 60-minute transport and processing time. Also, the tube decreases the many procedural manipulations required during conventional blood culture collections.

■ GLUCOSE TOLERANCE TEST

For patients who have symptoms suggesting problems in carbohydrate metabolism, such as diabetes mellitus, the **glucose tolerance test** can be an effective diagnostic tool. The test is performed by first obtaining fasting blood and urine specimens, giving the fasting patient a standard load of glucose, and obtaining subsequent blood and urine samples at intervals, usually during a 3 to 5-hour-period. Each specimen is then analyzed for its glucose

Figure 12–11. Wampole Isolator adult microbial tube.

(Courtesy of Wampole Laboratories, Cranbury, NJ.)

Figure 12–12. Wampole Isolator pediatric microbial tube.

(Courtesy of Wampole Laboratories, Cranbury, NJ.)

content. In general, glucose levels should return to normal within 2 hours after ingestion of the glucose. With diabetic patients, the test must be carried out for 4 to 5 hours to observe how the patient metabolizes the glucose.

Clinical Alert !

When a glucose tolerance test is to be performed, the patient should be given complete instructions about the procedure so that his or her cooperation can be ensured (Box 12–1). For best results, the patient should eat normal, balanced meals for at least 3 days prior to the test. Twelve hours prior to the beginning of the test, the patient should fast completely.[13] Water intake is strongly encouraged because frequent urine specimens are required throughout the procedure. Other beverages, including unsweetened tea or coffee, are not allowed. Smoking, tobacco chewing, and gum chewing (including sugarless gum) should be discouraged until the completion of the test because they may stimulate digestion and interfere with the interpretation of the results. If a patient is chewing gum prior to or during the test, note this on the requisition slip.

During the test, the patient drinks a standard dose of glucose, 75 g for adults or approximately 1 g/kg of body weight for children and small adults. A dose of 50 g or 75 g is recommended for diagnosis of gestational diabetes.[14] Commercial preparations are available as flavored drinks to make the glucose more palatable. The patient must start and finish the drink within 5 minutes. Water intake is encouraged throughout the procedure. If the patient should vomit at any point in the procedure, the physician should be notified immediately to decide whether the test should be continued or stopped.[13]

When the patient finishes drinking the solution, the time is noted, and 30-, 60-, 120-, and 180-minute blood and urine specimens are obtained. Thus, if the glucose is administered to the patient at 7:30 A.M., at 8:00 A.M. the 30-minute blood and urine specimens are obtained from the patient. This collection is followed by collections of blood and urine specimens at 8:30 A.M. (60 minutes), 9:30 A.M. (120 minutes), and 10:30 A.M. (180 minutes) (Fig. 12–13). The tubes should be labeled with the time, as well as "30 minutes," "1st hour," and so on. If blood is obtained initially by venipuncture, all succeeding specimens must also be venous blood. Similarly, if capillary blood is used, all specimens should be collected by microtechnique because the values and methods of analysis may vary between the two types of samples. Venous blood is the preferred specimen since glucose normal values are determined on venous blood. If serum samples are used instead of plasma samples with a preservative, the tubes should be centrifuged immediately after collection, then the serum should be separated from the blood cells and placed in the refrigerator to inhibit glucose use by the blood cells.

■ POSTPRANDIAL GLUCOSE TEST

The 2-hour **postprandial glucose test** can be used to screen patients for diabetes because glucose levels in serum specimens drawn 2 hours after a meal are rarely elevated in normal patients. In contrast, diabetic patients usually have increased values 2 hours after a meal.

BOX 12–1. SAMPLE PATIENT INFORMATION CARD

Patient Information Card Glucose Tolerance Test

Introduction

A glucose tolerance test (GTT) has been ordered by your physician. The purpose of a GTT is to test the efficiency of your body's insulin-releasing mechanism and glucose-disposing system.

You must prepare your body for the GTT by changing your eating and medication routines slightly for 3 days before the test. It is very important that you follow the instructions below in order for accurate results to be obtained.

Basically, you will need to follow these three guidelines to prepare for your GTT test:

1. Your carbohydrate intake must be at least 150 g per day for 3 days prior to the GTT.
2. Do not eat anything for 12 hours before the GTT, but do not fast for more than 14 hours before the test.
3. Do not exercise for 12 hours before the GTT.

Preparation: Medication

Before proceeding with the GTT, you must tell your physician if you are currently using any of the following medications because they may interfere with test results:

- Alcohol.
- Anticonvulsants (seizure medication).
- Blood pressure medication.
- Clofibrate.
- Corticosteroids.
- Diuretics (fluid pills).
- Estrogens (birth control pills or estrogen replacement pills).
- Salicylates (aspirin, pain killers)—only if taken in high doses, such as for rheumatoid arthritis.

Preparation: Diet and Exercise

Remember that for 3 days prior to your test, your diet must contain at least 150 g of carbohydrates per day. The following is a list of high carbohydrate foods:

- *Milk and milk products*—12 g of carbohydrates per serving. One serving is equal to 8 oz of milk (whole, skim, or buttermilk), 4 oz of evaporated milk, or 1 cup of plain yogurt.
- *Vegetables*—5 g of carbohydrates per serving. One serving is equal to 1/2 cup of any vegetable, excluding starches (e.g., potatoes, corn, or peas).
- *Fruits and fruit juices*—10 g of carbohydrates per serving. One serving is equal to 1/2 cup of juice, 1 small piece of fresh fruit, or 1/2 cup of unsweetened canned fruit, with the following exceptions:

Apple juice	⅓ cup
Grape juice	¼ cup
Raisins	2 tbsp
Watermelon	1 cup
Prunes	2 medium
Banana	½ small
Dates	2
Cantaloupe	¼ 6-in. melon
Honeydew melon	⅛ 7-in. melon

BOX 12–1. *(continued)*

- *Breads and starches*—15 g of carbohydrates per serving. One serving is equal to 1 slice of bread or 1 small roll. Other one-serving sizes are:

Bagel, English muffin	½
Tortilla	1
Cooked cereal	½ cup
Dry cereal	¾ cup
Cooked rice, noodles, pasta	½ cup
White potatoes, dried beans, and peas	½ cup
Yams	¼ cup
Corn	⅓ cup
Crackers	5–6

- *Meats, cheeses, and fats*—These foods contain few or no carbohydrates.
- *Miscellaneous*

Ice cream	½ cup	15 g of carbohydrates
Sherbet	½ cup	30 g of carbohydrates
Gelatin	½ cup	30 g of carbohydrates
Jams, jellies	1 tbsp	15 g of carbohydrates
Sugar	1 tsp	4 g of carbohydrates
Carbonated beverage	6 oz.	20 g of carbohydrates
Hard candy	2 pcs	10 g of carbohydrates
Fruit pie	⅙	60 g of carbohydrates
Cream pie	⅙	50 g of carbohydrates
Plain cake	⅒	30 g of carbohydrates
Frosted cake	⅒	38 g of carbohydrates

Preparation: General Health

The following physical conditions should be reported to your doctor because they too may affect the results of your test:

Acute pancreatitis.

Adrenal insufficiency.

Diabetes mellitus.

Hyperinsulinism (excess insulin secretion, resulting in hypoglycemia).

Hyperthyroidism.

Hypopituitarism (decreased function of pituitary gland).

Pregnancy.

Stress.

If you have any difficulty making the necessary alterations in your diet or medication schedule, please inform your doctor. For accurate test results, the instructions on this card must be followed.

(Courtesy of Division of Laboratory Medicine, U.T. M.D. Anderson Cancer Center, Houston, TX.)

Figure 12–13.   Graph of glucose tolerance test results.

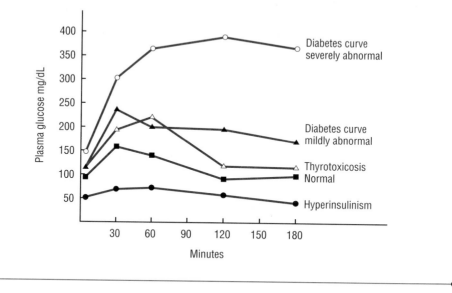

For this test, the patient should be placed on a high carbohydrate diet 2 to 3 days before the test. The day of the test, the patient should eat a breakfast of orange juice, cereal with sugar, toast, and milk to provide an approximate equivalent of 100 g of glucose. A blood specimen is taken 2 hours after the patient finishes eating breakfast. The glucose level of this specimen is then determined, and the physician can decide whether further carbohydrate metabolism tests (such as a glucose tolerance test) are needed.

■ LACTOSE TOLERANCE TEST

Some otherwise healthy adults experience difficulty in digesting lactose, a milk sugar. They appear to lack a mucosal lactase enzyme that breaks down the lactose into the simple sugars glucose and galactose. Instead, gastrointestinal discomfort may result, followed by diarrhea. These patients usually show no further symptoms if milk is removed from their diet.

To determine if a patient suffers from lactose intolerance, a physician may order a **lactose tolerance test**. A 3-hour glucose tolerance test should be performed 1 day in advance to determine the patient's normal glucose curve. A lactose tolerance test should be performed the next day in the same manner as the glucose tolerance, substituting the same amount of lactose for the glucose given the previous day. Fasting, 1-hour, 2-hour, and 3-hour blood samples are drawn and tested for glucose. When the results are graphed, the curve should be similar to that obtained from the glucose tolerance test, if the patient has the mucosal lactase enzyme and digests the sugar properly. If the patient is intolerant to lactose, his or her blood glucose level will increase by no more than 20 mg/dL from the fasting sample level.

The health care worker should be sure that a bathroom is located near the patient testing area because patients who are lactose intolerant may experience severe discomfort during the testing.

False-positive lactose tolerance test results have been known to occur in 25 to 33 percent of the patients tested who had normal lactase activity in small intestine biopsy specimens. Such results have been attributed to slow gastric emptying, not to the absence of the lactase enzyme.

■ THERAPEUTIC DRUG MONITORING (TDM)

Therapeutic drug monitoring (TDM) is used to monitor the serum concentration of certain drugs. It is an important laboratory assessment tool in the following circumstances:

- If the drug is highly toxic.
- When underdosing or overdosing can have serious consequences.
- If use of multiple drugs may alter the action of the drug being measured.
- If individual patients metabolize drugs at different rates.
- If the effectiveness of the drug is questionable.

TDM is often used for patients taking anticonvulsant drugs, tricyclic antidepressants, digoxin, theophylline, lithium, chemotherapeutic agents, such as methotrexate, or antibiotics, such as gentamicin.

Laboratory drug monitoring of therapeutic agents is a complex endeavor that requires much coordination among laboratory, nursing, and pharmacy personnel. A basic understanding of the variables, information needed, and definitions of terms is important to obtain accurate laboratory results. For most drugs, either plasma, serum, or whole blood is used to determine circulating levels of the drug.[15]

To adequately evaluate the appropriate dosage levels of many drugs, the collection and evaluation of specimens for trough and peak levels are necessary. The trough level is the lowest concentration in the patient's serum; that is, the specimen should be collected immediately prior to administration of the drug to ensure that the medication level stays within the therapeutic (effective dosage) range. The peak level is the highest concentration of a drug in the patient's serum. The time required to reach the highest concentration varies with the mode of administration (intramuscular injection v. IV infusion) and the rate at which the drug is infused. In addition, random levels may be appropriate for monitoring the drug dosage if the drug is administered by continuous infusion and if enough time has elapsed for the drug to reach equilibrium.

As a result of all these factors, laboratory personnel must acquire and document additional information when performing these tests. A health care worker may be asked to acquire the following information: patient's name; patient's identification number; patient's location; test ordered; requesting physician; collection time and date; mode of collection (venipuncture, central venous catheter collection) whether the order is for a peak level, a trough level, or a continuous-infusion random level determination; time and date of last dose; time and date of next dose; and a unit nurse's verification that the dose was administered. Specific specimen guidelines for each drug should be established by pharmacy and laboratory staff and strictly adhered to.

Clinical Alert

The time of collection is much more critical for drugs with shorter half-lives (e.g., gentamicin, tobramycin, and procainamide) than for those with longer half-lives (e.g., phenobarbital and digoxin). Certain drug levels (e.g., aminoglycosides) in the blood can be falsely altered if collected through a central venous catheter.[16] Also, blood should not be taken from the arm into which drugs or other fluids are being infused.[17]

Blood specimens for TDM should be maintained in an upright position during transportation. In addition, because falsely low levels of lidocaine, phenytoin, and pentobarbital occur with the use of gel serum separator tubes, this type of evacuated blood collection tube should be avoided in TDM unless the gel serum separator tube has been evaluated and determined not to cause interferences.[18,19]

Most TDM assays should be performed on clotted blood. The National Committee for Clinical Laboratory Standards (NCCLS) has devised toxicology and drug-monitoring requirements for blood collection containers; these requirements can be helpful to the pharmacy and laboratory personnel who are responsible for establishing specific specimen guidelines for each drug.

■ COLLECTION FOR TRACE METALS (ELEMENTS)

Testing for **trace metals** involves the use of specially prepared trace metal-free evacuated blood collection tubes. Also, special acid-washed plastic syringes are usually suitable for trace metal testing. For aluminum level determinations, a needle that is free of aluminum must be used. For lead level determinations, lead-free heparinized evacuated blood tubes equipped with sterilized stainless steel needles should be used for blood collection.[20] Specific specimen collection guidelines should be established as part of the clinical laboratory's technical procedures for trace metal testing. The NCCLS guidelines entitled *Control of Preanalytical Variation in Trace Element Determinations* are very helpful in the preparation of procedures to collect trace elements.[21]

■ GENETIC MOLECULAR TESTS

The proper collection of a blood specimen for genetic molecular tests is critical to obtain accurate results. To collect for molecular testing requires special informed consent forms to be signed by the patient and collection of the specimen in acid citrate dextrose (ACD) or EDTA—depending on laboratory protocol. In addition to the blood specimen, the patient's correct demographics (i.e., vital statistics such as age, place of birth, parents' ethnicity/race, etc.) must be obtained, which is more essential for genetic laboratory tests than for other types of assays. The genetic material (e.g., RNA) is only viable for approximately 6 to 24 hours, and thus the specimens must be sent to the laboratory immediately. This new type of testing will become increasingly popular and expansive in genetic assays. Thus the health care worker needs to stay up-to-date on the necessary blood collection protocols for genetic molecular tests.

■ IV LINE COLLECTIONS

Drawing blood specimens through intravenous (IV) or central venous catheter (CVC) lines requires special techniques, training, and experience. A CVC, also called a **central intravenous line**, is one of numerous **vascular access devices (VADs)**. The CVC is usually inserted into the (1) subclavian vein, which is in the chest area below the clavicle; (2) jugular vein; or (3) superior vena cava at or above the junction of the right atrium. A dressing covers the tubing that extends above the skin. Another type of VAD is a **peripherally inserted central catheter (PICC)**, which is inserted into the peripheral venous system with a lead into the central venous system. A PICC is usually placed in the arm in the basilic or cephalic vein. The PICC should not be used for blood collection because it may collapse during aspiration. An **implanted port** is another VAD that is a small chamber attached to an indwelling line. This port is surgically implanted beneath the skin. Ports must only be accessed with specially designed noncoring needles called Huber needles.

A **heparin or saline lock**, a device that can be inserted into a VAD, is used for medication administration and blood collection. This device is flushed with a heparin solution (Fig. 12–14) on a scheduled basis to prevent blood clots from developing in the line. If a heparin solution is used in this device, coagulation specimens must not be collected from it; otherwise, the solution will falsely alter coagulation test results. Many facilities have shifted to the use of saline in lieu of heparin.

Figure 12–14. Heparin lock flush solution. Many facilities have discontinued use of heparin and now use sterile saline.

> ⬡ **Clinical Alert**
>
> Usually, managers of health care facilities require nursing or laboratory personnel to take specialized training courses prior to allowing them to collect blood from a central venous line. The IV line is a direct pathway into the patient's bloodstream. Each time the IV system is entered, the possibility of contamination and infection exists. If aseptic technique is strictly adhered to, this procedure can provide a relatively safe means of access to the VAD and can save the patient some of the trauma of undergoing frequent venipunctures for laboratory studies. It has been determined, however, that hemolysis of blood samples obtained by an IV collection is significantly higher than when blood is obtained through venipuncture with the evacuated blood collection tube system. A lower incidence of hemolysis occurred with larger catheter diameters (i.e., 20 gauge, 18 gauge, 16 gauge, 14 gauge).[22] In regard to the CVC line, its use should be limited to once daily unless other instructions are received from a physician. Specific criteria must be established at each health care facility for obtaining blood through a CVC line.

DRAWING BLOOD THROUGH A CVC

> ⬡ **Clinical Alert**
>
> To draw blood through a CVC, a 20-mL syringe is the largest syringe recommended for use with a soft-wall catheter because larger sizes may collapse the catheter wall. The patient should be positioned with the catheter hub at or below the level of the patient's heart to prevent possible air emboli when the CVC is entered. Nursing or medical staff should be consulted before opening the CVC line to avoid interrupting medication, which is extremely vital to the maintenance of the patient's care. When drawing blood from multilumen catheters, the lumen(s) not being drawn should be clamped during the procedure to prevent dilution of the blood sample being drawn. With multilumen catheters, blood specimens should be obtained from the most proximal lumen whenever possible.

The following equipment and supplies should be prepared prior to the procedure: laboratory requisition forms, tubes, and labels for the specimen; sterile gloves; two or three 20-mL disposable syringes; one 10-mL disposable syringe; one 10-mL syringe filled with injectable normal saline used for flushing the catheter; two or three sterile needles; a 4 × 4-in. piece of sterile gauze; a linen protector to provide a clean work area; a plastic or paper container for wastes or soiled items; adhesive tape; a sterile heparin cap; alcohol wipes; and 100 U/mL heparin (optional).

The procedure may involve the following steps but is subject to differences among hospitals and must be performed by *authorized personnel only.*[23]

1. Check patient's chart for physician's order to draw blood through CVC.
2. Obtain laboratory requisitions and labels that reflect patient location and tests for which blood is needed.
3. Check labels against slips and patient's identification bracelet as described in Chapter 8.
4. Determine amount of blood to be drawn so that correct size of syringe(s) can be used.
5. Assemble equipment, wash hands, and put sterile gloves on.
6. Aseptically draw up to 10 mL injectable normal saline and cap with sterile needle cover to maintain sterility. Take all supplies to bedside in a tray or other enclosed container to avoid a needle stick.
   Note: Take *only* tubes for the patient, no others.
7. Identify patient by armband ID, noting full name and hospital number. Check against preprinted labels.
8. Explain procedure to patient.
9. Provide adequate room and light for procedure.
10. Position patient by elevating the bed to a comfortable working level and making the bed flat, and have catheter hub at or below the level of the patient's heart.
11. After placing linen protector on the bed, place tray of supplies on protector. Place sterile 4 × 4-in. gauze under connection site.
12. If IV is infusing, clamp off mainline IV tubing if appropriate to do so. Close slide clamp on short microbore tubing.
13. Loosen IV tubing connection or heparin cap. Aseptically disconnect IV tubing or injection cap from short microbore tubing, holding short microbore tubing and IV tubing "up" to avoid contamination.
14. Aseptically disconnect IV tubing and cap with sterile needle cover, and aseptically insert 10-mL syringe in short microbore tubing.
15. Unclamp short microbore tubing. Aspirate (slowly and steadily) the following amount of blood for discard:

   - Pediatrics, 2 mL; adults, 5 to 7 mL.
   - Coagulation studies: withdraw 20 mL of blood (13 mL may be used for testing after discarding 7 mL); collect 3 mL in a separate syringe. This process is only required when the CVC has been used to infuse heparin or has been heparin locked.

Close clamp, remove syringe with blood, and place in tray in order to discard later.

Clinical Alert

Since the possibility exists for transferring an infectious agent or causing a blood clot in the CVC line, most health care facilities do *not* allow reinfusion of the discarded blood.

An alternative to collecting a discard sample is to flush the catheter with 0.9 percent sodium chloride (saline) and then aspirate/flush back and forth several times to clear the catheter. Blood specimens may be obtained for most laboratory tests.

16. Aseptically insert syringe of correct size for needed blood specimen into short microbore tubing.
17. Open the slide clamp on short microbore tubing and slowly aspirate blood in the quantity needed.
18. Close slide clamp on short microbore tubing. Remove syringe and place sterile needle on syringe.
19. Quickly and aseptically insert the 10-mL syringe with normal saline into the short microbore tubing. Open slide clamp on short microbore tubing.
20. Gently irrigate catheter with 5 mL normal saline.
21. Close slide clamp on short microbore tubing; temporarily leave syringe with 5 mL normal saline in place.
22. Place blood into blood collection tubes using the correct order of draw.
23. Open slide clamp on short microbore tubing. Complete irrigation of catheter with remaining 5 mL normal saline. Close slide clamp on short microbore tubing.
24. Aseptically reconnect IV tubing to short microbore tubing. Open clamp on IV tubing and slide clamp on short microbore tubing.
25. Determine that IV fluids are infusing properly at rate set by unit nurse. *Note:* If pump is being used, make certain pump is ON and alarm is ON. If the rate of IV flow appears altered, the unit nurse should be notified *immediately.* Retape connection between short microbore tubing and IV tubing.
26. Make sure the patient is in a safe and comfortable position with the bed down, siderails up, and bedside table and call light accessible to patient. Place used equipment and supplies in appropriate discard containers. The needles should NOT be recapped before discarding.
27. Always immediately label the blood specimens according to NCCLS guidelines as discussed in Chapter 8 and place tubes of blood with the correct lab requisitions. Dispatch to laboratory in usual manner.
28. Document completion of procedure and any problems in the patient's medical record. *Note:* The uncapped used needles should NOT be placed on the patient's bed, but rather in an appropriate container until they can be properly discarded.

POSSIBLE INTERFERING FACTORS

❗ Clinical Alert

Heparin Interference

If possible, protime (PT) and partial thromboplastin time (PTT) levels should not be performed on blood specimens obtained from CVCs that have been heparin locked or heparin-coated or into which heparin is infusing. If a successful venipuncture is improbable,

> ## Clinical Alert (*continued*) ⊗
>
> however, coagulation studies may be collected from a heparinized catheter as explained earlier in the procedure. The description of the collection process and possible heparin contamination needs to be documented via computer, laboratory requisition slip, or medical record forms dependent on the documentation requirements of the health care facility.[24]

Benzalkonium Salts

If benzalkonium salts are present in a catheter, use a discard tube before blood collection of analytes. These salts contain chloride and may interfere with chloride measurements.

Catheter Interference in Blood Collection

The position of the catheter tip within the vein can lead to interference in blood collection. As two examples, if the tip of the catheter is against the wall of the vein or if the tip is positioned within a valve, the aspiration of blood from the IV line will be affected. If possible, attempt to reposition the catheter or extremity and try the blood collection procedure again.

Vein Interference in Blood Collection

Excessive vacuum pressure from the blood collection syringe or blood collection tubes can cause enough negative pressure to collapse the vein around the tip of the catheter and decrease or cut off blood flow through the catheter line. Complications associated with long-term indwelling lines may also result in the inability to collect blood specimens from the line. Examples of these complications include (1) thrombus development preventing a free flow of blood within the vein and limiting the amount of blood for collection; (2) phlebitis, which is the swelling of the tissues due to an inflammatory process, preventing a free flow of blood within the vein; (3) a fibrin sheath can develop over the tip of the catheter that results in less blood flow to the syringe or blood collection tubes; (4) sclerosis can occur in which the lumen of the vein narrows and slows venous blood return and blood flow for collection; (5) catheter has a kink outside or inside of the vein; and (6) lipid deposits have developed, preventing a free flow of blood.[24] Some strategies to use when it is difficult to draw blood from a CVC include (1) repositioning the patient; (2) having the patient cough and/or (3) flushing the line with 0.9% sodium chloride.[25]

Patient Interference in Blood Collection

If the patient has a cold external temperature, then he or she may have vasoconstriction that can lead to poor blood flow through the IV line for collection. Another possible complication can be low venous pressure in a patient. This low pressure increases the tendency of the vein to collapse during the collection procedure and lowers the amount of blood collected. Most likely, the tubes will be partially filled, increasing the likelihood of poor sample quality and bad laboratory results.

■ CANNULAS AND FISTULAS

A **cannula** is a tubular instrument that is used in patients with kidney disease to gain access to venous blood for dialysis or blood collection. Blood should be drawn from the cannula of these patients only by specially trained personnel because the procedure requires special techniques and experience.

A **fistula** is an artificial shunt in which the vein and artery have been fused through surgery. It is a permanent connection tube located in the arm of the patients undergoing kidney dialysis. Only specialized personnel can collect blood from a fistula. The health care worker should use extreme caution when collecting a blood specimen from these patients and avoid using the arm with the fistula as the site for venipuncture. If no other location can be found for the venipuncture site, the patient's arm must be cleaned *thoroughly* prior to blood collection. If the venipuncture site in this arm becomes infected, the inflammation in the blood vessels of the arm may shut down all the veins, requiring surgery to place a new shunt in the patient.

■ DONOR ROOM COLLECTIONS

Properly trained health care providers may be employed in a regional blood center or a hospital blood donor center to screen and collect blood from donors. This section summarizes the procedure outlined by the American Association of Blood Banks (AABB).[26] Only an experienced, properly trained health care worker or technologist should be considered for this function because a physical, emotional, or traumatic experience may keep a donor from volunteering in the future.

DONOR INTERVIEW AND SELECTION

Not everyone who wants to donate blood is eligible, so the interviewer must determine the eligibility of each potential donor. Carefully determining donor eligibility not only helps prevent the spread of disease to blood product recipients but also prevents untoward effects on the potential donor.

The following information should be kept on file on every donor indefinitely and is initially obtained from every prospective donor, regardless of the acceptability of his or her donation:[26]

1. Date and time of donation.
2. Name: last, first, and middle initial.
3. Address.
4. Telephone number.
5. Gender.
6. Age and birth date. (Donors should be at least 17 years of age; however, minors may be accepted if written consent is obtained in accordance with applicable state law. Elderly prospective donors may be accepted at the discretion of the blood bank physician.)
7. Written consent form signed by the donor (1) allowing the donor to defer from being a donor if he or she has risk factors for HIV, the causative agent of acquired immunodeficiency syndrome (AIDS), or (2) authorizing the blood bank to take and use his or her blood.

8. A record of reasons for deferrals, if any.
9. Social security number or driver's license number (may be used for additional identification but is not mandatory).
10. Name of patient or group to be credited, if a credit system is used.
11. Race (not mandatory, but this information can be useful in screening patients for a specific phenotype [chromosomal makeup]).
12. Unique characteristics about a donor's blood. (Donated blood that is negative for cytomegalovirus or that is Rh-negative group O blood is used for neonatal patients.)

To help minimize the incidence of dizziness, fainting, or other reactions to blood loss, donors are encouraged to eat within 4 to 6 hours of donating blood. Eating a light snack just before the phlebotomy may help prevent these reactions, but a donor should not be required to eat if he or she does not want to do so.

Blood bank records must link each component of a donor unit (red blood cells [RBCs], white blood cells [WBCs], platelets, etc.) to its disposition. If the donation is a "replacement for credit" for a particular patient, the donor must supply the patient's name or the group name that is to be credited.

A brief physical examination is required to determine whether the donor is in generally good condition on the day that he or she is to donate blood. The physical examination entails a few simple procedures easily mastered by the health care worker:

1. *Weight.* Donors must weigh at least 110 lb (50 kg); if the weight is less, the volume of blood donated must be carefully monitored and care taken that not too much blood is collected. Also, the anticoagulant in the bag must be modified for the lesser donation. Most blood banks will not routinely accept donors who weigh less than 110 lb.
2. *Temperature.* The donor's oral temperature must not exceed 37.5°C (99.5°F).
3. *Pulse.* The donor's pulse should be regular and strong, between 50 and 100 beats per minute. The pulse should be taken for at least 15 seconds.
4. *Blood pressure.* The systolic blood pressure should measure no higher than 180 mm Hg, and the diastolic blood pressure should be no higher than 100 mm Hg. People with blood pressure outside these limits should be deferred as donors and referred to their physicians for evaluation of a possible health problem.
5. *Skin lesions.* Both arms should be examined for signs of drug abuse, such as needle marks or sclerotic veins. The presence of mild skin disorders, such as a poison ivy rash, does not necessarily prohibit an individual from donating unless the lesions are in the antecubital area or the rash is particularly extensive. Donors with purulent skin lesions, wounds, or severe skin infections should be deferred, as should anyone with purplish-red or hemorrhagic nodules suggestive of Kaposi's sarcoma (an HIV-associated clinical sign). The skin at the site of the venipuncture must be free of lesions.
6. *General appearance.* If the donor looks ill, excessively nervous, or under the influence of alcohol or drugs, he or she should be deferred.
7. *Hematocrit or hemoglobin values.* The hematocrit value must be no less than 38 percent for donors. The hemoglobin value must be no less than 12.5 g/dL. A finger stick is commonly used to draw blood for such determinations. The health care worker may either collect blood in a plastic hematocrit tube for centrifuging and reading, measure hemoglobin spectrophotometrically, or use the copper sulfate method, in which the hemoglobin is qualitatively determined. (For further details on the copper sulfate method, please refer to the AABB technical manual.)[26]

An extensive medical history must be taken on all potential donors, regardless of the number of previous donations on record. Most blood bank donor rooms have a simple card listing all the questions to be asked and "yes" or "no" columns that are used to indicate the donor's responses. The health care provider should refer to the protocol of the donor room at the institution's blood bank or the AABB technical manual, which sets guidelines for donor screening and acceptance.

COLLECTION OF DONOR'S BLOOD

The health care worker in a donor room must operate under the supervision of a qualified, licensed physician. Blood should be collected by using aseptic technique; a sterile, closed system; and a single venipuncture. If a second venipuncture is needed, an entirely new, sterile donor set is necessary; the first is discarded according to the contaminated material disposal protocol of the institution.

A donor should never be left alone either during or immediately after blood collection. The health care worker should be well versed in donor reactions, equipment safety precautions, first-aid techniques, and location of first-aid equipment in case it is needed in the course of donation.

The health care worker should prepare the antecubital portion of the donor's arm in the same manner as for collection of a blood culture specimen (Box 12–2). The blood-collecting bag should be placed conveniently, and the tubing should be extended to ensure that it has no kinks that would prevent a free flow. After the arm is properly prepared, the tourniquet should be replaced and the donor given instructions to open and close the hand during the course of the phlebotomy. A 15-gauge regular or 17-gauge thin-walled needle is used most often. The 17-gauge thin-walled needle is preferable because it has the internal diameter of a 15-gauge needle and the outside diameter of a 17-gauge needle; that is, it has the large-bore size of a 15-gauge needle, but the smaller total size of the 17-gauge needle. The sterile needle is uncapped, and with a quick, sure motion, the needle is slipped under the skin and into the vein. As the collection begins, the needle and tubing should be taped in place and a dry, sterile gauze sponge laid on top. The health care worker should encourage the donor to continue to open and close the hand slowly and to report any discomfort or dizziness that occurs.

The health care worker should make sure that the blood in the bag mixes the anticoagulant during the collection, either manually or by placing it on a mechanical agitator. If the collection process takes more than 8 minutes to complete, platelet concentrates or antihemophilic factor preparations may not be possible. As long as the flow is constant and the bag contents continue to be mixed well, however, no time constraints are necessary.

Once the proper amount of blood is collected (405 to 495 mL), the phlebotomy should be stopped, the tubing clamped off with a hemostat or some other temporary clamp, the tourniquet or blood pressure cuff released, the needle removed, and pressure placed over the site for several minutes. It is advisable that the donor be instructed to raise his or her arm over the head while holding the gauze with pressure over the puncture site. This method minimizes bleeding into the site and surrounding tissues, but also helps restore the integrity of the vascular tissue. The donor should not be allowed to bend the arm until the bleeding stops; otherwise, the tissue may be further traumatized by bleeding into the area below the skin, as well as encouraging the vascular tissue to overlap and form scar tissue on the site during the healing process. A pressure bandage may be placed over the site once the bleeding stops.

BOX 12–2. PHLEBOTOMY

Purpose

To provide instructions for the following:

- Preparation for phlebotomy: confirmation of donor's identity, final pre-phlebotomy check of the donor record, inspection of collection bags and vacutubes, BUI verification
- Selection and preparation of venipuncture site
- Preparation of collection bag(s)
- Proper performance and documentation of the venipuncture procedure
- Discontinuing a phlebotomy, including removal of the needle from the donor's arm; filling test sample tubes; rechecking the labels on the donor record, primary and satellite bags, and sample tubes; and documenting the end of the phlebotomy
- Post phlebotomy cleaning of the donor's arm, and providing proper information for post donation instructions
- Performing and documenting a second phlebotomy when the first venipuncture on a particular donor is unsuccessful
- Recognizing, handling, and documenting whole blood and apheresis collections that do not meet the standards established for acceptable collections (QNS, overdraw, difficult, and QUCs)

Scope

This procedure should be performed by trained Donor Collections personnel prior to the platelet apheresis donation at the facility locations.

Materials

- Donor form
- Black or blue pen
- Black indelible marker
- Sterile gauze
- Gloves
- Lab coat
- Face mask (optional)
- Rubber bands
- Tape
- HOMS scale
- Test tube rack
- Plastic bags
- New blood bag set
- Hematron
- Hemostats
- Bio-sharps container
- Quarantined component tag
- Designated blood cooler
- Blood pressure cuff
- New red and purple top sample vacutubes

Procedure

Preparation for Phlebotomy (Whole blood and apheresis procedures)

(continued)

BOX 12–2. *(continued)*

1. Greet the donor as he/she enters the phlebotomy area and show him/her to a donor chair or bed.

2. Ask the donor, "What is your name?" or "Please state your full name," or a similar statement that helps to establish positive identity of the donor. Verify that the name is the same as the one on the **Donor Form.** If you cannot understand the donor's pronunciation, ask him/her to spell the name.

   If the donor has to leave the room between the completion of the screening process and phlebotomy, upon the donor's return, verify the donor's identity as described above.

3. Review the following parts of the **Donor Form** for completeness, accuracy, and legibility: donor demographics (including the recorded weight of the donor), **Donor Disqualification Directory** or computer check, medical history interview, physical examination, and blood unit identification number. Ensure that the donor has signed the informed consent statement and that the interviewer has signed and placed his/her employee ID # in the appropriate area of the **Donor Form.**

   If any section is incomplete, *confidentially* ask the donor for or obtain the missing information, where applicable, and generate a **Quality Improvement Report** (hereafter referred to as a **"QIR."** SEE: Quality Assurance SOP "Reporting An Incident.")

   a. If vital signs are missing, incomplete, and/or illegible, retake the vital signs and generate a **QIR.**

Note: Ensure all documentation is in accordance with Document Preparation and Review Standards.
If any reason for deferral is identified that was not identified by the screener, document this in the deferral section of the **Donor Form** and defer the donor according to the appropriate SOP.
Note: If the discrepancy is discovered during or after the collection procedure, quarantine the unit as appropriate.

4. Once the review is done, place the **Donor Form** near the donor for the duration of the phlebotomy procedure.

5. Inspect the blood bags and vacutubes for expiration date, defects, cracks, or contamination.

6. Verify that all bar coded and eye-readable labels on the **Donor Form,** blood/component bags, and vacutubes are identical and have been appropriately placed on the tubes.

   Note: It is the responsibility of the phlebotomist to ensure that this information is identical.

Selection of Venipuncture Site (Whole Blood and Apheresis)

Apply a tourniquet or pressure cuff snugly around the donor's arm. Have the donor squeeze a hand gripper intermittently. Select a vein for venipuncture.
Note: Avoid areas that are scarred or that have pits or dimples associated with prior phlebotomies since these areas are difficult to clean and bacteria are harder to remove.

1. Ask the donor if he/she is allergic to iodine.

   a. If the donor is not allergic to iodine, use the Routine Scrub (PVP Iodine Solutions) procedure.

   b. If the donor is allergic to iodine, refer to the non-routine scrub procedure.

2. You may mark the location of the vein with the stick end of an iodine scrub, so that the vein can be easily located.

3. If a vein is located, loosen the tourniquet or blood pressure cuff and proceed to clean the intended venipuncture site with the appropriate solutions as defined in this SOP.

4. If you are not able to find an adequate vein, ask another phlebotomist for assistance. If no veins can be found, defer the donor and document the deferral. Record in the Comments section of the **Donor Form,** "suitable vein not located" or a similar statement.

BOX 12–2. *(continued)*

Preparation of Venipuncture Site (Whole Blood and Apheresis)

Note: Proper preparation of the venipuncture site helps to assure that the phlebotomy procedure will be as aseptic as possible. The scrub process helps remove possible contaminates such as dead skin cells and bacteria, leaving an aseptic area.

Routine Scrub
PVP Iodine Solutions

Using the 0.75% PVP-iodine scrub solution, scrub the intended phlebotomy site and an area approximately 3 inches in diameter around the site, continuously and randomly for *at least* 30 seconds. Using the 1% PVP-iodine solution swab, start at the intended venipuncture site and move the swab in an outward spiral. Cover the entire 3″ diameter area that was initially scrubbed, and DO NOT reswab any area that has already been swabbed. You may cover the venipuncture area with a sterile gauze if the venipuncture is not going to be performed immediately.
Note: When applying the gauze, take precautions to avoid contamination of the side covering the intended venipuncture site, and avoid applying pressure during application and/or removal of gauze.

1. Allow the iodine solution to stand for at least 30 seconds; this allows time for the iodine to properly decontaminate the venipuncture site.
2. DO NOT touch or repalpate the area after it has been cleaned. Do not wipe the iodine off the scrubbed area. If the area is touched or otherwise compromised, repeat the entire arm prep procedure.

Povidone-Iodine Topical Gel

Dispense a 1 ml drop (approximately the size of a penny) directly from the bottle onto the intended venipuncture site.

1. Using a sterile applicator, scrub the intended venipuncture site for a total of 30 seconds. Hold the applicator at an approximate 30-degree angle to provide optimal surface contact. Work in a concentric circle scrubbing the phlebotomy site for 30 seconds; then, work from the inside out until the entire site is prepped. Approximately a 3″ circle should be prepped. Do not return to the center of the site with the same applicator.
2. Using a second sterile applicator, remove any excess gel (a thin film of gel should remain).
3. Allow site to air dry approximately 30 seconds.
4. If venipuncture procedure will not be performed immediately after prep procedure is completed, cover site with sterile gauze. Do not touch prepared site or procedure must be repeated.

Non-Routine Scrub (Soap/Alcohol Solutions)

Using the tincture of green soap swab, scrub the intended phlebotomy site and an area approximately 3″ in diameter around the site continuously and randomly for *at least* 2 minutes.
Using the acetone alcohol swab, start at the intended venipuncture site and move the swab in an outward spiral. Cover the entire 3″ diameter area that was initially scrubbed, and DO NOT reswab any area that has already been swabbed. Cover the venipuncture area with a sterile gauze.
Note: When applying the gauze, take precautions to avoid contamination of the side covering the intended venipuncture site, and avoid applying pressure during application and/or removal of gauze.

1. Allow the alcohol to stand for one minute or until dry; this allows time for the alcohol to properly decontaminate the venipuncture site.
2. DO NOT touch or repalpate the area after it has been cleaned. If the area is touched or otherwise compromised, repeat the entire arm prep procedure.

(continued)

BOX 12–2. *(continued)*

Prepare the Bag (Whole Blood) (May be performed prior to performing scrub)

Write "ASA" on the upper right side of the primary bag base label if it is indicated in the medical history section of the **Donor Form** that the donor has taken aspirin or Piroxicam or medications containing either of these drugs. Do not write over the bar code on the base label.

Write the blood type, if known, in the appropriate area of the primary bag base label. Do not write over the bar code on the base label.

Record the lot number of the blood bag pack in the appropriate area of the **Donor Form.**

If the donor presents himself/herself as a "Rare Donor" verbally or with a rare donor card, write "Rare Donor," or a similar statement on a manilla tag and attach the tag to the appropriate primary bag of the appropriate unit.

After properly labeling the bag, place the bag on a HOMS scale, shaker, or weight monitor depending on the donor's weight and the donation location.

1. **Platform (HOMS) Scales**—If the donor weighs between 110 pounds and 121 pounds, place the primary bag on the HOMS scale.

2. **Shakers**—If the donor weighs 122 pounds or over, place the primary bag flat on the shaker platform.

   a. Thread the two (2) standing metal leg supports attached to the platform through the side loop of the bag closest to the donor bed and thread the metal leg support located at the end of the metal platform through the slit at the bottom of the bag.

   b. Hang the satellite bags on the leg support located at the back of the shaker platform.

   c. Secure the labeled vacutubes through the side loops of a satellite bag.

3. **Weight Monitors**—If the donor weighs 122 pounds or over, hang the bag on the weight monitor from the slit at the bottom of the bag; this will allow the blood to travel from the tubing up into the bag through the anticoagulant.

   a. Thread the tubing through the cut-off groove on the Fenwal weight monitor (trip scale) or adjustable knob weight monitor and pull the tubing back and forth through the groove to ensure that it is not pinched.

   b. Hang the satellite bags from the peg on the end of the weight monitor.

   c. Secure the labeled vacutubes through the side loops of a satellite bag.

   d. Fold the tubing at approximately the fifth segment from the needle and clamp the tubing with a hemostat.

Preparation for Apheresis Collection

See the appropriate SOP for proper installation of the kits/sets for each apheresis procedure.

Venipuncture (Whole Blood)

Put on a clean pair of gloves.

Note: This step may be performed before or after the donor's arm has already been scrubbed as per SOP.

Apply the tourniquet or blood pressure cuff snugly around the donor's arm and inflate, and have the donor open and close his/her hand around the gripper, then make a clenched fist. Do not touch the scrubbed area.

Carefully remove the sterile gauze cover; avoid touching the scrubbed area.

Ensure the hemostat is occluding the blood tubing between the needle and the primary bag, at approximately the fifth segment, (or X).

Remove the cap from the needle, retract the skin firmly below the scrubbed area, and insert the needle through the skin and into the vein in one smooth motion.

Note: During the collection process, the donor should be in a reclined position. If the donor is unable to be placed in a reclining position, contact the Medical Director for instructions.

Release the hemostat, instruct the donor to unclench his/her fist, and watch for blood flow into the tubing.

BOX 12–2. (continued)

1. If the initial venipuncture does not produce blood flow or an adequate blood flow, adjust the needle or ask for assistance. Do not probe in the donor's arm.

   a. When stripping the unit to observe blood flow, strip the tubing away from the donor in a downward motion. **Never** strip toward the donor.

2. If the adjustment is unsuccessful, discontinue the phlebotomy. (See Repeat Phlebotomy— Double Stick Procedure.)

Secure the needle by taping the hub and tubing to the donor's arm.
Re-cover the venipuncture site with the gauze.
Ask the donor to open and close his/her hand slowly and continuously throughout the collection.
Perform the following functions as appropriate for the type of collection device being used:

1. *If using an electric bag shaker,* turn the shaker on.

2. *If using a Weight Monitor (trip scale), platform (HOMS) scale or adjustable knob weight monitor,* mix the blood and anticoagulant immediately after blood flow begins by gently inverting the bag several times. Mix the bag several times during the collection.

Refer to chart below for the approximate unit range (after hematroning). The weight of the primary bag should not differ significantly from the target unit range listed.
Note: For autologous donors who weigh less than 110 pounds, see: Special Procedures SOP.

Donor Weight	Target Unit Range after Hematroning
110 - 121 lbs	590 g - 635 g
122 lbs – over	590 g - 696 g

1. To identify the target weight for each apheresis procedure, see the specific apheresis procedure SOP.

Loosen/readjust the tourniquet, if necessary, for the donor's comfort.
Monitor the flow of blood. The frequent gentle inversion/agitation of the bag to mix the blood and anticoagulant, during a whole blood phlebotomy, is essential to prevent clots and to provide quality blood components.

1. If it appears the blood flow has slowed or stopped, use strippers to check the flow. DO NOT USE HEMOSTATS. Excessive stripping of tubing can cause the vein to collapse and can hemolyze cells.

2. If palpation of the vein after the insertion of the needle is necessary, it is recommended that the procedure be done only with a GLOVED finger above the site of insertion.

3. Adjust the needle, if necessary, to restore blood flow. Turning the needle slightly will often be adequate.

   a. If an adequate blood flow cannot be restored, discontinue phlebotomy as described in this SOP and refer to procedure for repeat phlebotomy.

Monitor the donor throughout the procedure, and observe for signs of an adverse reaction.
Note: Always observe donors for adverse reactions during and after their phlebotomies.

Documentation of Venipuncture

Document whole blood venipuncture appropriately according to the *Donor Form Documentation* SOP. Also document apheresis venipuncture appropriately according to the *Apheresis Procedure Documentation* SOP.
Write the time, in military time, that the whole blood collection began on the upper right side of the primary bag base label. Do not write over the bar code on the base label.

1. If satellite bags are attached to the primary bag, also write the time, in military time, the collection began on the upper right side of the appropriate satellite bag.

Note: On "double" bags, the time will be placed on the satellite bag with the paper label. On "triple" or "quad" bags, the time will be placed on the satellite bag with the preservative solution.

(continued)

BOX 12–2. *(continued)*

Discontinuation of Phlebotomy and Collection of Sample Tubes

Note: This process is performed following collection of the appropriate amount of blood in the primary bag. WEAR GLOVES ON BOTH HANDS.
Needle Removal.

1. At the completion of the phlebotomy procedure, release the tourniquet or pressure cuff and hemostat the tubing somewhere around the fifth segment away from the needle.

   a. If a blood shaker is being used, turn off the shaker.

2. Remove the tape from the donor's arm while gently holding the needle in place.

3. Holding a folded piece of gauze over the needle site, remove the needle and then apply pressure to the site using the gauze.

4. If the donor is able, have the donor raise his/her arm straight up and hold pressure over the venipuncture site with his/her other hand for approximately two minutes. If the donor is not able to apply pressure, hold pressure for him/her. If venipunctures were performed in both arms, the donor may bend both arms for approximately 2 minutes.

Fill Test Sample Tubes.

1. Obtain a Needle/Tube Sampling Protector.

Note: Whole Blood Procedures only. Do not use the protector device for apheresis procedures.

2. While holding the base of the needle, carefully insert the needle through the opening in the center of the Needle/Tube Sampling Protector.

3. Press firmly and twist until there is an audible snap, which indicates the needle is seated properly. When properly seated, the needle cannot be removed.

   a. **Do not place finger inside the cylinder portion of the used protector device.**

   b. Do not remove the needle from the protector device once it has been inserted.

4. If the weight monitor/trip scale is being used, dislodge the tubing from the cutoff groove of the monitor/trip scale.

5. Remove the red-top vacutube and purple-top vacutubes from the satellite bag(s).

   a. Remove the hemostat, and allow the sample tube to fill.

   b. When filling the next vacutube, (first purple vacutube), reapply the hemostat, remove the tube, and insert the next tube. Remove hemostat and allow the sample tube to fill. Repeat this process as many times as necessary for the number of tubes to be collected. Gently invert the purple-top vacutube(s) several times after filling.

   c. After filling the final vacutube, (purple), to avoid a back splash of blood, do not re-apply the hemostat.

Whenever blood cannot be collected in the vacutube(s), send the labeled vacutube(s) back with the unit as normal. Note in the Comment Section of the **Donor Form** what has occurred with the vacutube(s).

Note: 1. Always fill the test sample vacutube(s) while still at the donor's bedside.

2. If any tube does not fill at least halfway, get another tube of the same type and fill it. Apply a bar coded number sticker to the tube. If an extra sticker is not available, remove the label from the tube that did not fill; and apply it to the new tube. Have the supervisor or another person witness as you apply the bar code to the additional tube(s). Clear adhesive tape may be used to secure the number. Dispose of the first tube in a biohazard sharps container.

3. Do *not* place any separated blood segments from the unit in the labeled vacutubes. It is important that the blood segments remain attached to the unit.

BOX 12–2. *(continued)*

    6. Insert the red vacutube, stopper first, through the cylinder portion of the device so that the needle pierces the concave center of the vacutube. The tube stopper MUST be centered on the needle to avoid loss of vacuum and to avoid blood spills during removal.

Hold the needle protector device in an upright position when collecting samples or when removing sample tubes. Slowly twist and pull the sample tube to remove it from the needle protector device. It is imperative that the red vacutube be filled first and always attempt to completely fill all sample tubes.

Note: If the red-top vacutube is NOT drawn first, receiving the non-anticoagulated blood in the tubing between the needle and the bag only (so it can clot in the vacutube), or if there is not enough blood to test in the vacutube, the entire unit could be lost due to the inability to properly test it.

    7. Double loop the red- and purple- top tubes to the primary and satellite blood bags.

Sample tubes collected for apheresis are usually obtained at the beginning of the procedure, just after the phlebotomy. See the appropriate apheresis procedure SOP for the specific method of obtaining sample tubes.

Note: Remember, always attempt to fill the tubes at least halfway and gently invert the purple-top tubes several times after filling.

If there is a blood spill or needle injury, follow guidelines in Appendix Q for cleaning and reporting a blood spill or needle injury.

The biohazard containers for the protection device may be used until full.

Note: The Needle Protector Device should be placed in a downward position in the sharps container.

Recheck Labeling

At the donor's bed, check the bar coded unit identification numbers on the **Donor Form,** primary and satellite bags, and test sample tubes. Verify that all numbers are identical and present in each required location.

1. If an omission is noted, call the team leader or supervisor. Have him/her witness as you apply a bar code to the appropriate area and generate a QIR.

2. If a discrepancy that cannot be corrected at the bedside is noted, initiate an investigation to determine the cause. Attach a **Quarantined Component Tag** to the unit(s) that may be implicated in the discrepancy and generate a QIR.

Documentation of Discontinuance of Phlebotomy

Document the discontinuation of the phlebotomy appropriately according to the *Donor Form Documentation* SOP and/or *Apheresis Procedure Documentation* SOP.

1. When applicable, appropriately complete and attach a **Quarantined Component Tag.**

Note: If a Doublestick is performed, indicate this on the Donor Form and write "DS" in the upper right hand corner, on the base label of the primary bag from the first venipuncture.

2. Take the unit, test sample tubes, and **Donor Form** to the hematroning area.

One employee should not perform all the procedures involved in the collection of a unit of whole blood (screen, collect, and hematron). However, in circumstances when it is necessary for one employee to perform all of these procedures, another employee must be available to review the **Donor Form,** the unit of blood, and the test samples for potential discrepancies or errors.

Post-Phlebotomy Care

Check the venipuncture site after at least two minutes of applied pressure to see if the bleeding has stopped and if a hematoma is apparent. In the event of an arterial stick or a hematoma (see: Donor Collections Donor/Visitor Incidents: Recognition, Treatment, and Documentation procedures).

(continued)

BOX 12–2. *(continued)*

1. If bleeding has not stopped, reapply pressure to the site.
2. Once bleeding has stopped, clean the donor's arm around the venipuncture site with alcohol.
3. Apply a clean pressure bandage to the venipuncture site.
4. Once the donor has rested and exhibits no sign(s) of an adverse reaction, they may be released from the phlebotomy area. Assist the donor to a sitting position. **Do not leave a donor unattended!**
   a. If the donor feels ready and exhibits no symptoms of a donor reaction, assist the donor off the bed, supporting the arm in which the venipuncture was performed. Release and direct the donor to the refreshment area and recommend that he/she consume refreshments. If possible, escort the donor to the area.
   b. If the donor does not feel well or exhibits symptoms of a donor reaction, have the donor remain on the bed until symptoms subside. Follow instructions provided in "Recognition and Treatment of Adverse Reactions" procedures, as necessary.
   c. Thank the donor for his/her donation.

Note: A customer service evaluation form should be given to the donor following donation.

5. Prior to releasing the donor, explain the post donation instructions which are located on the **Information About Your Donation Process** leaflet. Verbally instruct the donor to call the Blood Center if he/she thinks his/her blood should not be used for transfusion.

Notes

None

References

1. Vengelen-Tyler, ed.: Technical Manual, 12th ed. Bethesda, MD: American Association of Blood Banks: 1996.
2. Code of Federal Regulations: Current edition. 21 CFR. Washington, DC: U.S. Government Printing Office.
3. American Association of Blood Banks Association Bulletin #96-6, regarding Bacterial Contamination of Blood Components, August 7, 1996.
4. AABB Monthly Newsletter, March 1997.
5. Baxter Fenwal Insert Needle/Tube Sampling Protector, 1988.
6. Reporting an Incident With the Quality Improvement Report Procedure—SOP #267.00.
7. Donor Deferment Procedure—SOP #301.05.
8. Special Procedures—SOP #301.09.
9. Review and Labeling Procedures—SOP #301.10.
10. Redi Product Suggested Procedure for Venipuncture Site Preparation (Operand Topical Povidone Iodine Gel).

Records, Reports, or Job Aids

1. Donor Record, GC 300
2. Donation History Sheet
3. Specific Apheresis Device Procedural Records
4. Quality Control of Plateletapheresis Components—GC 358

> **BOX 12–2.** *(continued)*
>
> ## Appendices
>
> Temperature Chart
>
> ### Appendix 1.0—Temperature Chart
>
> | | |
> |---|---|
> | Test Sample Tubes | 2°C–10°C |
> | Reagents | 2°C–8°C |
> | Whole blood intended for platelet production | 20°C–24°C *(Or in conditions that will allow the units to cool down to a temp of 20–24°C.)* |
> | Whole blood not intended for platelet production | 1°C–6°C *(See appropriate SOP for labeling units when applicable)* |
>
> (Courtesy of Gulf Coast Regional Blood Center, Houston, TX.)

The blood in the bag and tubing should be mixed well, properly labeled, and stored in accordance with blood bank standards.

If the donor complains of dizziness or other discomfort, he or she should be encouraged to remain seated or prostrate for 10 to 15 minutes or longer. If the donor appears to be well, he or she should be encouraged not only to drink more fluids than usual to replace the volume loss but also to refrain from strenuous exercise or work until after a full meal. Refreshments should be offered to the donor as a courtesy and as an opportunity for the donor to restore some of the lost body fluids. Any adverse reactions experienced by the donor should be recorded on the donor card. If the donor leaves before staff members recommend that he or she does so, this fact should also be noted on the donor's medical record.

■ THERAPEUTIC PHLEBOTOMY

Therepeutic phlebotomy is the intentional removal of blood for therapeutic reasons. It is used in the treatment of some myeloproliferative diseases, such as polycythemia, or other conditions in which there is an excessive production of blood cells. Records in the blood bank should indicate the patient's diagnosis, the physician's request for the phlebotomy, and the amount of blood to be taken. The medical director of the blood bank must decide whether the patient is to be bled in the donor room or in a private section of the blood bank. Some patients are visibly ill and weak, and their presence may have an adverse psychological effect on the healthy donors in the donor room. When a patient is obviously ill, his or her physician or the medical director of the blood bank should be present during the phlebotomy. Generally, the patient should be bled more slowly than a healthy donor, and the resting period should be extended.

The blood obtained through therapeutic bleeding may be used for homologous transfusion if the unit is deemed suitable by the director of the blood bank. If it is to be used, the recipient's physician must agree to use the blood for his or her patient, and a record of the agreement should be kept. The unit is then labeled and processed in the usual manner. The label must indicate that the blood is the result of a therapeutic bleed and must include the patient's diagnosis. If the unit is unsuitable for transfusion, the entire unit is disposed of in the usual manner for contaminated wastes.

■ AUTOLOGOUS TRANSFUSION

A practice that is frequently used is **autologous transfusion**: the patient donates his or her own blood before anticipated surgery. The reason for this type of transfusion is that the safest blood a recipient can receive is his or her own blood. The autologous transfusion prevents transfusion-transmitted infectious diseases (e.g., HIV, hepatitis) and eliminates the formation of antibodies in the transfused patient.

■ THE EMERGENCY CENTER

The atmosphere in an emergency center differs from that in any other area of the hospital. Most emergency rooms are chronically filled with people in pain whose medical problems range from relatively minor injuries or illnesses to major, traumatic injuries. In addition to those who come to the emergency center for immediate treatment of acute injuries or illnesses, some patients have no regular physician and use the local emergency center for treatment of acute illnesses, such as coughs and colds. Family members often accompany the patients and may be highly emotional and vocal about their concern for their loved ones.

This range of patients and families with varying needs who demand attention from the limited staff can create a highly charged atmosphere. In most emergency centers, the patients are prioritized in a central reception area, often referred to as a *triage area,* as they arrive. Those who need immediate attention are seen first, and those whose conditions are more stable are seen later. Even when the patients are prioritized according to their illnesses, however, the routine can be upset if a trauma patient arrives by ambulance and requires immediate life-saving measures. Although personnel at the triage desk may attempt to maintain a stable and orderly work flow in the emergency center, medical emergencies and critically ill or injured patients are unavoidable and must be handled professionally. The emergency center is an unpredictable setting; even though guidelines are placed on the flow of patients, the unexpected can occur at any moment.

Recognizing that the emergency center setting is stressful, the health care provider has two important responsibilities. First, he or she must be completely familiar with all the equipment and well versed in all blood-collecting procedures. If called on to collect STAT (immediate) blood specimens from a critically injured person about to go to surgery, the health care worker must respond quickly and must successfully obtain the correct specimen in the right volume. He or she may not have enough time to collect another specimen if the first one is unsuitable. Consequently, only experienced health care workers should accept positions in the emergency center, where skills must be well mastered and automatic. The second responsibility is to follow directions quickly and correctly. In a critical situation, the health care worker must be able to follow the orders exactly and not require extensive, time-consuming directions. Only an experienced, confident, mature health care worker is suited to the unpredictable emergency environment.

Another factor present in the emergency center, which may cause a great deal of stress in some persons, is the sight and sound of traumatically injured patients in pain. Profuse bleeding, disfigurement, moaning, and groaning are common occurrences in this setting.

Health care workers should be aware of their own reactions to critically injured patients. If they find the setting too stressful, they should opt for work on the general floors of the hospital or in a clinic where the sights and sounds are more predictable and controlled. The health care worker who chooses to work in an emergency center must learn to do his or her job with single-mindedness and to ignore anything that may distract from obtaining high-quality samples with speed and accuracy.

A career in emergency medicine is not for everyone; some people can work in the stressful setting for only a limited amount of time, whereas others would work nowhere else. The excitement of being part of a team of professionals who routinely provide life-saving treatment to critically injured patients has an attraction that cannot be easily duplicated in any other area of patient care. Health care workers must choose the environment that is best suited to their temperament and where they can best deliver quality patient care.

SELF STUDY

KEY TERMS

Allen Test
Arterial Blood Gases (ABGs)
Autologous Transfusion
Bacteremia
Bleeding-Time Test
Blood Cultures
Brachial Artery
Cannula
Capillary Blood Gas Analysis
Central Intravenous Line
Femoral Artery
Fevers of Unknown Origin
   (FUO)
Fistula
Glucose Tolerance Test
Heparin or Saline Lock

Implanted Port
Intravenous (IV) Catheter
Lactose Tolerance Test
Peripherally Inserted Central
   Catheter (PICC)
Postprandial Glucose Test
Radial Artery
Septicemia
Sodium Polyanethole Sulfonate
   (SPS)
Therapeutic Drug Monitoring
   (TDM)
Therapeutic Phlebotomy
Trace Metals
Vascular Access Devices (VADs)

STUDY QUESTIONS

For the following, choose the *one* best answer.

1. What is a cannula?

   a. the fusion of a vein and an artery
   b. a good source of arterial blood
   c. a tubular instrument used to gain access to venous blood
   d. an artificial shunt that provides access to arterial blood

2. Which of the following is a milk sugar that sometimes cannot be digested by healthy individuals?

   a. glucose
   b. glucagon
   c. lactose
   d. lactate

3. Which of the following is the preferred site for blood collection for ABG analysis?

   a. subclavian artery
   b. femoral artery
   c. ulnar artery
   d. radial artery

4. Which of the following supplies is *not* needed during an arterial puncture for an ABG determination?

   a. tourniquet   c. lidocaine
   b. heparin   d. syringe

5. What is the reason for performing the Allen test?

   a. to obtain the oxygen concentration of the patient
   b. to determine whether the patient's blood pressure is elevated
   c. to test for the possibility of a hematoma
   d. to determine that the ulnar and radial arteries are providing collateral circulation

6. When blood is drawn from the radial artery for an ABG determination, the needle should be inserted at an angle of no less than

   a. 20 degrees   c. 45 degrees
   b. 30 degrees   d. 65 degrees

7. Which of the following evacuated tubes is preferred for the collection of a blood culture specimen?

   a. yellow-topped evacuated tube
   b. green-topped evacuated tube
   c. light blue-topped evacuated tube
   d. red-topped evacuated tube

8. During a glucose tolerance test, which procedure is acceptable?

   a. a standard amount of glucose drink is given to the patient, then a fasting blood collection is performed
   b. the patient should be encouraged to drink water throughout the procedure
   c. the patient is allowed to chew sugarless gum
   d. all the patient's specimens are timed from the fasting collection

9. The bleeding-time test is used for what purpose?

   a. check for vascular abnormalities
   b. diagnose diabetes mellitus
   c. determine whether the patient's blood pressure is low
   d. assess liver glycogen stores

10. Autologous transfusion is to prevent which of the following possibilities?

   a. the transfused patient will develop diabetes mellitus
   b. antibodies will form in the transfused patient
   c. antigens will form in the transfused patient
   d. polycythemia will develop in the transfused patient

References

1. National Committee for Clinical Laboratory Standards (NCCLS): *Percutaneous Collection of Arterial Blood for Laboratory Analysis.* NCCLS Document H11-A2. Villanova, PA; NCCLS: vol Vol 12, no 8, 1992.

2. Okeson, GC, Wulbrecht, PH: The safety of brachial artery puncture for arterial blood sampling. *Chest.* 1998;114:748–751.

3. National Committee for Clinical Laboratory Standards (NCCLS): *Blood Gas Preanalytical Considerations: Specimen Collection, Calibration, and Controls.* NCCLS Document C27-A. Villanova, PA; NCCLS: 1993.

4. Smith, C: Surgicutt: a device for modified template bleeding times. *J Med Technol.* 1986:3(4).

5. International Technidyne Corporation: *Surgicutt: Package Insert of Procedure.* Edison, NJ: International Technidyne Corporation.

6. Balows, A (ed): *Manual of Clinical Microbiology,* 5th ed. Washington, DC; American Society for Microbiology: 1991.

7. Schifman, R, Pindur, A: The effect of skin disinfection material or reducing blood culture contamination. *Am J Clin Pathol.* 1993;99:536–538.

8. Koneman, E, Allen, S, Janda, W, et al. (eds): *Color Atlas & Textbook of Diagnostic Microbiology,* 5th ed. Philadelphia; Lippincott: 1997.

9. Isaacman, DJ, Karasic, RB: Lack of effect of changing needles on contamination of blood cultures. *Pediatr Infect Dis J.* 1990;9:274.

10. Krumholz, HM, Cummings, S, York, M: Blood culture phlebotomy: Switching needles does not prevent contamination. *Ann Intern Med.* 1990;13:290.

11. Schifman, R, Strand, C, Meier, F, Howanitz, P: Blood culture contamination. *Arch Pathol Lab Med.* 1998; 122: 216–220.

12. Baron, EJ, Peterson, LR, Finegold, SM (eds): *Bailey & Scott's Diagnostic Microbiology.* St. Louis; Mosby: 1998.

13. Report of the Expert Committee on the Diagnosis and Classification of Diabetes Mellitus. *Diabetes Care.* 2000; 23(suppl. 1). http://journal.diabetes.org.

14. American Diabetes Association: Gestational Diabetes Mellitus—Position Statement. *Diabetes Care.* 2000; *23* (Suppl. 1):1–6. http://journal.diabetes.org.

15. Kaplan, LA, Pesce, AJ (eds): Therapeutic drug monitoring. In: *Clinical Chemistry: Theory, Analysis Correlation.* 3rd ed. St. Louis; Mosby: 1996.

16. Franson, TR, Ritch, PS, Quebbeman, EJ: Aminoglycoside serum concentration sampling via central venous catheters: a potential source of clinical error. *JPEN.* 1987;*11*(1):77–79.

17. Guder, W, Narayanan, S, Wisser, H, Zawta, B: *Samples: From the Patient to the Laboratory.* Darmstadt: Git Verlag: 1996.

18. Quattrocchi, F, Karnes, H, Robinson, J, et al.: Effect of serum separator blood collection tubes on drug concentration. *Ther Drug Monit.* 1983; 5:359–362.

19. Dasgupta, A, Dean, R, Saldora, S, et al.: Absorption in therapeutic drugs by barrier gels in separator blood collection tubes. *Am J Clin Pathol* 1994; 101:456–461.

20. Meranger, J, Hollebone, B, Blanchette, G: The effects of storage times, temperature and container types on the accuracy of atomic absorption determination of Cd, Cu, Hg, Pb and Zn in whole heparinized blood. *J Anal Toxicol.* 1981;5:33–41.

21. National Committee for Clinical Laboratory Standards: *Control of Preanalytical Variation in Trace Element Determinations: Approved Guidelines.* Villanova, PA; Document C38-A. NCCLS: 1997.

22. Kennedy, C, Angermuller, S, King, R, et al.: A comparison of hemolysis rates using intravenous catheters versus venipuncture tubes for obtaining blood samples. *J Emerg Nurs.* 1996;*22*(6): 566–569.

23. U.T.M.D. Anderson Cancer Center—Division of Laboratory Medicine/General Services/Diagnostic Center: *Drawing Blood Through Central Venous Catheters.* Houston, TX; U.T.M.D. Anderson Cancer Center: 1997.

24. Baranowski, L, Lonsway, RA, Hedrick, C: *Intravenous Therapy: Clinical Principles and Practice.* Philadelphia; WB Saunders: 1996.

25. Becan-McBride, K, Baranowski, L: *BD Pre Analytix Training Program —Interactive Education Program for Health Professionals.* Franklin Lakes, NJ; Becton-Dickinson & Co.: 2000.

26. Vengelen-Tyler, V, (ed): *Technical Manual of the American Association of Blood Banks.* 13th ed. Bethesda, MD: 1999.

THIRTEEN

■

Elderly, Home, and Long-term Care Collections

CHAPTER OUTLINE

Chapter Objectives
Considerations for the Elderly
Considerations in Home Care
Glucose Monitoring
- Quality in Point-of-Care Testing (POCT)

Blood Gas and Electrolyte Analysis
Point-of-Care Testing for Acute Heart Damage

Blood Coagulation Monitoring
Hematocrit, Hemoglobin, and Other Hematology Parameters
Cholesterol Screening
Future Trends
Self Study
- Key Terms
- Study Questions

CHAPTER OBJECTIVES

Upon completion of Chapter 13, the learner is responsible for the following:

1. List two other terms that are synonymous with *point-of-care testing*.

2. Define five physical and/or emotional changes that are associated with the aging process.

3. Describe how a health care worker should react to physical and emotional changes associated with the elderly.

4. Identify four analytes whose levels can be determined through point-of-care testing.

5. Describe the most widely used application of point-of-care testing.

6. Given the abnormal and normal control values for glucose from a daily run, plot the control values on the appropriate quality control charts.

With new emerging technology, laboratory testing services and results delivery have expanded beyond the laboratory to the hospital bedside, the home, the nursing home, and any other direct-contact patient setting.[1] The terms used for these direct laboratory services include *decentralized laboratory testing, on-site testing, alternate-site testing, near-patient testing,* **patient-focused testing, point-of-care testing,** and *bedside testing.* With the increasing health care requirements of the growing U.S. elderly population and the innovations in point-of-care instrumentation, nurses, laboratorians, and other health care providers will increasingly perform additional on-site laboratory testing to obtain various types of laboratory test results. The demand for point-of-care testing is increasing because rapid turnaround of laboratory test results is necessary for prompt medical decision making.

■ CONSIDERATIONS FOR THE ELDERLY

The elderly or geriatric population comprises about 15 percent of the U.S. population and uses 31 percent of the nation's health care services.[2] In 25 years, the geriatric population will have reached 20 percent of the total U.S. population. Physical conditions, such as arthritis, **Parkinson's disease** (i.e., a disease causing tremors), and other debilitating diseases in the elderly will continue to increase point-of-care testing by skin puncture due to the difficulty of obtaining blood by venipuncture. In addition, this patient population will increasingly need point-of-care testing and other health care services in their homes, nursing homes, rehabilitation centers, and other long-term care facilities (where the length of stay is over 30 days). Estimates suggest that there are over 1 million elderly in nursing homes and institutions.

The process of aging presents physical and emotional problems that can be challenging for health care workers. Whatever the case, elderly individuals should be treated with the utmost respect and dignity. Age-related changes develop in each person in a unique way, and normal aging includes both gains and losses. It does not always mean the patient is in a declining state of health. There are many elderly individuals who are healthy. However, physical problems that are common include the following:

- Hearing loss may cause embarrassment and frustration. Repeating instructions or adjusting one's position to speak in the "good" ear may be necessary for the patient to truly understand a procedure.
- Failing eyesight is common, so the health care worker should take care to guide the elderly individual to the appropriate seat for blood collection or to the bathroom for urine collections.
- Loss of taste, smell, and feeling can accompany the aging process. Elderly people may lack an appetite, which may lead to malnourishment. They may tend to drop things or not be able to make a fist due to muscle weakness. The health care worker should make a note of these clues, particularly if the patient is homebound without a caregiver.
- Memory loss can affect the patient's ability to take medications or to remember the last time he or she ate. These factors may interfere with the interpretation of laboratory results.
- Epithelium and subcutaneous tissues become thinner, thereby making venipuncture more difficult. The phlebotomist must hold the skin extra taut so that the vein does not "roll." Also, the arm should not be "slapped" when trying to locate the vein. This causes bruising. Use of heated compresses can be helpful.

- Muscles become smaller, so the angle of penetration of a venipuncture needle may need to be more shallow.
- Increased susceptibility to accidental hypothermia (a subnormal drop in body temperature) can make the elderly patient feel cold. Thus, specimen collection may require warming of the site.
- Increased sensitivities and allergies. Therefore patients should be asked if they are allergic to anything.

Emotional problems that are associated with aging include the possible loss of career, spouse, close friends, or relatives and can be reflected by depression or anger at life in general. Health care workers should remember to address the elderly with dignity and respect by using "Mr./ Mrs./ Miss," etc. Respect for privacy should also be considered.

■ CONSIDERATIONS IN HOME CARE

Factors related to the physical setting can also affect a phlebotomist's work. If specimens are to be collected in homes, all procedures are similar except that extra care must be taken for the following:

- Extra supplies and equipment, including biohazard containers for disposables and a specimen transport container, should be taken into the home.
- The patient should be positively identified if possible. If not possible, then procedures of the health care organization should be developed and followed.
- The patient should be placed in a comfortable, preferably reclining, position in case of fainting.
- The phlebotomist should locate the nearest bathroom, sink, and clean towels for washing hands. It is advisable for home care workers to use hand disinfectants that are easily transportable. These are commercially available in creams and foams.
- The health care worker should carefully inspect the area after the procedure to assure that all trash and used supplies have been properly discarded.
- Specimens should be carefully labeled and placed in leakproof containers. Appropriate temperatures for transport should be checked.
- Health care workers who are working in high crime areas should take security precautions, travel with a mobile phone, and carry maps of the area to avoid getting lost on the way to or from the patient's home.
- Delays in returning specimens to the laboratory should be carefully documented.

■ GLUCOSE MONITORING

One of the most widely used applications of point-of-care testing is blood glucose monitoring, in which commercially available instruments, such as the one shown in Figure 13–1, are used to determine blood glucose levels. Such determinations allow the physician to choose appropriate treatment regimens for patients with **diabetes mellitus,** a chronic disease in which the pancreas cannot produce enough **insulin** or cannot use the insulin that it does produce. Insulin is a chemical that is released into the bloodstream by the pancreas when glucose levels in the blood increase after meals. Insulin causes the glucose to be absorbed from the blood into the body tissues, where it is used for energy. Because of the lack

Figure 13–1.   HemoCue β-Glucose analyzer.

(Courtesy of HemoCue, Inc., Mission Viejo, CA.)

Clinical Alert

If the blood glucose levels become too elevated, the diabetic patient can enter a state of metabolic acidosis (ketoacidosis), which can result in shock and then death. Because research has shown that strict glucose control in patients with diabetes mellitus is necessary to prevent serious complications, pocket-size glucose meters are used in point-of-care testing to help these patients monitor and maintain glucose levels within the acceptable range.[3]

of insulin in patients with diabetes mellitus, glucose is not properly absorbed by the tissues, and the glucose levels within the blood increase.

During the past decade, small glucose-monitoring instruments, such as those described in Table 13–1, became commonplace in the home, in the nursing home, and at the hospital bedside.

Table 13–1.   Blood Glucose Monitors

INSTRUMENT (MANUFACTURER)	FEATURES	TEST TIME	SAMPLE VOLUME (μL)
Glucometer Encore QA+ (Bayer Corp., Tarrytown, NY)	Quality Control (QC) management capability Memory function includes date and time; thus, no timing Above average accuracy No wiping required Easy to operate	15–60 seconds	4
Accu-Chek Complete Roche Diagnostics Corp., Indianapolis, IN)	QC data management capability Memory function includes data, time, and patient identification number Above average accuracy Setting Insulin Pump Option	15–60 seconds	4
One Touch Profile (Life Scan,Inc., Milpitas, CA)	QC data management capability Automated QC features Available for use in 19 languages Memory function includes date and time Above average accuracy Easy to use	45 seconds	10
β-Glucose analyzer (HemoCue, Inc., Mission Viejo, CA)	Refrigerated temperature required for test cuvettes Above average accuracy Memory capability is available Easy to operate	15–45 seconds	5
ExacTech RSG (Abbott Laboratories, Abbott Park, IL)	No wiping, blotting, or timing Credit care size and shape Blood does not enter sensor, so cleaning not required Memory function includes last reading recall and calibration code recall	30 second	10

These "rapid" methods require whole blood samples collected by skin puncture from the finger, heel (for infants), or a flushed heparin line. As for any blood collection procedure, appropriate safety protocols must be followed (e.g., wearing gloves), and disposal of potentially contaminated waste must be part of the quality control and safety guidelines. These bedside procedures are handy for quick screening in a hospital or outpatient setting. *Extreme caution* must be taken, however, to provide a rigid, up-to-date, quality control and training program for personnel before they begin to implement such procedures. Variance in methodology and lack of quality control on reagents and equipment may lead to serious medical consequences for patients being tested.[4,5] Therefore, careful adherence to manufacturers' instructions, a thorough evaluation of the monitoring devices, and strict adherence to daily quality control procedures will ensure a more accurate and precise screening tool. In addition, careful recording of the results must include the date, time, and health care worker identification, as well as verification that the results are from the bedside (or patient's home) rather than the clinical laboratory. In some health care facilities, bedside test results are recorded on special bedside testing written or computer forms or in a separate section of the patient's medical record.

To perform the blood glucose determinations, health care providers need to gather the appropriate supplies (Box 13–1) and must be aware of the total quality assurance procedures that are required to obtain accurate and precise results. A skin puncture is customarily performed to obtain the blood for these bedside glucose assays. The patient's finger should be cleansed with alcohol and allowed to dry. A microcollection safety lancet is used to puncture the finger. The first drop of blood is wiped away with a dry, sterile gauze pad, and the next drop is allowed to fall from the finger onto the reagent strip or pad. After the specified time indicated on the instrument's instruction sheet or electronic display elapses, the blood drop is removed by blotting or washing, and the strip is placed in the instrument to obtain a glucose reading. The timing of the reaction is critical, and most of these instruments call the time to the attention of the operator by buzzing, sounding an alarm, or digitally displaying the glucose result.

The HemoCue β-Glucose analyzer (HemoCue, Inc., Mission Viejo, CA) (Fig. 13–1) is an instrument used for bedside glucose testing. This instrument can obtain test results from capillary, venous, or arterial whole blood. It uses a microcuvette rather than a test strip and does not require blotting. Also, it can be used to monitor blood glucose in neonates.

QUALITY IN POINT-OF-CARE TESTING (POCT)

Some glucose-monitoring instruments should be calibrated with glucose standards (calibrators). The glucose values must be monitored daily with **quality control material,** and whenever a battery is changed, or the meter is cleaned. This control material should be similar to the patient's specimen in order to determine if the analytic system is working properly. For example, the glucose control material should be based on the use of whole blood because this type of body fluid is used for measurements with bedside glucose-monitoring instruments.

BOX 13–1.   SUPPLIES AND EQUIPMENT FOR BLOOD GLUCOSE MONITORING

Blood glucose testing monitor.

Strips (or cuvettes) appropriate for the monitor.

Calibrators and controls.

Tissues, gauze, or cotton balls.

70 percent isopropyl alcohol.

Safety blood collection lancets.

Gloves (nonlatex if allergic to latex).

Biohazard disposal container for lancets.

(Timing device for visual testing.)

Biohazard disposal trash can.

In addition, some instruments have automatic or "electronic quality control" (EQC). The purpose of EQC is to test the electronics—the internal and analyte circuits of the instrument. Both the liquid and electronic QC should be performed.

For each day the glucose assay or other point-of-care test is performed on patients' blood specimens, control material must be analyzed. The control value obtained each day is plotted on a chart under the appropriate date, and the daily plots are joined with a straight line (Fig. 13–2). Interpretation of this chart is based on the fact that for a normal distribution, 95 percent of the values about the mean, or average ($\bar{x}$), should be within ±2 standard deviations (SD) of the mean (average), and the fact that 99 percent of the values are within ±3 SD of the mean. Tolerance limits are determined by pooling the data obtained during a 20-day test period and referring to the mean ±2 SD. If a daily control value exceeds the tolerance limits, corrective action must occur according to the manufacturer's directions and be documented for future reference.

Another quality control measure that can be taken when point-of-care monitoring instruments are used is purchasing the reagent strips and controls in quantities that enable health care workers to use constant pools of the same lot number. This leads to reproducibility of the results. Required preventive maintenance of each point-of-care instrument is critical for accurate results.

Some point-of-care testing instruments can store and download calibrators, controls, and patients' results and can, thus, provide a complete instrument log for quality assurance interpretation. Table 13–2 provides a list that will help lead to quality results through *avoidance* of these problems.

■ BLOOD GAS AND ELECTROLYTE ANALYSIS

Blood gas analysis for critical patient care needs can also be accomplished through patient-focused testing using the Nova Biomedical Stat Profile pHOx analyzer (Fig. 13–3). Blood gas analysis involves measurement of the partial pressure of oxygen (pO_2), partial pressure of carbon dioxide (pCO_2), and pH. The pO_2 and pCO_2 are analyzed whenever a patient has a heart or lung disorder. The blood pH determines whether the blood is too acidic or too alkaline. All of these analytes must be closely monitored in emergency care situations, critical care units, cardiac intensive care units, and other units requiring immediate patient diagnosis and treatment.

In addition to monitoring blood gases, point-of-care instruments, such as the Nova Stat Profile pHOx Plus, can measure blood electrolyte levels—sodium (Na^+), potassium (K^+), chloride (Cl^-) or calcium (Ca^{++})—plus glucose, and calculate bicarbonate (HCO_3^-) and total carbon dioxide (TCO_2) levels. These electrolyte measurements, as well as blood gas analysis, are needed immediately in critical care situations.

Another POC blood gas and electrolyte analyzer, the i-STAT system, is shown in Figure 13–4.

These instruments require preventive maintenance and quality control similar to the glucose-monitoring instruments; however, these instruments measure more than one analyte and thus have more complex operational, quality control, and maintenance needs than the glucose monitors. Consequently, as a health care professional involved in collecting blood and determining the analytes' results with these instruments, it is extremely important to be thoroughly trained in their use prior to actually testing patients' blood.

Figure 13–2. Quality control record.

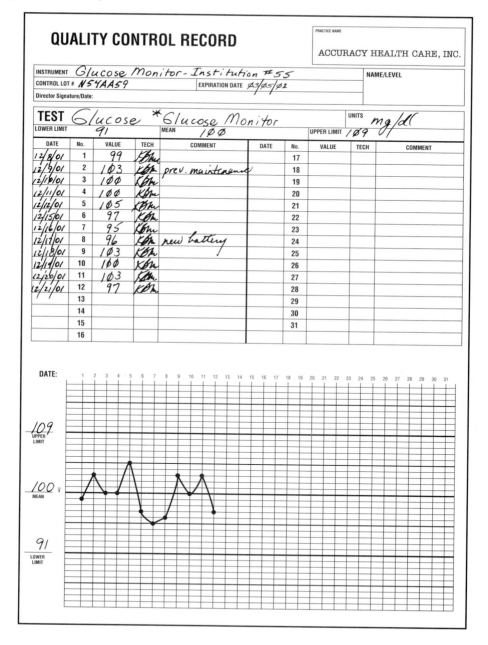

QUALITY CONTROL RECORD

PRACTICE NAME

ACCURACY HEALTH CARE, INC.

INSTRUMENT *Glucose Monitor- Institution #55*

CONTROL LOT # *N54AA59*   EXPIRATION DATE *03/05/02*

NAME/LEVEL

Director Signature/Date:

TEST *Glucose* *Glucose Monitor*   UNITS *mg/dl*

LOWER LIMIT *91*   MEAN *100*   UPPER LIMIT *109*

DATE	No.	VALUE	TECH	COMMENT	DATE	No.	VALUE	TECH	COMMENT
12/8/01	1	99	BM			17			
12/9/01	2	103	KBM	prev. maintenance		18			
12/10/01	3	100	KBM			19			
12/11/01	4	100	KBM			20			
12/12/01	5	105	BM			21			
12/15/01	6	97	KBM			22			
12/16/01	7	95	BM			23			
12/17/01	8	96	KBM	new battery		24			
12/18/01	9	103	KBM			25			
12/19/01	10	100	KBM			26			
12/20/01	11	103	BM			27			
12/21/01	12	97	KBM			28			
	13					29			
	14					30			
	15					31			
	16								

DATE:

1 2 3 4 5 6 7 8 9 10 11 12 13 14 15 16 17 18 19 20 21 22 23 24 25 26 27 28 29 30 31

109
UPPER LIMIT

100 x̄
MEAN

91
LOWER LIMIT

Table 13–2. Problems to Avoid in Point-of-Care Testing

Specimen is inappropriately stored.

Contamination of the blood with alcohol. (After alcohol is used to cleanse the skin puncture site, the skin must dry *completely* before puncturing the site.)

Wrong volume of specimen is collected.

Instrument blotting/wiping technique is not performed according to manufacturer's directions.

Instrument is not clean.

Reagents are outdated.

Timing of the analytic procedure is incorrect.

Reagents are not stored at the proper temperature, leading them to deterioration.

Patient has not dieted properly for procedure.

Patient's result/time/date/etc., are mislabeled.

Recording of result is incorrect.

Battery for instrument is weak or dead.

Calibrators and/or controls are not properly used and/or recorded.

Results are not sent to appropriate individuals in timely manner.

Figure 13–3. Nova Biomedical Stat Profile pHOx® analyzer.

(Courtesy of Nova Biomedical, Waltham, MA.)

Figure 13–4.   i-STAT system for point-of-care testing.

(Courtesy of i-STAT Corporation, Princeton, NJ.)

■ POINT-OF-CARE TESTING FOR ACUTE HEART DAMAGE

! Clinical Alert

Troponin T is a protein released and detected after a myocardial infarct (heart attack). Troponin T is elevated only when heart (cardiac) damage has occurred. Roche Diagnostics (Indianapolis, IN) has developed a point-of-care STAT test for determination of cardiac troponin T. The blood test results can be read from this rapid assay in 1 to 15 minutes, depending on the troponin T concentration in the patient's sample. If the test is positive, it indicates that the patient has had a myocardial infarction and should immediately be admitted to the hospital's coronary care unit (CCU).

Another cardiac point-of-care test is the CARDIA STATus from Spectral Diagnostics (Toronto, Ontario, Canada) for the measurement of troponin I, myoglobin, and creatine kinase–MB (CK-MB). These assays use whole blood, plasma, or serum. A positive test result is indicated by an observable purple-colored line, which identifies an increase in troponin I, myoglobin, and CK-MB as a result of cardiac damage.

■ BLOOD COAGULATION MONITORING

Similar to glucose monitoring, monitoring blood coagulation through point-of-care testing provides immediate results that can be used in controlling bleeding or clotting disorders in patients.[6] A blood coagulation instrument, such as the CoaguChek System (Roche Diagnostics Corp., Indianapolis, IN), is a hand-held instrument that can measure prothrombin time (PT) from an unmeasured drop of whole blood, providing results in 2 minutes (Fig. 13–5). The CoaguChek System can be used by home health care providers or other outpatient clinic providers to monitor long-term anticoagulation therapy in patients. The immediate test results allow rapid dose adjustments. Again, the health care provider using these instruments must be trained appropriately in the preventive maintenance and quality control parameters in order to obtain accurate results. Also, reading the manufacturer's directions is essential. For example, the CoaguChek System is calibrated to use the *first* drop of blood in skin puncture. The ProTime (International Technidyne Corp., Edison, NJ) measures prothrombin time, using one or two drops from a finger stick. The blood is collected directly into the disposable cuvette.

Figure 13–5.   CoaguChek System.

(Courtesy of Roche Diagnostics Corp., Indianapolis, IN.)

Figure 13–6. Actalyke Activated Clotting Time Test (ACT) System.

(Courtesy of Helena Laboratories, Beaumont, TX.)

Other point-of-care coagulation systems are the Actalyke Activated Clotting Time Test (ACT) System (Fig. 13–6) above (Helena Laboratories, Beaumont, TX), the Hemochron Jr. Instrument (International Technidyne Corp., Edison, NJ), the INRatio system (HemoSense, Milpitas, CA), and the Rapidpoint Coag analyzer (Bayer Corp., Diagnostics Division, Tarrytown, NY). These instruments are designed for use at the patient point-of-care (i.e., home, intensive care unit, physician's office) to monitor anticoagulation therapy such as heparin or warfarin sodium (Coumadin).

■ HEMATOCRIT, HEMOGLOBIN, AND OTHER HEMATOLOGY PARAMETERS

The hematocrit (Hct, packed cell volume [PCV], Crit) represents the volume of circulating blood that is occupied by red blood cells (RBCs). It is expressed as a percentage; thus, a hematocrit value of 38 percent indicates that 38 mL of each 100 mL of peripheral blood is composed of RBCs. Hematocrit values are obtained to aid in the diagnosis and evaluation of anemia, a less than normal number of erythrocytes, and may be used to evaluate blood volume and total RBC mass. Blood collection usually occurs by skin puncture. For accurate test results, remember not to squeeze the tissue to obtain capillary blood because doing so will dilute the sample with tissue fluid. It is very important to follow the healthcare facility's procedure. *Plastic* microcapillary tubes must be used to avoid the possibility of blood-borne pathogen exposure from a broken tube. A Federal Advisory has been issued on this important safety precaution.[7]

Determining a patient's hemoglobin level is another test to aid in the diagnosis and evaluation of anemia and other blood abnormalities. The hemoglobin test has been determined

Figure 13–7.   HemoCue β-Hemoglobin analyzer.

(Courtesy of HemoCue, Inc., Mission Viejo, CA.)

by the American Medical Association (AMA) to be more accurate than the hematocrit test in diagnosis and treatment. Also, the hemoglobin procedure is a safer method to detect anemia. A point-of-care analyzer that can be used to measure hemoglobin is the HemoCue β-Hemoglobin System (HemoCue, Inc., Mission Viejo, CA) (Fig. 13–7). A patient's venous, capillary, or arterial whole blood sample placed in the microcuvette and inserted into this instrument provides the patient's hemoglobin value.

The Ichor automated cell counter (Helena Laboratories, Beaumont, TX) is an instrument for hematology analysis in acute patient management (Fig. 13–8). It is the first system that became available for use at the point of patient care (e.g., ICU) to determine the hematology parameters that include platelet count, hemoglobin, hematocrit, WBC count, RBC count, and platelet aggregation results. The results are available in about 1 minute. In blood transfusion triage, Ichor can quickly provide results to guide clinical decisions about needed blood components. Since only 12 μL of whole blood is required per analysis, the analyzer can accommodate standard, pediatric, and microsample blood collection tubes for a variety of patient populations.

■ CHOLESTEROL SCREENING

Another laboratory testing procedure that health care providers are performing through point-of-care testing is cholesterol screening. Using a finger stick drop of blood, total cholesterol (TC)

Figure 13–8. Ichor automated cell counter.

(Courtesy of Helena Laboratories, Beaumont, TX.)

values can be monitored with the Cholestech L-D-X System (STAT Technologies, Golden Valley, MN). In addition, the Cholestech point-of-care analyzer can measure levels of other lipids (fats) in the blood, such as triglycerides and HDL cholesterol, with only a finger stick drop of blood.

The Accu-Chek InstantPlus (Roche Diagnostics, Indianapolis, IN) monitors total cholesterol (see Fig. 13–9). It uses test strips that provide cholesterol results via the monitor in 3 minutes using a finger stick drop of blood.

■ FUTURE TRENDS

Additional point-of-care testing procedures that have evolved include the ALT (alanine aminotransferase) liver enzyme assay tested by the Cholestech L-D-X System to test for liver damage; the hemoglobin A_{1c} procedure to test for maintenance of blood glucose levels

Figure 13–9.   The Accu-Chek® InstantPlus.

(Courtesy of Roche Diagnostics, Indianapolis, IN.)

using the Bayer Diagnostics DCA 2000+ Analyzer (Bayer Corp. Diagnostics Division, Tarrytown, NY); the handheld Bili*Check* (SpecRx, Norcross, GA) that noninvasively measures the concentration of bilirubin in the forehead skin of 1- to 8-day-old newborns; and a rapid HIV point-of-care test—the Murex Single-Use Diagnostic System (SUDS) (see Chapter 17 on Legal and Regulatory Issues) manufactured by Abbott Diagnostics (Abbott Park, IL).

More point-of-care testing procedures are evolving that will inevitably involve phlebotomists, nurses, patient care technicians, and others who are providing care at the hospital bedside, nursing home, and/or home. For each new procedure, the health care worker must make a point of learning in detail the blood collection requirements, preventive maintenance, quality control, ethical and legal implications of doing such a test (e.g., HIV testing), recordkeeping, and calibration requirements in order to provide accurate and precise test results.

KEY TERMS

Blood Gas Analysis
Diabetes Mellitus
Insulin
Parkinson's Disease

Patient-Focused Testing
Point-of-Care Testing
Quality Control Material
Troponin T

STUDY QUESTIONS

For the following, choose the *one* best answer:

1. Insulin is released into the bloodstream in which of these circumstances?
   a. blood cholesterol levels decrease
   b. blood glucose levels decrease
   c. blood glucose levels increase
   d. blood cholesterol levels increase

2. Diabetes mellitus is caused by the inability of the pancreas to make or to use which substance?
   a. glucose
   b. cholesterol
   c. sodium
   d. insulin

3. In which of the following organs is insulin produced?
   a. gallbladder
   b. pancreas
   c. liver
   d. kidney

4. What is the next step after the skin is punctured to obtain blood for glucose monitoring?
   a. use the first drop of blood for the glucose test
   b. use an alcohol pad to remove the first drop of blood
   c. use a dry, sterile gauze pad to remove the first drop of blood
   d. squeeze the patient's finger to make a big first drop of blood for the monitor

5. What should the blood collector do prior to using reagent strips and/or controls in point-of-care testing?
   a. check the date when the bottle was opened
   b. check the expiration date
   c. verify that they were stored at the appropriate temperature
   d. all of the above

6. How can a phlebotomist increase the blood flow from the skin puncture site for patient testing?

   a. squeeze the punctured finger
   b. massage the area
   c. puncture another site adjacent to the first puncture site
   d. none of the above

7. What do blood gas analyses measure?

   a. Na^+ and K^+
   b. pCO_2, pO_2, and pH

   c. Cl^- and HCO_3^-
   d. pCO_2, Na^+, and Cl^-

8. Which tests are measured through blood coagulation monitoring by point-of-care testing?

   a. PT and APTT
   b. PT and pCO_2

   c. pO_2 and pCO_2
   d. PT, APTT, and pH

9. Which of the following is a blood glucose monitor?

   a. One Touch Profile (Life Scan, Mountain View, CA)
   b. i-STAT (i-STAT Corporation, Princeton, NJ)
   c. AccuMeter
   d. AccuMonitor

10. Which tests can be measured by electrolyte monitoring through point-of-care testing?

   a. Na^+, K^+, PT, and APTT
   b. Pco_2, Po_2, and Na^+

   c. Na^+, K^+, Cl^-, and HCO_3^-
   d. Pco_2, Cl^-, HCO_3^-, and Po_2

References

1. Tsai, WW, Nash, DB, Last, JV: Point-of-care testing: barriers and facilitators to implementation. *Clin Lab News.* 1994; October: 14.
2. Faulkner, WR, Meites, M: *Geriatric Clinical Chemistry: Reference Values.* Washington, DC; AACC Press: 1994.
3. National Committee for Clinical Laboratory Standards (NCCLS): *Blood Glucose Testing in Settings Without Laboratory Support; Proposed Guideline.* NCCLS Document AST4-P. Villanova, PA; NCCLS: 1996.
4. National Committee for Clinical Laboratory Standards (NCCLS): *Ancillary (Bedside) Blood Glucose Testing in Acute and Chronic Care Facilities.* NCCLS Document C30-T. Villanova, PA; NCCLS: 1994.
5. Joint Commission for Accreditation of Healthcare Organizations (JCAHO): *Accreditation Manual for Pathology and Clinical Laboratory Services.* Oakbrook Terrace, IL; JCAHO: 2000.
6. Despotis, GJ, Sontoro, SA, Spritznagel, E, et al.: Prospective evaluation and clinical utility of on-site monitoring of coagulation in patients undergoing cardiac operation. *J Thorac Cardiovasc Surg.* 1994;*107*(1):271–279.
7. Joint FDA/NIOSH/OSHA Advisory. Glass Capillary Tubes: *Joint Safety Advisory About Potential Risks.* 2/99.www.cdc.gov/niosh.

FOURTEEN

■

Urinalysis and Body Fluid Collections

CHAPTER OBJECTIVES

Upon completion of Chapter 14, the learner is responsible for the following:

1. Identify the types of body fluid specimens, other than blood, that are analyzed in the clinical laboratory, and the correct procedures for collecting and/or transporting these specimens to the laboratory.

2. Identify the various types of specimens collected for microbiological, throat, and nasopharyngeal cultures and the protocol that health care workers must follow when transporting these specimens.

3. List the types of patient specimens that are needed for gastric and sweat chloride analyses.

4. List three types of urine specimen collections and differentiate the uses of the urine specimens obtained from these collections.

In addition to collecting and transporting blood specimens, health care workers usually are involved in the collection and/or transportation of urine and other body fluid specimens. The health care worker should be careful when transporting body fluids because they are difficult to obtain and because the quality of the clinical laboratory test result is only as good as the specimen that is collected and transported to the testing site as quickly as possible under appropriate environmental conditions. Also, because such specimens may be biohazardous, the health care worker must adhere to universal standard precautions (see Chapter 4, Infection Control, and Chapter 5, Safety and First Aid) during collection and transportation of these specimens. Just as for blood collections, the laboratory request slip must accompany the specimen, which must be properly labeled with the patient's name, the patient's identification number, the date, the time of collection, the type of specimen, and the attending physician's name. The label should be affixed on the container, not the lid.

■ URINE COLLECTION

Routine urinalysis (UA) is one of the most frequently requested laboratory procedures because it can provide a useful indication of body health. It can be performed on a "first morning" or "random" urine specimen. Various diseases and disorders, such as those listed in Table 14–1, can be detected through a routine UA. Some of the more common types of urine specimen collections and their uses are provided in Table 14–2.

The routine UA includes a physical, chemical, and sometimes microscopic analysis of the urine sample. The physical properties include the following: color, transparency v. cloudi-

Table 14–1. Abnormal Urine Test Results and Associated Conditions

ABNORMAL URINE TEST RESULT	ASSOCIATED CONDITION
Presence of protein urine (proteinuria)	Kidney disease
	Prolonged exercise
	Chemical poisoning
Presence of hemoglobin in urine (indicates blood destruction)	Kidney disease
	Malaria
	Severe burns
	Chemical poisoning
Presence of bilirubin in urine	Liver disease
	Obstructive jaundice
Presence of glucose in urine (glycosuria)	Diabetes mellitus
Presence of leukocytes in urine (white blood cells)	Infection of the kidney
	Infection of the urinary bladder
	Infection of the urethra
Presence of ketone bodies in urine (ketosis)	Diabetes mellitus
	Starvation

Table 14–2. Types of Urine Specimen Collections and Their Uses

SPECIMEN TYPE	REASON FOR COLLECTION	USE
Random	This type of specimen is most convenient to obtain.	Routine urinalysis (UA) Quantitative and qualitative
First urine of the morning	This urine excretion is the most concentrated.	Protein, nitrate, microscopic analysis Routine Urinalysis (UA)
Fasting	Metabolic abnormalities are suspected	Glucose level determinations for diabetes mellitus testing
Clean-catch midstream	The specimen is free of contamination.	Culture for bacteria and/or microscopic analysis
Timed (e.g., 2 hour, 4 hour, 24 hour)	The excretion rate of the analyte can be determined.	Creatinine clearance test, urobilinogen determinations, hormone studies
Tolerance test	Timed blood and urine specimens are obtained to detect metabolic abnormalities.	Glucose tolerance test (GTT) and other tolerance tests

ness, odor, and concentration as detected through a specific gravity measurement. The chemical analysis for abnormal constituents is determined by using plastic strips impregnated with color-reacting substances that test for the presence of glucose, protein, blood (red blood cells [RBCs] and hemoglobin), white blood cells (WBCs), bacteria, bilirubin, and other constituents. The plastic strip, which has a separate reagent pad for each chemical test, is dipped into the urine briefly. The color of each reagent pad is compared to a color chart usually shown on the outer label of the reagent strip container. The results are reported according to the reagent label specifications (e.g., trace, $1+$, $2+$, and so on for a positive result, or negative when no reaction occurs). The strip is discarded after it is used one time. As for all types of point-of-care testing, quality control monitoring must be used to ensure accurate results. As an example, a point-of-care urine dipstick control, The Dropper Plus (Quantimetrix Corp., Redondo Beach, CA) (see Fig. 14–1) is used to monitor dipsticks such as the Multistix, Chemstrip, Uriscan, and other urinalysis reagent strips. The urine may also be viewed microscopically for the presence of blood cells, bacteria and other pathogenic microorganisms, crystals, and casts.

Other tests that can be performed on urine specimens are the pregnancy, myoglobin, and porphyrin tests. Urine is also the specimen of choice for drug abuse testing. Other laboratory procedures associated with the urinary system include the **creatinine clearance test** to determine the ability of the kidneys to remove creatinine from the blood and the **blood urea nitrogen (BUN) test** to measure the amount of urea in the blood.

PREGNANCY TEST

Human chorionic gonadotropin (HCG) is the first detectable analyte produced in pregnancy. Thus, its determination in the urine or serum is the basis of pregnancy tests. HCG is

Figure 14–1.   The Dropper Plus point-of-care urine dipstick control.

(Courtesy of Quantimetrix Corp., Redondo Beach, CA.)

a hormone produced by the placental cells beginning approximately 10 days after conception (implantation of the ovum).

The urinary excretion of HCG peaks during the first trimester of pregnancy at approximately 10 weeks. Several types of assays are used to determine urinary HCG levels. An example of a frequently used enzyme immunoassay for HCG is the ICON II HCG urine assay (Beckman Coulter Inc. Primary Care Diagnostics, Fullerton, CA). The procedure for this assay follows:

1. Obtain a **random urine sample** from the patient. If possible, use the first urine specimen of the morning because it has the highest concentration of HCG.
2. Drop five drops of the patient's urine onto the center of the Icon II HCG membrane, allowing each drop to absorb into the membrane before adding the next.
3. Drop three drops of the antibody–enzyme conjugate reagent (bottle A) in rapid sequence onto the Icon II membrane so that the reagent covers the entire surface.
4. Wait 1 minute.
5. Dispense wash solution (buffer in kit) by directing flow toward the inner wall of the test cylinder. Fill the cylinder to the fill line and wait for drainage of the wash solution before proceeding.
6. Dispense three drops of the substrate reagent (bottle B) in rapid sequence onto the membrane so that the reagent covers the entire surface of the membrane.
7. Wait 2 minutes.
8. Stop the reaction by filling the cylinder to the fill line with wash solution.
9. With the indicator mark facing the user, observe the color development at the test zone and the positive reference zone. Formation of a circular blue dot in the test

area confirms the presence of HCG. A built-in negative control indicates when a test result is invalid because of interfering substances.

Pregnancy tests are performed not only because of inquiry regarding pregnancy, but also for other medical reasons. Some of these reasons include the following:

- Certain surgical and diagnostic procedures (e.g., X-rays, colon surgery) are postponed or reconsidered if the patient is pregnant.
- Genetic counseling and/or plans to investigate, through cytogenetic and genetic studies, the possibility of any familial defects in the infant that may occur if the pregnancy test is positive.
- The HCG level is elevated in the urine of persons having various types of neoplasms and tumors (e.g., lung carcinoma).

SINGLE-SPECIMEN COLLECTION

The preferred urine specimen for most analyses is the first voided urine of the morning, when urine is the most concentrated. The urine collection containers must be clean and dry prior to the collection process. For routine UA procedures, appropriate containers include plastic disposable cups or bags (for infants) with a capacity of 50 mL. The containers must be properly labeled (label on container, not the lid), free of interfering chemicals, able to be tightly capped, and leakproof. The specimen should be transported to the UA section promptly for analysis within 2 hours after the patient voids. If transportation or analysis cannot occur within this time period, the urine should be refrigerated.

Another type of single-specimen urine test is the urine **culture and sensitivity (C&S)**. This specimen requires a **clean-catch midstream** urine collection. The patient is instructed to void approximately one half of the urine into the toilet, a portion is collected in a readily available sterile container (Fig. 14–2), and the rest is allowed to pass into the toilet.[1]

If asked, "What is a *clean-catch urine specimen?*" the procedure should be described, stating that this type of specimen is used to detect the presence or absence of infecting organisms. The specimen must be free of contaminating matter that may be present on the external genital areas. Thus, the steps in Box 14–1 should be explained to a female patient who is to obtain a clean-catch midstream urine specimen. For a male patient, the procedure in Box 14–2 should be adhered to for obtaining a clean-catch midstream urine specimen.[2]

The urine specimen must be transported to the microbiology section promptly. If it cannot be taken to the area for microbiological culturing within 1 hour of collection, the specimen should be refrigerated to prevent an overgrowth of contaminate bacteria. Figure 14–3 (Courtesy of GKR Industries, Inc., Crestwood, IL) provides an example of a latex-free urine collection container that has an extra-wide funnel opening, making it easy to use, especially for women and children. It seals in urine to protect the health care worker from infectious fluids and thus complies with OSHA universal standard precautions.

TIMED COLLECTIONS

For some laboratory assays, such as the creatinine clearance test, urobilinogen determinations, and hormone studies, 24-hour (or other timed period) urine specimens must be obtained. Incorrect collection and improper preservation of this type of specimen are two frequent errors affecting timed collections. Thus, the health care worker should be aware of the protocol for

Figure 14–2. Midstream urine collection catch kits.

(Courtesy of Evergreen Scientific, Los Angeles, CA.)

BOX 14–1. CLEAN-CATCH MIDSTREAM URINE COLLECTION INSTRUCTIONS FOR WOMEN

1. After washing her hands, the woman should separate the skin folds around the urinary opening and clean this area with mild antiseptic soap and water or special towelettes.
2. Holding the skin folds apart with one hand and after urinating into the toilet, the patient should urinate into a sterile container. The container should not touch the genital area. It must be covered with the lid provided after urination. It is extremely important not to touch the inside or lip of the container with the hands or other parts of the body.
3. The health care worker, or sometimes the patient, will label the container with her name and the time of collection and deliver it to the requested location.
4. Health care personnel should refrigerate the urine specimen immediately.

BOX 14–2. CLEAN-CATCH MIDSTREAM URINE COLLECTION INSTRUCTIONS FOR MEN

1. The man should wash his hands and the end of his penis with soapy water or special towelettes and then let dry.
2. After allowing some urine to pass into the toilet, the patient should collect the urine in the sterile container. The container should not touch the penis. Steps 3 and 4 are the same as those for a woman.

Figure 14–3. VOID-EASE urine collection bag.

(Courtesy GKR Industries Inc., Crestwood, IL.)

collecting a 24-hour urine specimen so that he or she can assist other health care professionals and the patient in preventing collection errors. The steps in Box 14–3 should be followed for a 24-hour urine collection.[3]

TOLERANCE TESTS

The glucose tolerance test (GTT) (see Chapter 12 for detailed steps) requires individual urine specimens collected serially at times that correlate with the timing of the blood specimens (i.e., fasting, 30 minutes, 60 minutes). The diagnosis and treatment regimen depend on the interpretation of the timed specimens. Thus, specimens must be collected according to the schedule established for the patient. Each specimen must be labeled appropriately, including the time of collection and the specimen type (i.e., fasting, 30-minute collection). This protocol also applies to other tolerance tests.

■ CEREBROSPINAL FLUID

Cerebrospinal fluid (CSF) is obtained by a physician through a spinal tap or lumbar puncture. The fluid is usually collected in three sterile containers numbered in the order in

BOX 14–3.   INSTRUCTIONS FOR A 24-HOUR URINE COLLECTION

1. The patient should be given a chemically clean, wide-mouthed, 3- to 4-L container with a tight-fitting lid. The laboratory personnel should add any required preservatives to the container prior to giving it to the patient. Patients should not be allowed to submit urine specimens in their own jars because the jars might not be chemically clean and would not contain the required preservatives. The preservative and any associated precautions should be written on the collection container label. The label should be placed on the container, not on the lid. Other information on the label should include the following:

   - Patient's name.
   - Patient's identification number.
   - Starting collection date and time.
   - Ending collection date and time.
   - Name of the requested laboratory test.

Other information that may be required by the facility includes:

   - Physician's name.
   - Patient's location (e.g., hospital room, outpatient).

2. The patient should be instructed verbally that the collection of the 24-hour urine specimen begins with emptying the bladder and discarding the first urine passed. This first step in the collection process should start between 6 and 8 A.M., and the exact time should be written on the container label.

3. Except for the first urine discarded, all urine should be collected during the next 24-hour period. The patient should be reminded to urinate at the end of the collection period and to include this urine in the 24-hour collection. The patient should be told to urinate before having a bowel movement because fecal material in the urine specimen will make the specimen unacceptable for collection.

4. Because urine is an ideal culture medium for microorganisms that decompose chemical constituents, the patient should be instructed to refrigerate the entire specimen after adding each collection during the 24-hour period, except for urate testing.

5. Some preservatives for 24-hour urine collection are corrosive if accidentally spilled or if the patient comes in contact with them during collection. Thus, the patient should be warned of any preservatives in the container.

6. The patient should be informed not to add anything except urine to the container and not to discard any urine during the collection period.

7. A normal intake of fluids during the collection period is desirable unless otherwise indicated by the physician.

8. Some laboratory assays require special dietary restrictions; these instructions should be given to the patient.

9. If possible, medications should be discontinued for 48 to 72 hours preceding the urine collection as a precaution against interference in the laboratory assays.

10. The 24-hour urine specimen should be transported to the clinical laboratory as soon as possible. The specimen should be placed in an insulated bag or a portable cooler to maintain the cool temperature.

11. Following the verbal instructions for the 24-hour urine collection, the patient should be provided with written instructions (non–English speaking patients should receive instructions in their native language) as a reminder.

which they were collected. The first tube is usually contaminated with blood or tissue debris. Thus, the first tube is usually transported to the clinical chemistry or serological testing area of the laboratory. The second tube is used for clinical microbiology testing, and the third tube is usually used for cytological and microscopic analysis. Tests commonly performed on CSF include total protein level, glucose level, cell count, microbiological, chloride level, and cryptococcal antigen determinations. Wearing gloves, CSF must be *immediately* transported at room temperature to the clinical laboratory for stat analysis. Transportation can occur to a reference laboratory if the CSF is maintained in an ice slurry;[4] however, it should not be frozen.

■ FECAL SPECIMENS

Stool (fecal) specimens are commonly collected in order to detect parasites (e.g., **ova and parasites [O&P]**), enteric disease organisms (e.g., *Salmonella, Shigella, Staphylococcus aureus*), and viruses. The specimen is collected in a wide-mouthed plastic or waxed cardboard container with a tight fitting lid. If the patient is to collect the stool specimen at home, he or she should be given a collecting container and instructed to avoid urinating in the container because urine can kill the microorganisms in the collected stool specimen. For children, the container can be placed under the toilet seat so that the child can sit on the toilet. The patient should be instructed to wash the outside of the specimen container after collection and to wash his or her hands thoroughly. The specimen container must be properly sealed to prevent leakage and contamination because fecal material from patients with infectious intestinal diseases is extremely hazardous. The specimen must be transported to the laboratory immediately and maintained at body temperature (37°C) for detection of parasitic infections.

In addition to the collection of stool specimens for microorganism detection, feces are collected to detect invisible (occult) quantities of blood that do not alter the appearance of the stool. Laboratory determination of **occult blood** assists in the confirmation of the presence of blood in black stools and can be helpful in detecting gastrointestinal (GI) tract lesions and colorectal cancer. Feces for occult blood tests are often collected by the patient using special test cards, such as Hemdetect (DIPRO Diagnostic Products, Louisville, KY). The cards can be mailed or brought to the health care facility after collection. Manufacturers have also developed occult blood tests that can be performed at home without collecting a stool specimen. A chemically impregnated pad is dropped into the toilet by the patient after he or she has a bowel movement. The patient watches for a color change that he or she reports to the physician via a special test result card supplied with each patient kit. The health care workers involved in specimen collection and transportation should be aware of the procedural steps for these occult blood tests to instruct the patient for proper collections.[5] Many factors can contribute to false-negative or false-positive test results (i.e., patient's ingestion of aspirin, corticosteroids, ibuprofen, anticoagulants, and/or rare meats).

■ SEMINAL FLUID

Semen is examined in the clinical laboratory to (1) determine the effectiveness of a vasectomy, (2) investigate the possibility of sexual criminal charges, and (3) assess fertility. Before collection of a semen specimen, the patient should be given clear instructions for proper specimen collection. Semen must be collected in containers that are clean and free of trace detergents. Condoms can be used but must be washed free of spermicidal substances prior to use. Specimens must not be exposed to extremes of temperature or light prior to being submitted to the clinical laboratory and should be transported within 2 hours of collection.

■ AMNIOTIC FLUID

Fluid that bathes the fetus within the amniotic sac is called **amniotic fluid**. It may be collected by a physician when the pregnant patient is at approximately 16 weeks' gestation so that fetal abnormalities can be detected through chromosomal analysis and chemical tests, such as the alpha-fetoprotein (AFP) assay. Occasionally, amniotic fluid is obtained in the last trimester of pregnancy to determine the lung maturity of the fetus. In addition to wearing gloves when transporting amniotic fluid to the laboratory, the specimen must be protected from light and transported immediately.

■ OTHER BODY FLUIDS

In addition to the fluids just discussed, other types of body fluids that sometimes must be transported to the laboratory include **synovial fluid**, which is extracted aseptically from joint cavities, and fluid aspirated from body cavities (e.g., **pleural fluid** obtained from the lung cavity, **pericardial fluid** from the heart cavity, **peritoneal fluid** from the abdominal cavity). Other specimens for forensic and toxicology studies are mentioned in Chapter 15.

Upon receiving any type of body fluid for transportation, it is important to verify that the container is properly labeled with the patient's name, the patient's identification number, the date, the time of collection, and the type of body fluid collected.[5] If the containers holding any type of body fluids are contaminated on the outside, it is extremely important to wear gloves when transporting them.

■ CULTURE SPECIMENS

Other specimens that the health care worker may be requested to transport to the clinical laboratory include **sputum** (fluid from the lungs containing pus), throat and sinus drainage cultures, wound cultures, ear or eye cultures, and skin cultures. The health care worker should be extremely careful while transporting each type of specimen because the specimens can easily become contaminated and may be biohazardous. For safety, the health care worker needs to wear gloves when handling and transporting these specimens in their containers.

■ OTHER NONBLOOD PROCEDURES

THROAT AND NASOPHARYNGEAL CULTURE COLLECTIONS

Nasopharyngeal cultures are often performed to detect carrier states of *Neisseria meningitidis, Corynebacterium diphtheriae, Streptococcus pyogenes, Haemophilus influenzae,* and

Staphylococcus aureus. For infants and children, from whom significant sputum cultures are difficult to obtain, nasopharyngeal cultures may be used to diagnose whooping cough, croup, and pneumonia. Throat cultures are most commonly obtained to determine the presence of streptococcal infections. Because coughing may force organisms from the lower respiratory tract into the nasopharynx, it may be best to perform a throat culture on a child or an infant and stimulate coughing in order to obtain a more significant nasopharyngeal culture. Health care workers should be thoroughly taught the correct procedures before they are allowed to acquire specimens from patients.

When a throat culture is ordered, the patient should be instructed to open the mouth wide, as if to yawn. A light source should be directed into the mouth and throat so that areas of inflammation, ulceration, exudation, or capsule formation can be readily seen. A tongue blade or spoon is used to depress the tongue and to prevent contamination with organisms from the oral cavity. A sterile cotton swab should be used to brush both tonsillar areas, the posterior pharynx, and all other areas of possible infection.[6]

The swab can then be placed in a special transport medium or the fluid on the swab can be inoculated directly onto agar in a Petri dish by rolling the swab across a small area of the medium. The specimen can then be transported to the laboratory, where it may be spread out, or "streaked," for distribution of the microorganisms. A Gram-stained smear is often useful to provide preliminary indications of infection and should be made with the swab by rolling it across a sterile slide before placing it in a transport medium or inoculating plate agar. The slide, the swab, and any inoculating media should be taken to the laboratory and processed as soon as possible after collection. The culture should be placed under optimal growth conditions for suspected pathogens (i.e., the culture should be incubated). Timely processing of the specimen helps prevent overgrowth of normal flora, which can inhibit or mask any pathogenic organisms present.

Nasopharyngeal specimens should be obtained with a Dacron- or cotton-tipped flexible wire that can be easily sterilized prior to use. Commercially packaged sterilized swabs are also available. The swab is passed gently through the nose and into the nasopharynx, where it is rotated. Then the swab is carefully removed and placed in a transport medium or the fluid on the swab is inoculated onto a medium for isolation. Again, the timely processing of all specimens is crucial for best results.

SKIN TESTS

On occasion, a nurse or other health care worker may be asked to perform a **skin test**. The health care worker should check the policies of the health care facility prior to performing the procedure. Skin tests are simple and relatively inexpensive. They determine whether a patient has ever had contact with a particular antigen and has produced antibodies to that antigen. A wide range of disease states stimulate antibody responses in individuals. Tests range from detection of ragweed and milk allergies in hypersensitive individuals, to detection of tuberculosis (TB) and fungal infections in persons who have had contact with these organisms.

The TB skin test can be administered using an automatic device or by pulling 0.1 mL of diluted antigen into a tuberculin syringe. All air bubbles should be expelled by holding the syringe vertically and tapping the sides of the barrel. The volar surface of the patient's forearm should be cleaned with alcohol and prepared in the same manner as for a venipuncture (see Chapter 8). The area should be devoid of scars, skin eruptions, and excessive hair.

Holding the syringe at a slight angle (approximately 20 degrees), the needle should be slipped just under the skin. The plunger should be pulled back to ensure that a blood vessel has not been entered. The fluid may be slowly expelled into the site. The needle should be promptly removed, and only slight pressure applied, with gauze, over the site. Care should be taken that the fluid does not leak onto the gauze or run out of the injection site. The patient should hold the arm in an extended position until the site has time to close and retain the fluid. A bandage should not be used over the site because it may absorb some of the fluid and distort the results of the skin test by causing skin irritation from the adhesive.

The patient should report any reaction, no matter how slight, to the physician. Also, a return visit for proper interpretation of the skin reaction should be scheduled with the physician. At some health care agencies, the patient is asked to note the exact size of the reaction site or to compare their reaction with pictures on a prelabeled card that can be mailed back to the institution. When this is the case, patients should be fully informed about how to read positive and negative reactions.

GASTRIC ANALYSIS AND HOLLANDER TEST

Gastric analysis and the **Hollander test** both involve gastric (stomach) fluid to determine gastric function in terms of stomach acid production. The gastric analysis measures gastric acid secretion in response to stimulation from histamine or pentagastrin, whereas the Hollander test uses insulin to stimulate gastric secretions. Both tests involve passing a tube through the patient's nose and into the stomach. Both tests also require intravenous (IV) administration of the stimulant. The health care worker may be asked to assist and collect specimens as required. The responsibility for properly intubating the patient (using fluoroscopic examination) and administering the stimulant intravenously usually rests with the physician or the nurse. The health care worker can be present to assist in patient care and to draw any required blood specimens, but under *no* circumstances should be expected to carry out the procedure unless properly trained. Improper placement of the tube poses a high risk to the patient and could result in a punctured lung if the tube enters the bronchial system instead of the esophagus. The health care worker can and should be responsible for proper labeling of gastric and blood samples when he or she is present and assisting during the procedure.

■ BREATH ANALYSIS FOR PEPTIC ULCERS

Helicobacter pylori is a bacteria that has been shown through research to alter the gastric lining, making it more vulnerable to damage by gastric acids and leading to peptic ulcers. Recently, a breath test, Meretek UBT, to detect *Helicobacter pylori* has been introduced by Meretek (Nashville, TN) to diagnose and monitor peptic ulcers. The health care worker should be aware of the procedural steps to assist the patient.

SWEAT CHLORIDE BY IONTOPHORESIS

The **sweat chloride test** is used in the diagnosis of cystic fibrosis.[7,8] Cystic fibrosis is a disorder of the exocrine glands, generally thought to be enzymatic in nature, that causes changes in mucus-producing glands in the body. Primarily affected are the lungs, upper respiratory tract, liver, and pancreas. Patients with cystic fibrosis produce chloride in their sweat at two to five times the level produced by healthy individuals.

For the laboratory evaluation, pilocarpine hydrochloric acid (HCl) is iontophoresed into the skin of the patient to stimulate sweat production. The sweat is absorbed onto preweighed gauze pads, then the weight of the sweat is determined. The pad is then diluted with deionized water, and the chloride is generally read by titration with a chloridometer.

When a health care provider receives an order to perform a sweat chloride test on a patient, he or she should properly prepare for the procedure under the supervision of a clinical laboratory scientist. Four cups and lids should be preweighed with two 2-in. square gauze pads in each cup. Only two cups are normally used, but the other two can be used as backups, if needed. The patient needs to be appropriately dressed for the climate and drinking fluids to be well hydrated.

Choosing a site with the largest surface area (in children and infants, the leg is best suited), the health care worker should wipe the surface of the skin with an alcohol prep and then with a gauze pad soaked in *deionized* water. Tap water must not be used. Next, the area is wiped dry with a sterile gauze pad. Another 2-in. square, eight-ply gauze pad is soaked in 0.07 moles/liter sodium bicarbonate and placed on the cleaned area. The negative electrode is placed on the gauze and taped securely to the skin. The electrode should not come into direct contact with the skin at any time when the current is on.

Another gauze square is soaked in 0.33 percent pilocarpine HCl and placed on the skin next to the sodium bicarbonate square but not touching it. The positive electrode should be placed on this piece of gauze and taped securely in place. Again, care should be taken that the electrode does not come into direct contact with the skin at any time during the procedure. Before the current is turned on, the area between and around the secured gauze squares should be wiped dry.

Next, the current is turned on and very slowly increased to 1 mA. The current must be incremented slowly because a sudden increase may electrically shock the patient. After 10 minutes, the current is decreased to zero. The switch is turned off, and the electrodes and gauze squares are removed and discarded. Reagent-grade water is used to wipe off the pilocarpine HCl area, which is then wiped dry.

A 2 × 2-in. square of thin waxed film, such as Parafilm, should be cut out and handled with clean forceps. Using the forceps, the film can be placed against the cleaned area and taped securely onto the skin on adjacent sides. Still using the forceps, two gauze pads from a preweighed cup are removed and placed between the Parafilm and the skin. The remaining side can be taped securely. Tape may also be applied across the top of the Parafilm to prevent it from tearing. A timer should be started for 1 hour. During that period, the procedure should be repeated on the other arm or leg.

After 1 hour, the tape should be carefully removed, and the gauze sponges removed with forceps and returned to the original cup. The lid must be placed tightly on the cup and the cup weighed again. After weighing, 200 μL of deionized water should be added to the cup. The lid should be replaced and wrapped securely with Parafilm. The gauze sponges should equilibrate 2 to 3 hours or overnight. The cups and a record of the weights measured during the procedure should be taken to the laboratory, where a clinical laboratory scientist will determine the chloride and calculate the results.

SELF STUDY

KEY TERMS

Amniotic Fluid
Blood Urea Nitrogen (BUN)
Cerebrospinal Fluid (CSF)
Clean-Catch Midstream
Creatinine Clearance Test
Culture and Sensitivity (C&S)
Gastric Analysis
Hollander Test
Occult Blood

Ova and Parasites (O&P)
Pericardial Fluid
Peritoneal Fluid
Pleural Fluid
Random Urine Sample
Skin Test
Sputum
Sweat Chloride Test
Synovial Fluid

STUDY QUESTIONS

For the following, choose the *one* best answer.

1. What type of urine specimen is needed to detect an infection?

   a. random
   b. clean-catch
   c. routine
   d. 24 hour

2. Which of the following types of specimens is most frequently collected for analysis?

   a. amniotic fluid
   b. urine
   c. CSF
   d. pericardial fluid

3. Which of the following body fluids is extracted from joint cavities?

   a. pleural fluid
   b. peritoneal fluid
   c. synovial fluid
   d. pericardial fluid

4. The O&P analysis is requested on what type of specimen?

   a. CSF
   b. amniotic fluid
   c. fecal
   d. synovial fluid

5. Fetal abnormalities are detected through analysis of which fluid?

   a. pleural
   b. peritoneal
   c. amniotic
   d. CSF

6. The occult blood analysis is frequently requested on what type of specimen?

   a. CSF
   b. fecal
   c. throat culture
   d. seminal fluid

415

7. Ketosis is frequently detected with which of the following conditions?

   a. liver disease
   b. diabetes mellitus

   c. chemical poisoning
   d. infection

8. Which of the following body fluids is obtained from the abdominal cavity?

   a. synovial fluid
   b. pericardial fluid

   c. peritoneal fluid
   d. CSF

9. Which of the following can be used in children and infants to diagnose whooping cough?

   a. CSF culture
   b. nasopharyngeal culture

   c. amniotic fluid culture
   d. pericardial fluid culture

10. What is the specimen of choice for drug abuse testing?

    a. CSF
    b. urine

    c. synovial fluid
    d. gastric fluid

References

1. Garza, D: Urine collection and preservation. In: Ross, DL, Neely, AE, (eds): *Textbook of Urinalysis and Body Fluids.* New York; Appleton-Century-Crofts: 1983, p. 61.

2. Free, AH, Free, HM: *Urinalysis in Clinical Laboratory Practice.* Cleveland; CRC Press: 1975.

3. National Committee for Clinical Laboratory Standards (NCCLS): *Routine Urinalysis and Collection, Transportation, and Preservation of Urine Specimens.* NCCLS Document GP16-T. Villanova, PA; NCCLS: December 1992.

4. Guder, WG, Narayanan, S, Wisser, H, Zawta, B: *Samples: From the Patient to the Laboratory.* Darmstadt, Germany; Git Verlag Pub.: 1996.

5. Jacobs, ES, Horvat, R, Demott, W et al., (eds): *Laboratory Test Handbook.* 4th ed. Cleveland; Lexi-Comp Inc.: 1996.

6. Becan-McBride, K, Ross, D: *Essentials for the Small Laboratory and Physician's Office.* Chicago; Mosby-Year Book: 1988.

7. National Committee for Clinical Laboratory Standards (NCCLS): *Sweat Testing: Sample Collection and Quantitative Analysis.* NCCLS Document C34-A. Wayne, PA; NCCLS: 1994.

8. Cystic Fibrosis Foundation: *Clinical Practice Guidelines for Cystic Fibrosis.* Bethesda, MD; 1997.

15

FIFTEEN

■

Specimen Collection for Forensic Toxicology, Workplace Testing, Sports Medicine, and Related Areas

CHAPTER OUTLINE

Chapter Objectives
Overview and Prevalence of Drug Use
Forensic Toxicology Specimens
Chain-of-Custody
Federal Workplace Drug Testing
Drug Testing in the Private Sector
Drug Use in Sports
Preferred Specimens for Drug Tests
Specimen Collection Sites

Specimen Collection Procedures
- Collecting Urine for Drug Testing
- Collecting Specimens for Alcohol Levels
Neonatal Drug Testing
- Tampering with Specimens
Self Study
- Key Terms
- Study Questions

CHAPTER OBJECTIVES

Upon completion of Chapter 15, the learner is responsible for the following:

1. Define *toxicology* and *forensic toxicology*.

2. Give five examples of specimens that can be used for forensic analysis.

3. Describe the role of the health care worker or "collector" in federal drug testing programs.

4. List security measures and minimum site requirements for urine collection for federal drug testing programs.

5. Describe the function of a chain-of-custody, and the Custody and Control Form.

6. List the basic steps in specimen collection for urine drug tests and blood alcohol levels.

7. Describe how to detect adulteration of urine specimens.

■ OVERVIEW AND PREVALENCE OF DRUG USE

The use of alcohol, tobacco, and **illicit drugs** (illegal drugs including opiates, cocaine, amphetamines, etc.) has been declining in recent years; however, a significant percentage of the U.S. population uses at least one of these substances. Alcohol is the most commonly used substance. In a 1992 survey, approximately 48 percent had consumed alcohol in the past month and approximately 11 percent acknowledged using illicit drugs in the past 12 months. Persons between the ages of 18 to 25 years are the most likely to use illicit drugs, and approximately 30 percent of high school seniors are classified as heavy users of alcohol (having five or more drinks in the previous 2 weeks). Teenagers use alcohol and tobacco more than any other drugs. They are sometimes referred to as **"gateway drugs"** because adolescents with substance abuse problems tend to begin with alcohol and cigarettes, progress to marijuana, and then move on to using other drugs or combinations of drugs.[1]

The leading cause of death among people between 15 to 24 years of age is violence, including accidents, homicides, and suicides. Often these deaths are attributed to the use of drugs and alcohol.[1]

Among pregnant women approximately 25 percent use nicotine and 5 to 8 percent are at risk for alcohol-related prenatal problems. It is estimated that 500,000 to 750,000 newborns are exposed to illicit drugs annually. Treatment of heroin addiction during pregnancy, however, is particularly important for the health of the mother and the baby. Heroin produces wide swings in blood levels, can lead to premature labor, spontaneous abortion, and other severe adverse effects. If an addicted mother is treated by methadone maintenance, pregnancy tends to increase methadone metabolism so some patients require two doses per day to maintain stable blood levels. Infants born to mothers on methadone therapy are dependent on opioids but are not addicted and are more easily treated. Approximately 11 percent of women in a 36-hospital study had taken illicit drugs during pregnancy.[1,2]

The development of modern collection devices, screening techniques, clinical laboratory automation, molecular advances, and computer technology have increased the variety of laboratory testing options available for the diagnosis and treatment of drugs of abuse and analysis of specimens in remote locations or from crime scenes. The following sections will provide basic guidelines and resources for further information.

The health care worker who is responsible for collecting the specimen plays a key role in ensuring the integrity of the specimen. The major responsibilities for the collector include:

- Identification of both the donor and the specimen
- Prevention of specimen adulteration or substitution
- Tamper proofing the collected specimen
- Initiation of the chain-of-custody
- Accurate and comprehensive documentation

■ FORENSIC TOXICOLOGY SPECIMENS

Toxicology is the scientific study of poisons (including drugs), how they are detected, their actions in the human body, and the treatment of the conditions they produce. **Forensic specimens** are those involved in civil or criminal legal cases. Forensic toxicology usually involves testing specimens for drugs of abuse in legal cases.

In toxicologic analysis, very small amounts of analytes are usually found in the blood, urine, or other specimens obtained for analysis. Thus, the type of specimen (e.g., venous blood, arterial blood, urine, hair, meconium), materials, and equipment used for collecting specimens for toxicologic analysis can greatly affect analytic results. The type of glass or plastic composing the collection tube, cover, or both may contain materials that will contaminate and/or react with or absorb the analytes. Even oils or bacteria from dirty fingers that handle specimens may cause contamination. Thus, for toxicologic specimens, the health care worker must strictly adhere to the facility's laboratory guidelines for collection of these types of specimens.

Extensive training, experience, and supervision are required for collecting specimens for forensic analyses. Box 15–1 includes types of specimens that may be used for forensic toxicology studies or other medical applications of a criminal investigation. Forensic laboratory analysis is completely different from other types of laboratory analyses in the following ways[3]:

- Specimens are very diverse, ranging from vaginal swabs in rape cases to contact lenses found on a sofa at a crime scene
- Specimens may be exposed to the elements (rain, mud, mixed blood from multiple individuals)
- Specimens may be available in only trace amounts (a single hair or one smudge of blood)
- Forensic scientists must perform analyses in all types of environments, and their results must be able to stand up to the most intense judicial scrutiny

Crime laboratories are involved in analyzing **trace evidence** (evidence found at the scene of the crime or on a person, e.g., fingerprints, shoe impressions, hairs, fibers, paint chips, glass fragments, soil samples); firearms and toolmarks (to analyze bullets and tool markings); drug chemistry (identification of drugs); toxicology (e.g., carbon monoxide, poisonings, drugs); arson and fire debris; biology and serology (e.g., semen stains, vaginal swabs

BOX 15–1.   FORENSIC SPECIMENS

Specimens that may be used in forensic analyses[4–7]:
- Anorectal swabs
- Arterial blood
- Bones
- Capillary blood
- Clothing
- Dried blood stains
- Hair
- Nails, nail scrapings or clippings
- Saliva
- Skin
- Sperm, semen residue
- Sweat
- Teeth, oral swabs
- Urine
- Venous blood
- Vaginal swabs

from sexual assaults, crime scene specimens, DNA analysis); documents (e.g., paper, ink, type of printing, gum marks, etc.); and computers.[3]

DNA testing has become particularly helpful because of its accuracy in identification. Many highly publicized trials hinge on the outcome of DNA testing, and recently several dozen inmates have been released because of a wrongful conviction proved by DNA testing. In sexual assault cases, only 20% to 45% of the victims show signs of bodily injuries; therefore, laboratory evidence is vital to support the victim's claims. In general, DNA analysis is useful for the following reasons[4,5]:

- It is the same in all parts of the body except eggs and sperm, which contain one-half of the DNA material
- It stays the same throughout life
- It is present in all cells
- It differs from one person to another except in the case of identical twins

All specimens must be labeled using permanent markers with the victim's name, sample, site, and if possible an identification number for reference. The evidence must pass directly from the medical examiner to the individuals who will process specimens using a chain-of-custody signature procedure. This provides a complete documentation system of all individuals who handle the specimen. Specimens should be kept in a locked area.

■ CHAIN-OF-CUSTODY

The **chain-of-custody** is a process for maintaining control and accountability of each specimen from the point of collection to final disposition of the specimen. The process documents the identity of each individual that handles the specimen and each time a specimen is transferred in the chain. A chain-of-custody form is also required that indicates specific identification of the patient or subject, the individual who obtained and processed the specimen, the date, the location, and the signature of the subject documenting that the specimen in the container is the one that was obtained from the person identified on the label. The specimen must be placed in a specimen transfer bag that is permanently sealed until it is opened for analysis. The seal ensures a "tamper-evident" transfer of contents until it reaches its destination for analysis.[2] Even after the specimen reaches its destination, each individual who handles every aliquot should sign and complete the chain-of-custody forms.

■ FEDERAL WORKPLACE DRUG TESTING

Workplace drug testing programs initially began in the mid-1980s when Mandatory Guidelines were published by the **Department of Health and Human Services (HHS).** This initiative established scientific and technical guidelines for federal drug testing programs, as well as standards for certification of laboratories engaged in urine drug testing for federal agencies, such as the **Department of Transportation (DOT).** The standards relate to the testing of specimens, quality assurance and quality control, the chain-of-custody form called the **Custody and Control Form (CCF),** personnel, and results reporting. They require that each certified laboratory be inspected at least twice a year to document performance. Box 15–2 indicates the classes of drugs that the DOT requires in initial testing and confirmatory testing, and Box 15–3 indicates the format of the CCF. The Substance Abuse and Mental Health Services Administration (SAMHSA) has published a useful

BOX 15–2. DRUG TESTS REQUIRED BY FEDERAL AGENCIES

Initial tests (using immunoassays):

- Marijuana metabolites.
- Cocaine metabolites.
- Opiate metabolites.
- Phencyclidine.
- Amphetamines.

Confirmatory tests (using gas chromatography/mass spectrometry techniques):

- Marijuana metabolite: delta-9-tetrahydrocannabinol-9-carboxylic acid.
- Cocaine metabolite: benzoylecgonine.
- Opiates: morphine and codeine.
- Phencyclidine.
- Amphetamines: amphetamine and methamphetamine.

BOX 15–3. USE OF THE OMB-APPROVED CUSTODY AND CONTROL FORM (CCF) TO DOCUMENT THE COLLECTION OF A URINE SPECIMEN[6]

The CCF is usually obtained from the laboratory performing the testing. The CCF consists of five copies:

1. Laboratory copy—must accompany specimen to laboratory.
2. Medical review officer copy.
3. Collector copy.
4. Employer copy.
5. Donor copy.

A copy of the CCF (OMB No. 0930-0158, Exp. Date: 6-30-2003) is on the SAMHSA Web site (www.health.org/workpl.htm).

Information (steps) required on the CCF.

1. Name, address, and identification number of the employer, specific name and address of the Medical Review Officer (MRO), donor's social security number or other employee identification number, reason for the test, and tests to be performed (e.g., random, pre-employment). (See the next page for special considerations for identification.)
2. Record temperature measurement of the specimen as "acceptable" or "unacceptable," whether it is a split or single specimen, whether it was an "observed" collection and why, and if no collection was obtained and why.
3. The collector seals the specimen bottle and has the donor initial the seal.
4. The donor provides a daytime phone number, evening phone number, date of birth, printed name, signature, and date of collection.

(continued)

BOX 15–3. *(continued)*

5. The health care worker provides the name and address of the collection facility, collector's business phone number, printed name and signature of the collector, date of collection, time of collection, and an indication of whether the collection was a single or split specimen collection.

6. This step is used to document the transfer and handling of the specimen at the collection site. On the first line, the collector records the date and prints and signs his or her name in the column labeled "Specimen received by." The collector should complete the first line immediately after receiving the specimen from the donor. A slight delay may be necessary while the temperature is being taken (within 4 minutes).

Special Considerations for Identification of Donor.

1. The donor must be positively identified by a photo identification, an authorized agency/employer representative, or any other identification specifically allowed under the agency's drug testing plan.

2. The following are *not* acceptable: identification by a co-worker or another donor or a single, nonphoto identification card. If the donor has no photo identification, the collector must document in the "Remarks" section of the CCF that none was available. If the donor can provide **two** items of identification bearing his or her signature (e.g., social security card, credit card, union or other membership cards, pay vouchers, voter registration card), the collector must confirm signature identification and may proceed with the collection process. If the signature identification is unconfirmed the collection may be discontinued. The collector must include ample information in the "Remarks" to help make a determination regarding the validity of the specimen collection process. A single nonphoto identification card is not an acceptable form of identification.

handbook for urine collection procedures in federal workplace drug testing programs.[6] It provides guidance to health care workers responsible for collecting urine specimens for these programs.

> The collector is the key to the success of a drug testing program and is the one individual with whom all donors will have direct, face-to-face contact. If the collector does not ensure the integrity of the specimen and adhere to the collection process, the specimen may not be considered a valid piece of evidence. If a specimen is reported positive for a drug or metabolite, the entire collection process must be able to withstand the closest scrutiny and all challenges to its integrity.[6]

■ DRUG TESTING IN THE PRIVATE SECTOR

Many private-sector employers also choose to have workplace drug testing procedures in place, and the testing guidelines may vary from the federal standards. However, private industries often elect to use laboratories that comply with the federal standards, so for purposes of this review the federal guidelines are discussed. Typically employees are screened without prior notice; therefore, the collection procedure, processing, analysis, and reporting are very strict and well-defined. Also, private employers may request that the certified laboratory test for several drugs or drug classes other than those required by the federal agencies (see Box 15–2), or they may use different testing levels for initial or confirmatory tests. Usually employers implement drug testing for the following reasons[7]:

- For contractor and vendor employees
- For designated positions
- Requirements by the government for airline pilots or bus drivers
- For safety or security sensitive positions
- For cause (i.e., sudden incidents or progressive incidents such as excessive unexcused absenteeism, tardiness, erratic behavior)
- After accidents
- Before promotions for specific positions
- Reasonable suspicion because of impaired functioning
- Clearance to return to work

The actual procedures for collecting a urine specimen for drug testing are discussed in the sections below.

■ DRUG USE IN SPORTS

Using drugs and performance-enhancing substances in sports has become more prevalent and highly publicized in recent years. At many levels of competitive sports, including collegiate, e.g., National Collegiate Athletic Association (NCAA); professional, e.g., National Basketball Association (NBA), the National Football League (NFL), and/or the Olympics, drug use is prominent. Even at the 2000 Olympics in Sydney, Australia, a new substance, **erythropoietin (EPO),** surfaced in athletes who tried to increase their endurance by overloading their system with erythrocytes through the transfusion of blood or the use of drugs such as EPO. EPO increases the body's production of RBCs, thereby increasing the oxygen-carrying capacity; the practice is also referred to as "blood doping." It leads to performance advantages in endurance sports such as cycling. However, it has also been associated with cardiovascular problems, strokes, and deaths. While EPO is harder to detect, recent advances in blood and urine testing should become strong deterrents.[8–10]

The NCAA alone tests more than 10,000 student athletes annually through drug testing programs. They test primarily for marijuana, cocaine, and amphetamines and employ a three-strike penalty for trying to treat and rehabilitate student athletes. After a third positive, the athlete is usually dismissed from athletic participation at his or her university or college. There are also indications that the use of anabolic steroids is on the rise.[9]

■ PREFERRED SPECIMENS FOR DRUG TESTS

Even though blood is the best specimen for alcohol and EPO testing, urine remains the preferred specimen in sports drug testing for the following reasons[9,10]:

- Drugs and their metabolites are present in higher concentrations in urine than in blood
- Large specimen volumes are easily obtainable
- There is no pain or discomfort to the athlete when collecting the specimen
- The process of collection is noninvasive

The downside of using urine specimens for drug testing is that it is easily adulterated, or altered by the donor. This is discussed further in a later section. Urine drug detection times are also limited from about 12 hours to 2 or 3 weeks, with most drugs being undetectable in 2 to 5 days. Detection times for drugs in human hair are longer, ranging from weeks to months; however, it is costly, and infrequent drug use will not likely be detected. Breath is a useful specimen when alcohol is suspected. There are numerous noninvasive **evidential breath testing (EBT)** devices on the market. These devices are often used in Emergency departments and law enforcement agencies since they are not regulated by CLIA '88. The Food and Drug Administration has also approved a saliva test for monitoring alcohol use.[10]

■ SPECIMEN COLLECTION SITES

According to federal guidelines, collection sites can be permanent or temporary facilities located at remote sites or in the workplace. The minimum site requirements are:

1. The site must allow the donor to have privacy while providing the urine specimen.
2. A source of water or moist towelettes must be available for washing hands.
3. There must be a work area for the collector.
4. The collector must be able to restrict access to the site during the collection.

Security measures should include:

1. Access should be restricted to authorized personnel only.
2. Only collection supplies/materials should be taken into the collection site.
3. Unobserved entrances/exits should be prohibited.
4. Secure handling/storage should be provided.
5. Access to water supply should be controlled by using tape to prevent opening/turning faucet handles, or closing the shut off valve for the water supply.
6. Bluing or other color-appropriate agents must be added to any tank or toilet bowl that is accessible to the donor.[6]

■ SPECIMEN COLLECTION PROCEDURES

COLLECTING URINE FOR DRUG TESTING

When a site has been selected, the health care worker should assure that the appropriate supplies are available. These are noted in Box 15–4.

The actual collection steps for a typical urine collection procedure for drug testing (noted in Box 15–5) under the HHS Mandatory Guidelines are extensive and highly regulated. Facilities that perform these tests and health care workers responsible for collecting the specimens must be adequately trained.[6]

Without appropriate documentation and meticulous attention to the details of the procedure, a specimen can be rejected for testing or results can be invalidated. This results in enormous losses, both financial and emotional, to the donor being tested, the agency or employer, and/or to the collector, who may lose his or her job. Box 15–6 indicates documentation errors that may result in specimen rejection.

If the specimen collector omits information, HHS recommends that laboratories retain specimens for a minimum of 5 days to allow the collector to provide a **Memorandum for Record (MFR),** a document that provides the appropriate correction, if possible. The laboratory should contact the collector immediately after a specimen is received to determine

BOX 15–4.   URINE COLLECTION SUPPLIES FOR DRUG TESTING[6]

The following supplies should be available to conduct proper collections:

1. Clean, single-use, wrapped or sealed specimen bottles with appropriate caps/lids.
2. Clean, single-use, wrapped or sealed collection containers for each donor to urinate into. These have wider bottle necks so they are easier to use.
3. Temperature strips that can be attached to the exterior surface of collection containers or specimen bottles to measure the temperature within 4 minutes after the donor gives the specimen bottle/container to the collector.
4. Temperature measuring devices that can be used to measure a donor's body temperature if the temperature of the specimen is outside of the mandatory range (32 to 38°C or 90 to 100°F).
5. Approved Chain-of-Custody Forms. The Office of Management and Budget (OMB) has approved Custody and Control Forms (CCFs), but they *cannot* be used by private sector companies for their workplace testing programs.
6. Tamper-evident labels/seals for the specimen bottles that have the same preprinted specimen ID number that appears on the CCF. Appropriate labels/seals are provided with each CCF.
7. Separate supply of tamper-evident seals in case the one provided does not properly adhere to the specimen container.
8. Leak-proof plastic bags in which sealed specimen containers are placed prior to shipment to the laboratory.
9. Absorbent material that is placed inside the leak-proof plastic bag in case the specimen container breaks or leaks during shipment.
10. Shipping containers/mailers that can be labeled for transporting specimens to the laboratory and that can be securely sealed to eliminate the possibility of undetected tampering.
11. Bluing or other coloring agent to add to the toilet bowl or tank to discourage adulteration/dilution of the specimen.
12. The health care worker should have appropriate identification. He or she is required to provide identification if requested by the donor. There is no requirement for the collector to have a picture ID or to provide his or her driver's license with an address. Also, the collector is not required to provide any certification or other documentation to the donor proving the collector's training in the collection process. It may benefit the health care worker to have his or her agency representative's name and telephone number to call should the donor request it.
13. Storage box, area, or place where specimens can be stored before shipment to the laboratory. It may be necessary to temporarily use a refrigerator or cabinet that can be secured. The health care worker should be within sight of the temporary storage area to ensure that no one has access to the specimens.
14. Single-use disposable gloves for use while handling specimens.

whether the collector can provide a means that would recover an error or omission in his or her documentation. If the collector indicates that the information can be recovered, the laboratory may test the specimen, but it may not report the results until the correction MFR is received.[6] Box 15–7 provides a sample MFR.

COLLECTING SPECIMENS FOR ALCOHOL LEVELS

Many states have provisions under which drivers suspected of being intoxicated by the arresting police officer must voluntarily give implied consent to the performance of certain laboratory assays to determine the level of blood alcohol. In some states, this statute applies

BOX 15–5. A TYPICAL URINE COLLECTION PROCEDURE FOR DRUG TESTING (FEDERAL MANDATORY GUIDELINES)[6]

1. The collector prepares the collection site to collect urine specimens. All collection supplies must be available, the area properly secured, water sources secured, and bluing agent placed in all toilets.

Note: If access to a water supply in the restroom cannot be controlled, the collector may tell the donor that he or she will be listening at the entrance to the restroom for any sounds associated with the donor attempting to use the available sources of water. Alternatively, the collector may enter the restroom with the donor if the collector is the same gender as the donor, but remains outside the toilet stall.

2. The collector begins the collection without delay after the donor arrives at the collection site.

Note: Do not wait because the donor is not ready, is unable to urinate, or an authorized employer or employee representative is delayed in arriving.

3. The collector requests the donor to present an acceptable form of identification as described previously.

Note: If the donor cannot satisfy the identification requirement, the collector may proceed with the collection if the donor can provide **two** items of identification bearing his or her signature. After the donor signs the certification statement, the collector should compare the donor's signature with signatures on the identification that was presented. If the signatures match, the collector lists on the "Remarks" line the two items of identification used to identify the donor and states that "signature identification was confirmed." The collector then continues with the collection process. If the signature does not match the signatures on the two items of identification presented, the collector should state on the "Remarks" line that "signature identification is unconfirmed," discontinue the collection, and notify the collection site supervisor and the agency.
Note: In situations where the donor does not have either a photo identification or two other appropriate items of identification that could be used to verify identity and signature, this should **not** be automatically considered a refusal to test. The collector should proceed with the collection. The collector should provide sufficient information on the "Remarks" line to help the Medical Review Officer (MRO) and the agency make a determination regarding the validity of the specimen and the collection process.
Note: If the donor asks the collector to provide identification, the collector must show the donor some form of identification. It must include the collector's name and the employer's name, address, and telephone number. It does not have to be a picture identification or include a home address.

4. The collector reviews the instructions on the back of the CCF with the donor.

5. The collector begins entering information and/or ensures that the required information is provided at the top of the CCF (the laboratory name and address and a pre-printed specimen ID number) and in Step 1 of the CCF (employer's name, address, and I.D. number (if applicable), MRO name, address, phone and fax number, donor SSN or employee ID number, reason for test, drug test to be performed, collection site information).

Note: A specific MRO's name and address must appear on the form rather than the name of the clinic or medical facility.

6. The collector asks the donor to remove any unnecessary outer clothing (e.g., coat, jacket, hat, etc.) and to leave any briefcase, purse, or other personal belongings he or she is carrying with the outer clothing. The donor may retain his or her wallet.

Note: The donor must not be asked to remove other articles of clothing, such as shirts, pants, dresses, or under garments. Additionally, the donor must not be requested or required to remove all clothing and wear a hospital or examination gown.

7. The collector directs the donor to empty his or her pockets and display the items to ensure that no items are present that could be used to adulterate the specimen. If nothing is there that can be used to adulterate a specimen, the donor places the items back into the pockets and the collection procedure continues.

Note: If an item is found that appears to have been brought to the collection site with the intent to adulterate the specimen, a direct observed collection procedure is used. If the item appears to be inadvertently brought to the collection site, secure the item and continue with the normal collection procedure.

BOX 15–5. *(continued)*

8. The collector instructs the donor to wash and dry his or her hands, preferably under the collector's observation, and told not to wash this or her hands again until after delivering the specimen to the collector.

Note: The donor must not be allowed any further access to water or other materials that could be used to adulterate/dilute the specimen.

9. The collector either gives the donor or allows the donor to select the collection container from the available supply. Either the collector or the donor, with both present, then unwraps or breaks the seal of the collection container.

Note: Do not unwrap or break the seal on any specimen bottle at this time.
Note: Do not allow the donor to take anything except the collection container into the room used for urination.

10. The collector directs the donor to go into the room used for urination, provide a specimen of at least 45 mL (split-specimen collection) or 30 mL (single-specimen collection), not to flush the toilet, and return with the specimen as soon as possible after completing the void.

Note: The donor is always permitted to provide a specimen in private unless a direct observed collection has been authorized.
Note: Pay close attention to the donor during the entire collection process to note any conduct that clearly indicates an attempt to substitute or adulterate a specimen. If you detect such conduct, immediately begin a new direct observed collection using a second CCF. Provide an appropriate comment on the "Remarks" line in Step 2 on the first CCF and submit it along with the specimen to the laboratory for testing. This will ensure that the laboratory knows that two separate specimens are being submitted for testing; the first one possibly being adulterated or substituted. Additionally, inform a supervisor that a collection took place under direct observation and the reason for doing so.

11. After the donor hands the specimen to the collector, the collector must measure the temperature of the specimen, check the specimen volume, and inspect the specimen for adulteration or substitution.

Temperature

Check the temperature of the specimen within four minutes after the donor hands you the specimen. The acceptable temperature range is 32°-38°C/90°-100°F. Temperature is determined by reading the temperature strip originally affixed to or placed on the outside of the collection container after the donor hands you the specimen.

1. If the temperature is within the acceptable range, the "Yes" box is marked in Step 2 on the CCF and the collector proceeds with the collection procedure.

2. If the temperature is outside the acceptable range, the "No" box is marked in Step 2 on the CCF and the collector immediately begins a direct observed collection procedure using a second CCF. The original specimen is sealed and sent with the first CCF to the laboratory with an appropriate comment on the "Remarks" line to indicate that a direct observed specimen was also being collected and submitted to the laboratory.

Specimen Volume

Check to make sure that the specimen contains a sufficient amount of urine (i.e., 30 mL for a single-specimen collection, 45 mL for a split-specimen collection).

A. Single-specimen collection. If the volume is less than 30 mL, the action taken will depend on whether the temperature of the specimen is in or outside the acceptable range.

1. If the temperature is in the acceptable range, the specimen is discarded and a second specimen is collected. The collector may use the same CCF for the second specimen, but must use a new specimen collection container. If the donor fails for any reason to provide 30 mL of urine for the second specimen collected, the collector will contact the agency to obtain guidance on the action to be taken.

(continued)

BOX 15–5. *(continued)*

2. If the temperature is **outside** the acceptable range, a second specimen is collected under direct observation and both specimens are sent to the laboratory for testing. The collector must use a separate CCF for each specimen and provide an appropriate comment on each CCF to indicate why two specimens were collected. If the donor fails for any reason to provide 30 mL of urine for the second specimen collected, the collector will contact the agency to obtain guidance on the action to be taken.

Note: In either case when a second specimen is to be collected, HHS permits giving the donor a reasonable amount of fluid to drink to provide a second specimen distributed reasonably through a period of up to 3 hours, or until the donor has provided a new sufficient amount of urine, whichever occurs first.

B. Split-specimen collection. If the volume is less than 30 mL, the action taken will depend on whether the temperature of the specimen is in or outside the acceptable temperature range.

1. If the temperature is in the acceptable range, the specimen is discarded and a second specimen is collected. The collector may use the original CCF for the second specimen, but should use a new specimen collection container.

   If the donor fails to provide 45 mL for the second specimen collected, the donor forfeits the right to the use of a split-specimen collection procedure and the collector submits the second specimen as a single-specimen collection with an appropriate comment on the "Remarks" line on the CCF.

2. If the temperature is **outside** the acceptable range, a second specimen is collected under direct observation and both specimens are sent to the laboratory for testing. The collector must use a separate CCF for each specimen and provide an appropriate comment on each CCF to indicate why two specimens were collected.

If the donor fails to provide 45 mL for the second specimen collected, the donor forfeits the right to the use of a split-specimen collection procedure and the collector submits the second specimen as a single specimen collection (regardless of the volume collected) with an appropriate comment on the "Remarks" line on the CCF.

Note: In either case when a second specimen is to be collected, HHS permits giving the donor a reasonable amount of fluid to drink to provide a second specimen distributed reasonably through a period of up to 3 hours, or until the donor has provided a new sufficient amount of urine, whichever occurs first.

C. Split-specimen collection. If the volume is between 30 and 45 mL, the action taken will depend on whether the temperature of the specimen is in or outside the acceptable temperature range.

1. If the temperature is in the acceptable range, all of the urine should be poured into one specimen bottle (Bottle A). Bottle A is sent to the laboratory along with the CCF. The collector should provide an appropriate comment on the "Remarks" line on the CCF that the donor did not provide a sufficient volume of urine for the split (Bottle B) specimen. The donor forfeits the use of a split-specimen collection procedure.

2. If the temperature is **outside** the acceptable range, a second specimen is collected under direct observation and both specimens are sent to the laboratory for testing. The collector must use a separate CCF for each specimen and provide an appropriate comment on each CCF to indicate why two specimens were collected.

If the donor fails to provide 45 mL for the second collection, the second specimen is submitted as a single-specimen collection and the collector should provide an appropriate comment on the "Remarks" line on the CCF that the donor did not provide a sufficient volume of urine for the split (Bottle B) specimen. The donor forfeits the use of a split-specimen collection procedure.

Note: In either case when a second specimen is to be collected, HHS permits giving the donor a reasonable amount of fluid to drink to provide a second specimen distributed reasonably through a period of up to 3 hours, or until the donor has provided a new sufficient amount of urine, whichever occurs first.

BOX 15–5. *(continued)*

Adulteration or Substitution

Inspect the specimen for unusual color, presence of foreign objects or material, or other signs of adulteration (e.g., if you notice any unusual odor). If it is apparent from this inspection that the donor has adulterated or substituted the specimen (e.g., the specimen is blue, exhibits excessive foaming when shaken, has smell of bleach), a second collection using direct observation procedures is conducted. The first specimen and the specimen collected using direct observation are both sent to the laboratory for testing. The first specimen is always sent to the laboratory even though it may have had an insufficient volume for either a single- or split-specimen collection.

If the donor does not provide the required amount of urine for the second collection using direct observation, the collector submits the second specimen as a single-specimen collection (regardless of the volume) and provides appropriate comments on the "Remarks" line on both CCFs.

Note: When a second specimen is to be collected, HHS permits giving the donor a reasonable amount of fluid to drink to provide a second specimen distributed reasonably through a period of up to 3 hours, or until the donor has provided a new sufficient amount of urine, whichever occurs first.

Note: Under no circumstance is the collector permitted to collect and add or combine urine from two separate voids.

12. The sealed specimen bottle is then unwrapped/opened in the donor's presence after the donor gives the specimen in the collection container to the collector. The collector or the donor may unwrap/open the specimen bottle.

Note: There will be two specimen bottles to be unwrapped/opened if a split specimen was collected.

Note: Both the collector and donor will maintain visual contact of the specimen until the label/seal is placed over the specimen bottle cap/lid.

13. The collector pours the specimen from the collection container into a specimen bottle, places the lid/cap on the bottle, and uses the "A" bottle tamper-evident label/seal. The "B" bottle label is discarded. If a split-specimen collection procedure is used, the collector pours 30 mL of urine into a specimen bottle, places the lid/cap on the bottle and uses the "A" bottle label/seal. The collector then pours the remaining urine (at least 15 mL) into a second bottle, places the lid/cap on the bottle, and uses the "B" bottle label/seal.

Note: The tamper-evident label/seal must be placed over the lid/cap to ensure that the lid/cap cannot be removed without destroying the label/seal. The donor must be present to observe the sealing of the specimen bottle(s).

14. The collector writes the date on the tamper-evident label(s)/seal(s). The donor is requested to initial the tamper-evident label(s)/seal(s).

Note: Occasionally, the tamper-evident label/seal provided with the CCF will not properly adhere to the specimen bottle because of environmental conditions (e.g., moisture, temperature, specimen bottle material). When this occurs, the collector should still apply the tamper-evident label/seal provided with the CCF and then apply a second, separate tamper-evident seal to seal the specimen bottle. This second seal should be placed perpendicular to the CCF label/seal to avoid obscuring information on the CCF. This second seal must be initialed and dated by the collector and should be initialed by the donor (i.e., if the donor is still present when it is apparent that the CCF label/seal is not properly adhering to the specimen bottle; however, a label/seal may appear to adhere when initially placed on the bottle, but after several minutes the label/seal begins to lift off along the edges). The collector must also provide an appropriate comment on the "Remarks" line (CCF, Step 2) stating why the second seal was used.

Note: If while sealing and initialing the CCF label/seal the collector or donor accidentally breaks/damages the seal, the collector must apply a second, separate tamper-evident seal to seal the specimen bottle. This second seal should be placed perpendicular to the CCF label/seal to avoid obscuring information on the CCF label/seal. This second seal must be initialed and dated by the collector and initialed by the donor. The collector must also provide an appropriate comment on the "Remarks" line (CCF, Step 2) stating why the second seal was used.

Note: Since the specimen bottle is now sealed with tamper-evident tape and does not have to be under the donor's direct observation, the donor is allowed to wash his or her hands if he or she desires to do so.

(continued)

BOX 15–5. *(continued)*

15. The donor reads the certification statement on Copy 2 of the CCF (Step 5), signs and dates the certification statement, provides date of birth, printed name, and day and evening contact phone numbers.

Note: If the donor refuses to sign the form, the collector must make a notation on the "Remarks" line to that effect. Otherwise, without the collector's comment, a CCF without the donor's signature could result in a canceled test. The same procedure should be followed if the donor refuses to initial the label(s).

16. The collector completes the chain of custody on the CCF (Step 4) by printing his or her name, signing where indicated, recording the date and time of the collection, and indicating the specific name of the delivery service to whom the specimen bottle(s) are being released.

17. The collector removes Copy 5 from the CCF and gives it to the donor. The donor may now leave the collection site.

Note: At this time, the collector can tell the donor to list any prescription and over-the-counter medications he or she may have recently taken on the back of the donor copy (Copy 5) of the CCF, but not on any other copy. This information will help the donor remember what medications he or she may have taken if a positive result is reported by the laboratory to the MRO.

18. The collector places the specimen bottle(s) and Copy 1 of the CCF inside the appropriate pouches of the leak-resistant plastic bag, seals the pouches, and initials and dates the seal.

19. The collector places the sealed plastic bag in an appropriate shipping container (e.g., express carrier mailer) and seals the shipping container as appropriate.

Note: If a collector is collecting several specimens within a short period of time, the sealed plastic bags may be placed into a single shipping container. The collector must maintain visual contact of the sealed plastic bags until all plastic bags are sealed in the single shipping container.
Note: The collector must ensure that each specimen is shipped to a laboratory as expeditiously as possible, the same day preferably.

Excerpted from "Urine Specimen Collection Handbook for Federal Workplace Drug Testing Programs" for Use with the New Federal Drug Testing Custody and Control Form OMB No. 0930-0158, Expiration date: June 30, 2003. Downloaded 2/19/01 from www.health.org/workplace/urinebook.htm.

BOX 15–6. DOCUMENTATION ERRORS ASSOCIATED WITH URINE DRUG TESTING

The following errors and omissions on the part of the collector may result in a specimen being rejected[6]:

1. The preprinted number on the custody form does not match the specimen ID number on the seal of the specimen bottle.
2. There is no specimen ID number on the seal.
3. There is an insufficient quantity of urine.
4. The seal is missing, broken, or shows evidence of tampering.
5. The specimen has been obviously tampered with (e.g., color, foreign objects, unusual odor).
6. The collector signed the certification statement but forgot to sign the line on the chain-of-custody.
7. The donor's social security number or ID number is omitted on the CCF, and the collector did not state that the "donor refused to provide information" in the "Remarks."
8. The donor's certification statement is not signed and there is no indication that the "donor refused to sign."

> ## BOX 15–7.   SAMPLE MEMORANDUM FOR RECORD[6]
>
> A *Memorandum For Record* is a statement prepared by an individual that provides or corrects information on any documents associated with a drug test.
>
> (*Use appropriate letterhead*)
>
> Memorandum For Record
>
> Date: _____
>
> From: _____ (*Collector's printed name*) _____
>
> To: _____ (*Drug Testing Laboratory Name and Address*) _____
>
> Subject: Memorandum to recover missing information
>
> Re: Specimen ID Number
>   Donor SSN or other ID Number
>
> On (*date of collection*) I served as the collector for the above specimen. While completing the custody and control form, I inadvertently forgot to (*insert appropriate phrase that describes the issue*). I have reviewed the collection procedure and am certain that I followed all other parts of the collection procedure (*may list other parts of the procedure here*) as required.
>
> To ensure that this omission will not happen again, I am planning to review the entire custody and control form before I separate the copies and seal the specimen bottles and the form in the leak-proof plastic bag.
>
> _____
>
>   (*Collector's signature*)
>
> cc: Medical Review Officer

only to the testing of urine and breath samples. Therefore, it is advisable to determine the medically acceptable manner for obtaining blood specimens from patients in each state. If blood alcohol specimens are collected by venipuncture, all procedures are similar to routine collections except that the health care worker performing the phlebotomy *must use a non-alcoholic disinfectant* to cleanse the site. If an alcohol wipe is used to cleanse the site it may interfere with test results. Correct identifications, precautions, and labeling procedures apply to these situations as well. The National Committee for Clinical Laboratory Standards (NCCLS) published *Blood Alcohol Testing in the Clinical Laboratory: Approved Guideline,* that provides technical and administrative guidance on laboratory procedures associated with blood alcohol testing, including specimen collection, analytic methods, quality assurance, and result reporting.[12,13]

■ NEONATAL DRUG TESTING

There are many health problems associated with neonatal drug exposure, including premature birth, low birth weight, impaired neurological functioning, and a higher risk of abuse and neglect.[2] Neonatal drug exposure is determined by using the maternal history, newborn clinical symptoms, and laboratory toxicology testing of the mother and infant. Cocaine is the drug most often identified in neonatal drug testing. Other drugs that are detected are opiates (including heroin, morphine, codeine, and other narcotics such as hydromorphone and hydrocodone), amphetamine and methamphetamines, and phencyclidine (PCP). Urine is the specimen most often used for neonatal drug exposure. Collection is possible by using neonatal urine collection bags and collecting the urine during the first 24 hours after birth. If the infant's urine is positive, it generally means that the mother used drugs 24 to 72 hours prior to childbirth. **Meconium,** the first intestinal discharge of a neonate, is greenish and consists of epithelial cells, mucus, and bile. Meconium is also used for drug analysis; the specimen is easier to collect than urine. Since meconium accumulates in the fetal bowel at approximately 16 weeks of gestation, a positive result indicates drug exposure to the neonate months before the birth. Other specimens used are amniotic fluids, cord blood, and gastric fluid; however, they are less suitable due to poor recovery of drugs from these samples.[2]

TAMPERING WITH SPECIMENS

Drug users have become very imaginative in ways to avoid a positive drug test result. **Adulteration** is a means of tampering with the specimen, usually urine, to make the specimen test negatively for drugs. It occurs in two ways: when substances are ingested by the patient to alter his/her own urine, and when substances are added or substituted for urine at the time of collection. Water is the most common substance added to the specimen or ingested to dilute the urine so that the drug concentrations are below the detection limit. Other substances that have been added to urine are liquid soap, bleach, salt, ammonia, vinegar, baking soda, UrinAid (glutaraldehyde), Klear (potassium nitrite), lemon juice, cologne, or other fluids.[11]

Detecting and deterring adulterants in urine can occur by:

- Sensory examination (odor and color) of the urine—e.g., bleach odor, foaming, or turbidity can be a sign of a liquid soap additive
- Simple tests such as specific gravity (if it is less than 1.003 or greater than 1.025); or urine creatinine less than 20 mg/dL and electrolytes (to determine values outside the physiologic range); Klear can be detected as a strong positive nitrite in a urine specimen with no bacteria present
- Working with the Substance Abuse and Mental Health Services Administration (SAMHSA) to seal off the water supply in the collection area, adding bluing to the toilet water, and preventing the patient from taking unneeded items into the collection stall

If tampering is suspected or observed, the health care worker must always seek approval to conduct another collection procedure under "direct observation." Federal guidelines are very strict about the circumstances for this measure; however, there are situations when it is required.[6]

SELF STUDY

KEY TERMS

Adulteration

Chain-of-Custody

Custody and Control Form
  (CCF)

Department of Health and
  Human Services (HHS)

Department of Transportation
  (DOT)

Erythropoietin (EPO)

Evidential Breath Testing (EBT)

Forensic Specimens

"Gateway Drugs"

Illicit Drugs

Meconium

Memorandum for Record (MFR)

Single-Specimen Collection

Split-Specimen Collection

Toxicology

Trace Evidence

STUDY QUESTIONS

The following questions may have *one* or *more* answers.

1. Persons in which of the following age categories are most likely to use illicit drugs?

   a. 12–17 years old
   b. 18–25

   c. 25–40
   d. 41–70

2. Specimens that can be used in forensic analysis include which of the following?

   a. hair
   b. urine

   c. blood
   d. nails

3. "Gateway drugs" include which of the following?

   a. alcohol
   b. tobacco

   c. heroin
   d. cocaine

4. Forensic specimens are those involved in which of the following?

   a. routine testing for diabetes
   b. legal cases/criminal
      investigations

   c. urine screening for
      pre-employment physicals
   d. Pap smears

5. What is the purpose of a chain-of-custody process?

   a. maintain control of the donor
      who gives the specimen
   b. maintain control and
      accountability of a specimen
      from point of collection to
      final results

   c. specimen identification
   d. provide privacy to the donor

6. Appropriate seal(s) on the specimen containers used in the chain-of-custody assures which of the following?

   a. tamper-evident
   b. privacy

   c. aliquot identification
   d. confidentiality

7. Which of the following agencies/organizations are likely to conduct drug testing programs?

   a. NFL
   b. DOT

   c. NBA
   d. international chemical company

8. Minimum requirements for a urine collection site for drug testing includes which of the following?

   a. privacy for the specimen donor
   b. water source for washing hands

   c. work area for the collector
   d. access to site must be restricted during collection

9. Skin preparation for blood alcohol levels must be cleansed with which of the following?

   a. 70 percent ethyl alcohol
   b. iodine

   c. 70 percent isopropyl alcohol
   d. nonalcoholic disinfectants

10. Which of the following is not acceptable for positive identification of a urine donor for drug testing?

    a. a co-worker
    b. nonphoto identification card

    c. social security card
    d. driver's license

References

1. National Institute on Drug Abuse (NIDA): *Diagnosis and Treatment of Drug Abuse in Family Practice—Epidemiology.* Web page: http//165.112.78.61/DiagnosisTreatment/Diagnosis3html. December, 1997.

2. Soo, VA: Neonatal Drug Testing, *Adv Med Lab Professional,* July 3, 2000; 19–23.

3. Weedn, VW: Elementary, My Dear Watson: Technological advances will fuel laboratory-based forensic science into the next millennium. *Adv Med Lab Personnel,* 8–11. February 8, 1999.

4. Weedn, VW, Rogers, GS, Henry, BE: DNA testing in the forensic laboratory, *Lab Med.* 1998; *29*(8): 484–489.

5. Collins, KA: The laboratory's role in detecting sexual assault. *Lab Med.* 1998; *29*(6): 361–365.

6. Substance Abuse and Mental Health Services Administration (SAMHSA): *Urine Specimen Collection Handbook for Federal Workplace Drug Testing Programs.* US Department of Health and Human Services. Downloaded Feb, 2001; OMB No. 0930-0158, Exp. date: June 30, 2001. Web page: www.samhsa.gov.

7. Massey, LD: Federal workplace drug testing, where urine specimen collection has a whole new meaning, *Adv Med Lab Professional,* September 25, 2000; 14–19.

8. Briefings: Industry. *Lab Med.* 2001; *32*(2):60.

9. Thomas, C, Olander, R: Keeping collegiate sports drug use in check, *Adv for Med Lab Professional.* October 9, 2000; 30–32.

10. Fuller, DC, Orsulak, PJ: The broader view of drug testing, *Adv Lab Professional.* April 10, 2000; 8–12.

11. Dufour, DR: Drugs-of-Abuse Testing Adulteration. *Med Lab Observ,* April, 1999; 10.

12. US Department of Transportation. Part 40: *Procedures for Transportation Workplace Drug Testing Programs.* US Government Printing Office. 49CFR40, October 1, 1997.

13. National Committee for Clinical Laboratory Standards (NCCLS): *Blood Alcohol Testing in the Clinical Laboratory: Approved Guideline.* T-DM6-A. (NCCLS; 940 West Valley Road. Ste. 1400, Wayne, PA 19087-1898, (610) 688-1100); 1997.

PHLEBOTOMY CASE STUDY

■

Home Care Collections

Mr. Albert A. Thomson, a 55-year-old white man, was released from Nicholson Community Hospital on March 25. He had been in the hospital for 14 days as a result of undergoing cardiac bypass surgery and experiencing some complications. On March 29, Ms. Terry Alright, a home health care phlebotomist from Nicholson Community Hospital, saw that her schedule included a visit to Mr. Thomson for blood collection for the following laboratory tests:

- Chemistry screen
- Protime
- CBC
- APTT
- Calcium, ionized

When she arrived at Mr. Thomson's home and began her preparations for blood collection, she noticed that Mr. Thomson had hematomas in both antecubital fossa areas of the left and right arms. Thus, she checked the right hand and found a vein that looked suitable for collecting blood with a safety winged infusion set with small blood collection vacuum tubes. She prepared the site for blood collection, and using a 23-gauge safety winged infusion needle, she inserted the needle into the vein and first collected blood in a red-speckled-topped vacuum tube, followed by a purple-topped tube, two light blue–topped tubes, and then a green-topped tube. As she collected each tube, she mixed the blood and additive in the blood collection tube. After completing the blood collection, she labeled the tubes, discarded the biohazardous blood collection items in her biohazardous disposal container, and left Mr. Thomson's home with the collected blood and her blood collection items.

 She traveled next to Ms. Jennifer Smith's home to collect blood from Ms. Smith for a digoxin assay and a plasma potassium level determination. Ms. Smith, an 85-year-old African American woman, was homebound because of arthritis and a cardiac arrhythmia problem. Collecting blood from the median cubital vein in Ms. Smith's left arm, the phlebotomist used a syringe because of the fragility of the vein. After collecting 5 mL of blood in the syringe, Ms. Alright placed 2 mL of blood in a small red-speckled-topped blood collection tube and 3 mL of blood in a small purple-topped blood collection tube. She labeled the tubes, discarded the biohazard blood collection items, and left Ms. Smith's house to travel to the hospital laboratory and drop off the blood specimens.

QUESTIONS

1. For each of the following laboratory tests, what color should the top of the blood collection tube be?

Laboratory Assay	Color of Blood Collection Tube Top
Calcium, ionized	
APTT	
CBC count	
Protime	
Chemistry screen	
Digoxin	
Plasma potassium	

2. Did the home health care phlebotomist use the proper order of draw for Mr. Thomson's laboratory tests? If not, what was the proper order of draw?

3. Did the phlebotomist use the proper order of draw to fill tubes for Ms. Smith's laboratory tests? If not, what was the proper order of draw?

See Answers in Appendix.

PHLEBOTOMY CASE STUDY

■

Bedside Glucose Testing

A 59-year-old Hispanic woman having non-insulin diabetes mellitus tested her glucose level at home on March 14, 1998, and obtained a glucose reading of 320 mg/dL using a test strip. Because she was having symptoms of sweating, feeling bad, and feeling lightheaded, the woman went to her physician the next day. Her physician immediately hospitalized her for treatment of uncontrolled diabetes. During the hospitalization, the following glucose meter v. clinical laboratory comparisons were performed:

DATE	GLUCOSE METER RESULTS (mg/dl)	LABORATORY TEST RESULTS (mg/dL)
3/15/98	151	198
3/16/98	192	238
3/17/98 (A.M.)	96	267
3/17/98 (P.M.)	120	246

From product performance specifications, hospital personnel determined that the comparisons for March 15 and March 16 were within the acceptable product performance variation range. The last two comparisons, however, fell outside the acceptable range. The patient indicated that she followed the preventive maintenance schedule described in the documentation packaged with the glucose meter. The calibration was checked weekly, and the last calibrator reading, which was performed on March 17, was in range. A control run on March 16 resulted in a reading of 129 mg/dL, with confidence limits of 90 to 120 mg/dL.

QUESTIONS

1. What is the problem in this case study?
2. What troubleshooting technique(s) should have been implemented to resolve this problem?

See Answers in Appendix.

PHLEBOTOMY CASE STUDY

■

Newborn Nursery Collections

Two health care workers oversee blood collections in the newborn nursery on Saturday and Sunday of each week. On Sunday morning, the clinical laboratory scientist (CLS) overseeing the clinical chemistry section noticed that the bilirubin value for Baby McPherson was as follows:

DAY	*TIME*	*BILIRUBIN VALUE (mg/dL)*
Friday		15
Saturday	8:15 P.M.	12
Sunday	7:10 A.M.	2

Knowing that the ultraviolet light on newborn Baby McPherson could not make the bilirubin value decrease that dramatically from Saturday to Sunday, the CLS called in the health care worker who had collected the Sunday morning blood sample to ask him questions regarding the collection.

QUESTIONS

1. What type of microcollection container should have been used to collect the bilirubin sample?
2. Does taking the blood immediately to the laboratory for testing make any difference?
3. Give two reasons why the Sunday bilirubin value for Baby McPherson was so different from the values of the previous 2 days.

See Answers in Appendix.

PHLEBOTOMY CASE STUDY

■

Collecting Blood from an Infant

The phlebotomist, Sherry Wiggins, had to collect blood from the infants in the critical care unit of the children's hospital. For Infant Jim Jenkins, the requested laboratory tests were hemoglobin, potassium, and thyroxine. The hospital protocol for this infant's age was to collect blood by skin puncture from the heel.

QUESTIONS

1. What blood collection equipment was required for this infant's blood collection?
2. What was the proper "order of draw" for this microcollection?

See Answers in Appendix.

QUALITY
MANAGEMENT
AND LEGAL ISSUES

HE FINAL PORTION OF THIS TEXTBOOK covers professional issues, such as assessment of the quality of services that are provided in phlebotomy practice, professional and ethical communication and management practices, and the sensitive issues of legal risk and regulatory matters.

Chapter 16, Quality, Competency, and Performance Assessment, describes the role of quality-monitoring activities in improving the practice of phlebotomy and related procedures. Specific examples are provided that demonstrate how quality-improvement tools (e.g., flowcharts, Pareto charts, cause-and-effect diagrams) can enhance services to customers, who include patients, families, physicians, nurses, and other health care professionals.

Chapter 17, Ethical, Legal, and Regulatory Issues, describes general ethical and legal issues related to phlebotomy and provides definitions of legal terminology. Also covered are the following legal issues that are particularly important to health care professionals who practice phlebotomy: confidentiality, human immunodeficiency virus (HIV) exposure, informed consent, implied consent, and legal claims. In addition, legal cases that are related to phlebotomy and laboratory practices are cited, and issues of how to manage legal risk, malpractice insurance, and protective equipment are highlighted.

SIXTEEN

■

Quality, Competency, and Performance Assessment

CHAPTER OBJECTIVES

Upon completion of Chapter 16, the learner is responsible for the following:

1. Define quality improvement and quality control.

2. Describe the "5 Ds" in terms of negative patient outcomes.

3. Identify steps in monitoring and evaluating a specimen collection process.

4. Give examples of improved patient outcomes for phlebotomy services.

5. Give examples of how phlebotomists can participate in quality improvement efforts.

6. Describe essential elements of a phlebotomist's performance assessment.

■ PERCEPTIONS OF QUALITY

The concern about the quality of health care services is not new. Many stakeholders have influenced the way health care quality is monitored and evaluated. **Stakeholders** are individuals, groups, organizations, and/or communities that have an interest in, or are influenced by, health care services. Internal stakeholders are individuals or groups within a health care organization itself; and external stakeholders are individuals or groups outside the organization. Box 16–1 lists examples of key stakeholders for a hospital, and a specimen collection service. Stakeholders are also considered to be "customers." The Joint Commission on the Accreditation of Healthcare Organizations (JCAHO), a key stakeholder in the health care industry, has been one of the most influential organizations in bringing quality improvement methodologies to health care as a requirement for accreditation. Other organizations/groups/agencies that have also significantly impacted the trends in quality assessment include Medicare, Medicaid, the College of American Pathologists (CAP), many professional organizations, and patient advocacy groups.

BOX 16–1.   EXAMPLES OF STAKEHOLDERS (CUSTOMERS) IN HEALTH CARE

External stakeholders (outside the health care organization)

- Local community
- Insurance companies that pay for services
- Employers who pay for services for their employees
- Grant agencies and/or foundations that provide funding
- Federal agencies—OSHA, CDC, etc.
- State agencies
- Accrediting agencies—JCAHO, CAP
- Advocacy groups—AARP

Internal stakeholders (within the health care organization and/or specimen collection services)

- Inpatients and outpatients
- Patient's families and friends
- Patient's support groups
- Blood donors
- Clinical laboratory staff
- Secretaries and clerks
- Pathologists
- Nurses
- Administrators
- Students
- Research staff
- Volunteers

Health care workers, including phlebotomists themselves, are concerned about the quality of their work as evidenced by the following:

- Educational programs have been established to teach basic skills.
- Certification examinations have been implemented to certify basic knowledge.
- Associations have been established to voice and publicize the issues related to phlebotomy practice.
- Codes of ethics have been designed.
- Competencies have been identified. (Refer to Chapter 1 for more information about competencies and certifying organizations for phlebotomists.)

The concept of "quality" can be described in a variety of ways. One way to describe quality is in terms of the technical aspects of care versus the interpersonal aspects of care. *Scientific or technical aspects of care* entail how well clinical skills are applied to the situation, e.g., are the correct procedures and therapies used for the patient. *The nontechnical or interpersonal aspects of care* involve how well the personal needs of the patient are satisfied, e.g., are communication skills adequate, are the services convenient and timely, are patients satisfied with the comfort and safety of the environment, were the health care workers professional and careful.

Another way to describe quality in health care uses three major concepts: efficacy, appropriateness, and caring functions.

Efficacy—the health care services provided have a positive impact on the patient's health, i.e., the health outcome is that the patient improves or gets well.

Appropriateness—the procedures performed on the patient were the correct ones for that particular condition or illness.

Caring functions—the services provided to the patient are available, timely, effective, safe, efficient, respectful, and sensitive to the patient's needs.

One of the more famous frameworks for quality was developed by a physician, Avedis Donabedian, and involves total quality management through continuous quality improvement. It focuses not only on meeting a minimum standard but also on the processes and assessments to constantly improve the services that are provided to customers. The major components and examples are listed below[1]:

Structure—Physical or organizational properties of the settings where care is provided. Assessments of structural components include:

- Physical structure—Facilities where services are provided, adequacy of supplies and equipment, safety devices, safety procedures, availability and condition of equipment, e.g., computers, sterilizers, refrigerators, thermometers, centrifuges, autoclaves, and glucose-monitoring devices.
- Personnel structure—Adequate numbers of personnel and support staff, ratios of staff to patients, qualifications of staff, and availability of the medical director or supervisors.
- Management or administrative structure—Updated, available procedure manuals, adequacy of systems for secure recordkeeping, open lines of communication throughout the organization.

Quality assessments of structural components may reveal potential problems that other assessments cannot. For example, the use of outdated blood collection tubes may cause faulty laboratory test results, even though the blood collection, testing, and reporting processes are perfect and the treatment plan for the patient is appropriate. Also, health care workers often confuse the terms *quality control, continuous quality improvement,* and *proficiency testing.* Box 16–2 distinguishes these terms and gives examples of their use.

Process—what is done to the patient or client. Process assessments are common throughout the specimen collection and clinical testing arenas and include procedures and skill assessment. This is where traditional QC measures are applicable. In addition to the normal laboratory data collection routines, however, other methods are effective for monitoring processes. These include evaluation of patient records for complications, correct technical skills, and correct documentation procedures; direct observation of practices; videotaping of health care interactions and practices; patient interviews; and questionnaires.

Outcomes—what is accomplished for the patient. The ultimate goal of CQI is to improve patient outcomes. Most outcomes assessments rely on information in the patient's medical record. Chart reviews usually evaluate the health status after services are provided. Timing is usually an important component of these measures. Outcomes assessments are typically the most difficult to measure and often relate to recovery rates, cure rates, nosocomial infection rates, return to normal functions, and so on. Poor patient outcomes have been described as the "5 Ds"[2]:

- Death
- Disease
- Disability
- Discomfort
- Dissatisfaction

BOX 16–2.   DEFINITIONS: CONTINUOUS QUALITY IMPROVEMENT (CQI), QUALITY CONTROL (QC), PROFICIENCY TESTING (PT)

Continuous Quality Improvement (CQI)

CQI is a theoretical framework and management commitment to improve health care structures, processes, outcomes, and customer satisfaction. It is ongoing and involves all levels of the health care organization.

Quality Control (QC)

QC monitors a process. It adjusts the analytic process to meet specific standards. It includes activities, such as developing technical policies and procedures, ensuring that supplies are functional and not outdated, calibrating and maintaining equipment, and performing temperature and function checks. QC also involves testing known samples (i.e., with high and low test values) in parallel with patient samples. It enables the laboratory to ensure accuracy and reliability of the results reported.

Proficiency Testing (PT)

PT is used as a measure of a clinical laboratory's performance and is required by CLIA, CAP, and JCAHO. A PT program is a system by which a laboratory subscribes to one of several organizations to provide blind samples for testing. After the laboratory analyzes the blind samples, the test results are sent back to the PT organization for comparison with the results from many other laboratories. Thus one laboratory can compare its results with others to see how it performs. It is a well-proved method to detect critical errors in testing procedures. If errors are detected, they must be corrected immediately.

Unfortunately, health care workers can have negative effects in each of these categories. For example, misidentification of a patient can result in an erroneous cross-match and blood transfusion, which could be fatal to a patient (death). Inappropriate cleansing techniques or hand washing could result in transmitting nosocomial infections (disease). Poor venipuncture techniques, such as improper needle insertion or excessive probing, could result in nerve damage (disability) or severe pain (discomfort). And lengthy waiting times, rude behavior, or messy work sites can contribute to an overall feeling of patient dissatisfaction. Even though these examples are extreme, they do exist in reality and need to be improved.

Quality improvement efforts for phlebotomy services often involve evaluating the following:

- The health care worker's technique
- Complications such as hematomas
- Recollection rates resulting from contamination
- Multiple sticks on the same patient

All these issues have the potential to result in a negative outcome for the patient. Thus, continuous improvement in minimizing these problems would be most beneficial to the patient and the health care worker.

CUSTOMER SATISFACTION

The study of satisfaction among patients and health care workers is usually accomplished by using questionnaires, mail outs, and telephone or personal interviews. Although the information gathered by using these techniques may be subjective, knowing *why* customers are dissatisfied and *which* customers are unhappy is extremely valuable. This information can be used to improve targeted services or aspects of a service. Health care workers must remember that positive patient outcomes usually result in positively satisfied customers.

■ TOOLS AND TRENDS FOR PERFORMANCE ASSESSMENT

In a laboratory, check sheets, run charts, and statistical tests can be used to review both the analytic and nonanalytic parts of the laboratory. In an analytic sense, clinical laboratory scientists and technicians use data collection to ensure test sensitivity, specificity, precision, and accuracy. In a nonanalytic sense, data can be used to assess the timeliness of responses to requests, turnaround time for reporting test results, and effective communication. Tools for implementing CQI include the following[1]:

- **Flowcharts.** Useful for breaking a process into its components so that people can understand how it works (Fig. 16–1).
- **Pareto charts.** Bar charts that show the frequency of problematic events; the Pareto principle suggests that "80 percent of the trouble comes from 20 percent of the problems" (Fig. 16–2).
- **Cause-and-effect (Ishikawa) diagrams.** Diagrams that identify interactions between equipment, methods, people, supplies, and reagents (Fig. 16–3).
- **Plan-Do-Check-Act cycle (PDCA).** A cycle for assessing and making positive changes, then reassessing (Box 16–3).
- **Line graphs, histograms, scatter diagrams.** Pictorial images representing performance trends.
- **Brainstorming.** Method used to stimulate creative solutions in a group.

Figure 16–1.   Flowchart[4].

(Adapted from Martin, BG, ed.: *The CLMA Guide to Managing a Clinical Laboratory.* Malvern, PA; Clinical Laboratory Management Association: 1991.)

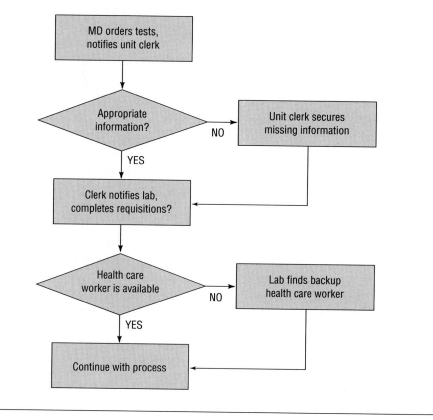

Westgard and associates suggest a **"5 Q" framework** for clinical laboratories that focuses on the following:[2]

- Quality planning (QP).
- Quality laboratory practices (QLP).
- Quality control (QC) of processes.
- Monitoring performance, quality assessment.
- Quality improvement (QI) when problems occur.

This is a self-perpetuating, cyclic process that should become a way of life for all employees in the laboratory. Each health care institution has different characteristics, however, and the laboratory's quality-management program will vary based on philosophy, mission, and tools selected for use.

There are many varied strategies for assessing performance of laboratories, most of which are highly effective. The role of the individual health care worker, through his or her

Figure 16–2. Pareto chart.

(From Martin, BG, ed.: *The CLMA Guide to Managing a Clinical Laboratory.* Malvern, PA; Clinical Laboratory Management Association: 1991, with permission.)

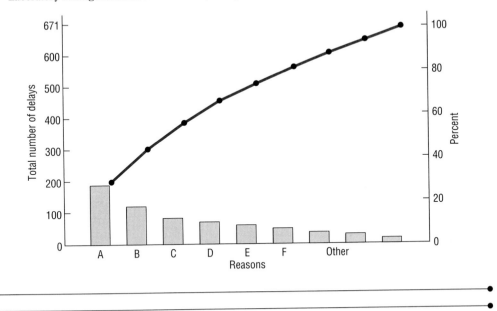

Figure 16–3. Ishikawa diagram. ER, emergency room.

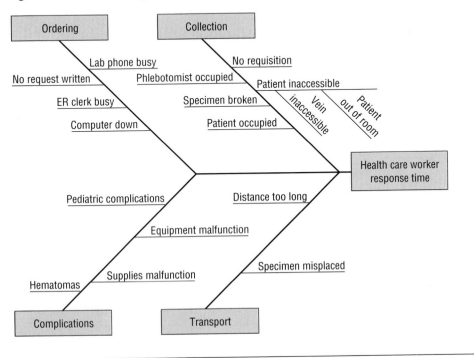

> **BOX 16–3.   PLAN–DO–CHECK–ACT (PDCA) CYCLE**
>
> **Plan** a change.
> **Do** the improvement, data collection, and analysis.
> **Check** the results to see the effect of the change.
> **Act** on what was learned by either rejecting the change, adjusting the change, or adopting the change as a standard part of the process.

technical competence, however, is equally important and should also be a routine part of quality and performance assessments. Basic competencies were covered in Chapter 1, but, in addition, each health facility may have its own additional required competencies.

■ CQI FOR SPECIMEN COLLECTION SERVICES

CQI studies for specimen collection services can be very revealing for laboratory employees, supervisors, and managers. A study by Howanitz and colleagues indicated that 98.6 percent of patients in a study group from numerous hospitals were satisfied with many aspects of the phlebotomy services that they received.[3] In this group, 97.3 percent of the patients had blood collected on the first phlebotomy attempt, and 16.1 percent of the punctures resulted in ecchymosis. In 25 percent of the cases, the time required for the phlebotomy procedure was 5 minutes or less. Each of these factors, in addition to numerous others, was analyzed, and areas for targeted improvement were identified. One of the general areas cited for suggested improvement was reduction of discomfort or pain caused by the puncture. Examples of CQI **assessments** that should be considered in specimen collection services are listed in Box 16–4.

> **BOX 16–4.   CONTINUOUS QUALITY IMPROVEMENT ASSESSMENTS FOR SPECIMEN COLLECTION SERVICES**
>
> - Health care worker response time (for inpatients).
> - Patient waiting time (for outpatients).
> - Time required for completion of the phlebotomy procedure.
> - Percentage of successful blood collections taken on the first attempt.
> - Number of phlebotomy attempts beyond the first attempt.
> - Number of phlebotomy attempts per patient by the medical service.
> - Volume of daily blood loss per patient due to venipunctures.
> - Number and size of hematomas.
> - Number of patients who faint.
> - Amount of time spent and number of telephone calls needed to acquire appropriate identification.
> - Number of redraws requested because of inadequate specimens.
> - Contribution of health care worker to turnaround times of designated laboratory tests.
> - Number of incomplete forms, documents, logs, and so forth.
> - Number of therapeutic drug monitoring tests that have incorrect documentation or timing.
> - Number of specimens received in incorrect tubes.
> - Contamination rate for blood cultures.
> - Results of patient satisfaction questionnaires or focus groups.
> - Frequency of complaints.

Monitors or indicators for quality assessment should fit specific criteria in order to be useful and valid. The **RUMBA model** is an easy check for determining the feasibility of monitoring a particular procedure or process.

- R—Relevant
- U—Understandable
- M—Measurable
- B—Behavioral
- A—Achievable

Before a study of a particular problem is begun, the RUMBA criteria should be applied. The following questions should be asked:

- Are the problems or variations in practices relevant to laboratory services or patient care?
- Are the items to be monitored understandable by those who will be collecting the data?
- Can measurable objective data be collected?
- Are there behavioral aspects that can be changed if necessary?
- Is the project realistic and achievable?

An important factor that can sometimes become a stumbling block for quality assessment is the data collection process. Most of the data can be collected from information already available in the patient care unit of the hospital or the laboratory, or by adding a brief tally to forms already in existence. In addition, there are many other accessible sources of information (refer to Box 16–5), although the use of some of these data sources may require special permission.

■ COLLECTION PROCEDURES TO ENSURE QUALITY

Health care workers can consider the clinical laboratory testing process in several phases. The primary goal of specimen collection is to obtain an accurate sample for analysis. Many variables exist, however, before the specimen is actually analyzed. Box 16–6 depicts preanalytic, analytic, and postanalytic phases in specimen collection, processing, and testing. For purposes of this text, the quality assessment efforts focus on the preanalytic phases. Analytic and postanalytic phases involve rigorous quality control procedures and other types of

---

BOX 16–5.   SOURCES OF INFORMATION FOR QUALITY ASSESSMENT

Medical records	Committee reports
Incident reports	Staff meetings
Accident reports	Marketing agents
Written complaints	Pathologists
Patient questionnaires	Attending physicians
Customer focus groups	Direct observation or videotape
Quality circles	Laboratory employees

BOX 16–6. PREANALYTIC, ANALYTIC, AND POSTANALYTIC PHASES IN SPECIMEN COLLECTION, PROCESSING, TESTING, AND REPORTING

Preanalytical Phase Outside the Laboratory

Patient identification and information
Isolation techniques
Correct venipuncture or skin puncture
Appropriate use of supplies and equipment
Appropriate transportation and handling

Preanalytical Phase Inside the Laboratory

Sample treatment
Specimen registration and distribution
Centrifugation
Identification of aliquots
Appropriate storage

Analytical Phase

Testing the specimen

Postanalytical Phase

Reporting the results
Appropriate follow-up or repeat testing

---

quality assessment procedures, including proficiency testing using specimens from outside approved sources, and periodic inspections from authorized agencies. Table 16–1 indicates examples of preanalytic processes that are subject to quality reviews and monitoring.

Each health care facility should target specific issues for quality assessment based on recognized concerns, incident reports, and/or recurring problems. A monthly review of the laboratory's collection procedures and policies is recommended to reduce collection errors. The clinical laboratory should provide the nursing staff with a floor book (online version or paper-based) that describes laboratory services, preparation of the patient, and special handling of patients' specimens. In addition, the phlebotomist should have access to a pocket-sized collection booklet that contains the same information as that found in the floor book, along with other useful information for specimen handling, transporting, and processing.

ANTICOAGULANTS AND PRESERVATIVES: QUALITY ASSURANCE

As discussed in Chapters 7 and 8, the health care worker uses various anticoagulants and preservatives in the collection of blood specimens. These tubes containing anticoagulants must be inverted promptly after blood is drawn to ensure mixture of the anticoagulant and the blood and, thus, to provide quality assurance of a perfectly collected specimen. As reviewed in Chapter 8, when several evacuated tubes of blood are collected from a patient, tubes containing anticoagulants should be filled in the appropriate order so that proper inversion can occur and carryover of anticoagulants to clotted tubes will not occur.

Table 16–1. Examples of Preanalytic Variables and Processes That Are Subject to Quality Control and Monitoring

PREANALYTIC VARIABLES AND PROCESSES	SUPPLIES AND MATERIALS
Patient preparation	Blood collection tubes
Identification	Urine containers
Dietary information (fasting)	Expiration dates on all supplies
Posture	Warming devices
Previous complications (syncope)	
Providing information to patient	
Warming the site of collection	
Preparation of specimen	Request forms
Entering requests	Sample identification
Appropriate labeling	
Specimen procurement	Needles
Timing	Collection tubes
Cleansing the site	Disinfectants
Vein selection	
Needle positioning	
Order of draw for multiple tubes	
Transporting specimen	Transport containers
Appropriate timing	Pneumatic tube systems
Transporting on ice	Cooling systems
Protection from light sensitivity	
Avoidance of leakage or breakage	
Processing the specimen	Identification and tracking software
Readiness for testing	Centrifuge
Aliquot preparation	Pipettes
Centrifugation	
Storing the specimen	Refrigerators
Timing	Freezers
Site and temperature	Containers
Preparation after storage	

For quality concerns, the anticoagulants and preservatives should meet the requirements established by the National Committee for Clinical Laboratory Standards (NCCLS). The manufacturer of the anticoagulants and preservatives must provide the shelf-life or expiration date of these additives on the packages so that the user will know how long these additives are effective. When restocking the supply of collection tubes, health care personnel should place the tubes with a shelf-life (expiration date) nearest the current date at the front of the shelf so that these tubes are used first. Manufacturers of collection tubes must test and verify draw and fill accuracy until the stated expiration date. The health care worker should be cognizant of expiration dates on any item used in specimen collection.

Accreditation standards require the health care institution to establish QC procedures for proper inspection of new lot numbers of evacuated blood collection tubes. In addition, quality can be obtained in specimen collection only with fresh specimens. If the blood specimen is not to be tested immediately, the health care worker must make certain that it is stored properly until the test is run.

REQUIREMENTS FOR A QUALITY SPECIMEN

The clinical competency of health care workers is ultimately linked to the quality of the specimen delivered.

! Clinical Alert

The requirements for a quality specimen include the following:

1. Using universal standard precautions, the patient is prepared properly and medication interference is avoided, if possible.
2. Collecting specimens from the correct patients and proper labeling are done. Because the policy of most clinical laboratories is to discard specimens that are unlabeled or labeled incorrectly, the health care worker must abide by the written laboratory policy describing acceptable identification of specimens. The potential errors in after-the-fact reidentification of a specimen by floor personnel can be extremely detrimental to the patient in question and must be avoided. (See Chapter 8 for identification and labeling procedures.)
3. The correct anticoagulants and preservatives must be used with the sufficient amount collected (see Chapters 7 and 8). Safety devices should be used.
4. Specimens should not be hemolyzed.
5. Fasting specimens should be collected in a timely fashion and should actually be fasting samples.
6. Timed specimens should be correctly timed and documented.
7. Specimens without anticoagulants should be allowed to stand a minimum of 30 minutes so that clot formation can occur completely. (Gel separator tubes will shorten the time of clot formation, depending on the manufacturer's tubes.)
8. Specimens should be transported to the clinical laboratory in a timely fashion to maintain freshness (within 45 minutes). If the laboratory does not have designated delivery times for specimens, the health care worker may suggest to his or her laboratory supervisor that such a system would ensure fresh specimens and, thus, high-quality laboratory test results. A list of the specimens that are delivered after the designated time limits should be maintained in a logbook. Such a list can usually help personnel detect the source of the problem so that quality assessments can be evaluated. The list reveals the number of specimens that were delivered after the allowable limits and how late they were. The supervisor of specimen control usually decides whether the late specimen should be discarded and a new one collected.

NUMBER OF BLOOD COLLECTION ATTEMPTS

Another way to provide quality services to patients is by monitoring and reducing the number of unsuccessful collection attempts. If the health care worker has had consecutively unsuccessful phlebotomy attempts on different patients, the supervisor and the health care worker will know that the problem in blood collection must be identified and solved to prevent future unsuccessful attempts. Most clinical laboratories have a written procedure on the inability to draw specimens that describes the steps that should be taken by the health care worker when (1) collection attempts are unsuccessful (no more than two sticks), (2) the patient is unavailable, or (3) the patient refuses to have blood drawn.

BLOOD LOSS DUE TO PHLEBOTOMY

For adults, blood loss due to venipuncture is usually well tolerated physiologically because the volume constitutes a small percentage of the total blood volume in the body. However, in some cases, patients are very ill and need to be closely monitored, so the frequency of blood collection and volumes needed may increase to a clinically significant level. Patients in intensive care units and/or those with arterial lines, and those with poor prognoses tend to have more total blood collected and more often. As discussed in Chapter 11, circumstances are also different for neonates and infants where even a small volume of blood may represent a large portion of the total blood volume. In these cases phlebotomists must realize that blood conservation is a priority to avoid anemia and other complications. In the laboratory, analytical variables that influence minimum blood volume requirements include the following[6]:

- Analytical instruments require a minimum volume to aspirate for testing
- Analytical instruments may require a standard test tube size to function automatically
- Special handling procedures for separating plasma or serum into sample aliquots for testing in different areas of the laboratory or for sending to a reference laboratory
- Repeat testing after a quality control failure
- Add-on testing ordered by a physician after the initial specimen is drawn
- Volume requirements by the tube manufacturers to ensure adequate dilution with an anticoagulant or other additive

Strategies to reduce phlebotomy volume losses usually focus on organizing and coordinating blood draws. More specifically, health care workers in a specimen collection department can have an impact by assisting with the following[5]:

- Coordinating all requests into a single phlebotomy event daily or by shift
- Schedule blood draws on a regular and frequent basis to eliminate the need for random STAT requests

Clinical Alert

If too much blood is withdrawn in a short period of time, a patient may require a blood transfusion. Therefore it is important to monitor daily blood loss if patients are neonates, have poor prognoses, or are being tested frequently. In these cases, the use of smaller test tubes and/or microcollection techniques might be warranted.

- Ask for a review of duplicate requests for tests that are already pending
- Maintain a daily tally of blood loss from each patient when clinically indicated and in the cases of neonates
- Suggest a review of standing orders that may no longer be needed because the patient has improved
- Assist the laboratory in reducing turnaround time for test results through efficient, accurate, and timely preanalytical processes

QC AND PREVENTIVE MAINTENANCE

The health care worker should be aware that QC checks and preventive maintenance of certain instruments and equipment most often occur in the specimen control section of larger clinical laboratories or by trained laboratory personnel in smaller facilities. Instruments that must be monitored and maintained for quality by blood collection personnel may include:

- Thermometers
- Sphygmomanometers
- Centrifuges

In addition to undergoing preventive maintenance procedures, the centrifuge that is used to spin down the blood must be checked for accurate speed. The speed of the centrifuge can be checked with a tachometer, which indicates the speed in revolutions per minute (RPM). The relative centrifugal force, or g value is then determined from a nomogram available in laboratories. The g value gives the efficiency of the instrument by determining the true force exerted by the centrifuge. A g force of approximately 1000 for 10 minutes is usually efficient for good separation of cells or clotted blood from plasma or serum. The health care worker, however, must be sure to follow the manufacturer's directions when using gel separator devices to separate blood specimens. These collection tubes usually require a specified force higher than 1000 g for complete separation. The NCCLS publishes a manual entitled *Procedures for the Handling and Processing of Blood Specimens,* which provides more information on centrifugation of blood specimens.

COMPETENCY AND PERFORMANCE ASSESSMENT

The goals of competency and performance assessment can include any of the following[6]:

- Evaluate individual performance
- Evaluate group (departmental) performance
- Meet standards set by regulatory agencies (CAP, JCAHO, etc.)
- Address problematic issues within the health care facility

The process is usually ongoing and often takes on characteristics identified by each health care organization. The process often entails the following major categories:

- Responsibility—what needs to be done that relies on one person to complete; and the scope of work defined by the job description.
- Authority—the right to act and make decisions, i.e., collect data, identify patients, perform clinical procedures such as skin puncture or venipuncture, make recommendations, and take action in defined situations.
- Accountability—measurable assessment of consequences; success or failure in duties as defined by the job description.

This chapter has provided numerous examples of the types of activities that are involved in producing a high quality specimen and reducing errors. Certainly many of these activities can be incorporated into competencies and performance assessments for phlebotomists, e.g., monitoring the number of hematomas or redraws, monitoring the number of contaminated blood culture specimens, etc. Also, Chapter 1 provides examples of minimal competencies expected of entry-level phlebotomists, and Chapters 8 through 15 provide detailed descriptions of technical procedures that phlebotomists may encounter in the course of their jobs. Successful performance of these procedures should also be a part of the competency assessment of each individual, based on their specifically assigned duties. Suggestions and examples are available for specific checklists.[7] However, using all the information in this textbook, it is up to each facility to tailor their competencies and performance assessments to their own needs and required duties.

SELF STUDY

KEY TERMS

Assessments
Brainstorming
Cause-and-Effect (Ishikawa)
    Diagrams
Continuous Quality
    Improvement (CQI)
"5 Q" Framework
Flowcharts
Histograms
Line Graphs
Outcomes

Pareto Charts
Plan-Do-Check-Act Cycle
    (PDCA)
Process
Proficiency Testing (PT)
Quality Control (QC)
RUMBA Model
Scatter Diagrams
Stakeholders
Structure

STUDY QUESTIONS

The following questions may have *one* or *more* answers.

1. Of the following, which are examples of customers for phlebotomy services?

   a. outpatients
   b. patient's family members
   c. attending physicians
   d. nursing staff

2. Examples of unfavorable patient outcomes include which of the following?

   a. excessive probing for a vein
   b. multiple sticks on the same patient
   c. nosocomial infections
   d. hematomas

3. Which of the following are examples of structural components of quality that should be periodically checked?

   a. expiration dates
   b. condition of supplies
   c. adequacy of supplies
   d. nosocomial infections

4. Which of the following are examples of process components of quality that should be checked?

   a. documentation procedures
   b. hematomas
   c. multiple sticks
   d. use of incorrect anticoagulants

5. Why is rapid delivery of specimens important?

   a. because cells should not remain in contact with sera for excessive periods
   b. so that the health care worker can hurry to the next patient
   c. to reduce turnaround time for results
   d. because laboratory test results are most accurate when fresh specimens are used

References

1. Graham, NO: *Quality in Health Care: Theory, Applications, and Evolution.* Gaithersburg, MD; Aspen Publishers: 1995.

2. Westgard, JO, Barry, PL, Tomar, RH: Implementing TQM in health care laboratories, *Clin Lab Manage Rev.* 1991; *5*(5):354.

3. Howanitz, PJ, Cembrowski, GS, Bachner, P: Laboratory phlebotomy—CAP Q-probe study of patient satisfaction and complications in 23,783 patients, *Arch Pathol Lab Med.* 1991; 115:867–872.

4. Martin, BG (ed): *The CLMA Guide to Managing a Clinical Laboratory.* Malvern, PA; Clinical Laboratory Management Association: 1991.

5. McPherson, RA: Blood sample volumes: Emerging trends in clinical practice and laboratory medicine, *Clin Leader Manage Rev.* Jan/Feb., 2001; 3–10.

6. Wright, D: *The Ultimate Guide to Competency Assessment in Healthcare,* 2nd ed. Minneapolis, MN; Creative Healthcare Management: 1998.

7. Phelan, S: *Phlebotomy Techniques: A Laboratory Workbook.* Chicago; American Society of Clinical Pathologists: 1993.

SEVENTEEN

■

Ethical, Legal, and Regulatory Issues

CHAPTER OUTLINE

CHAPTER OBJECTIVES

Upon completion of Chapter 17, the learner is responsible for the following:

1. Define basic ethical and legal terms and explain how they relate to the health care setting.
2. Define risk and describe the major elements in a risk management program.
3. Describe the basic functions of the medical record.
4. Define *informed consent.*
5. Describe how to avoid litigation as it relates to specimen collection in a health care environment.
6. Describe CLIA '88 in perspective to blood collection and transportation responsibilities.

The topics of **law, ethics,** and **bioethics** are all interrelated and difficult to discuss without referring to one another. "Laws are societal rules or regulations that are advisable or obligatory to observe. Laws protect the welfare and safety of society, resolve conflicts in an orderly and nonviolent manner, and constantly evolve in accordance with an increasing pluralistic society."[1] Ethics are the moral standards of behavior or conduct that govern an individual's actions. Bioethics (*bio* refers to life) are the moral issues or problems that have resulted because of modern medicine, clinical research, and/or technology. Usually, bioethics refers to "life-and-death" issues, e.g., abortion, when a patient should be allowed to die, or who receives organ donations.

■ ETHICS OVERVIEW

Health care workers must act professionally and in a manner of respect for others and themselves. Recently, the Joint Commission on the Accreditation of Healthcare Organizations (JCAHO) has placed greater emphasis on ethical behavior in health care facilities. Ethical standards are designed to protect clients and create a positive climate for relationships between the health care worker and the client. In most larger health care facilities, Ethics Committees have been established to deal with ethical dilemmas before they happen or to make decisions when unusual cases arise. Professional codes of ethics have evolved in most professional organizations. The code of ethics defines how members of that profession should behave. Other codes deal more with the rights of patients such as the American Hospital Association's Patient's Bill of Rights. (Codes of ethics are also discussed in Chapter 1.)

All health care workers are faced with ethical decisions at one time or another. Each individual should reflect on their own standards of behavior and those of their professional affiliations. The simple set of questions listed below can serve as an "ethics check" for individuals facing an ethical dilemma or decision. To evaluate a difficult situation it involves simply asking oneself[1]:

- Is this legal or does it comply with institutional policy?
- Does it foster a "win-win" situation with the patient/supervisor or other individuals?
- How would I feel about myself if I read about this decision in the newspaper? How would my family feel?
- Can I live with myself after making this decision?
- Is it right?

An example of ethical behavior for a phlebotomist could be related to a mistaken patient identity. If the phlebotomist realizes that he or she has made a mistake in identifying a patient and specimens, the phlebotomist faces an ethical decision about whether or not to report her/his own mistake. Reporting it may result in disciplinary action against him or her. Each phlebotomist should go through the ethics check questions to help in deciding that the right ethical decision to make would be to report her or his own mistake as soon as possible to avoid any clinical and/or treatment decisions based on the wrong test results. This is the right decision because it complies with policy, it fosters a "win-win" situation for the patient and doctor, it would be embarrassing and hurtful to see this reported in the newspaper, and, above all, it is just the right thing to do. In addition, legal risk is minimized for the phlebotomist and the health care facility if the error is appropriately corrected and documented.

■ BASIC LEGAL PRINCIPLES

The laws governing medicine and medical ethics complement and overlap one another. For many years, even centuries, the decision of the physician or health care professional was unquestioned. This has changed. Health care consumers and patients have become more aware, more critical, and much more willing to sue anyone that their lawyer believes has been at fault, including health care workers who are collecting blood specimens.

The legal system in the United States falls under legislative, regulatory, and judicial procedures at the federal, state, and local levels.

STATUTORY LAW

Statutes are written laws enacted by state legislatures and the US Congress. Legislative activities performed by local governments lead to written laws referred to as *ordinances*. Statutes and ordinances are **statutory laws** that are binding but in certain instances may require the courts (judicial law) to interpret how the statutory law applies to a given set of facts. For example, a statute may state that no sexual harassment will be allowed in the workplace. A court then may be called on to decide whether certain actions by a person are considered sexual harassment and, therefore, violate the law.

ADMINISTRATIVE LAW

Once enacted, statutes and ordinances must be implemented; this is **administrative law.** This process is performed by the executive branch, which has numerous departments and agencies. Administrative agencies (e.g., Health Care Financing Administration) write regulations that enforce the laws created through the legislative body. One department under the executive branch that has a major effect on administrative laws regarding health care workers is the US Department of Health and Human Services (HHS). The HHS is the main source of regulations affecting the health care industry.

JUDICIAL LAW

The function of the judicial branch of local, state, and federal governments is to resolve disputes in accordance with law. Most of the nation's **judicial law** actions occur at the state level. State and federal systems have trial courts, which are the first level. The second level within the court system includes intermediate courts (appeals courts), which review the decisions of the trial courts. The highest level within the judicial system is the supreme court of each state and of the federal system; these courts will hear only specific cases. Most of the written legal decisions occur from the appeals and supreme courts. More than 90 percent of all lawsuits are settled out of court, however, and many that are tried are settled before a final verdict is rendered.[2] Usually, phlebotomy cases are tried in state courts. If federal laws or regulations pertain to the case, however, the federal court system is used.

LEGAL TERMINOLOGY

If a health care worker understands basic legal concepts, this understanding can help to define how personnel involved in the specimen collection process can be liable for activities that may occur in this field of health care. Such understanding can also reduce the conflicts between law and the health care workers. Liability for the lack of a proper standard of health care may be imposed on any health care worker, including health care institutions, physicians, nurses, laboratorians, patient care technicians, and phlebotomists. The number of substantial awards against health care workers as a result of improper care has grown in recent years as patients have become more sensitive to treatment complications.

Lawyers have become advisers to health care professionals and institutions in matters ranging from termination of treatment to approval of experimental protocols. Some lawyers specialize in hospital law or food and drug law; personal injury lawyers handle malpractice claims, and others are especially knowledgeable about Medicaid and workers' compensation benefits. No one lawyer can master all these areas. William J. Curran defined *health law* as a "specialty area of law and law practice related to the medical and other health fields—such as dentistry, nursing, hospital administration, and environmental law."[3]

To grasp the legal implication of health care, the health care provider must have some knowledge of basic legal terminology. The avoidance of legal conflicts through education and planning is called **preventive law.** Thus, there is a need to understand basic legal definitions and, it is hoped, to develop a preventive law approach in the procedures and techniques of blood collection. A few major definitions with health care examples can be found in Box 17–1.

BOX 17–1.   LEGAL TERMINOLOGY

- **Assault.** The unjustifiable attempt to touch another person or the threat to do so in such circumstances as to cause the other to believe that it will be carried out, or to cause fear. An assault may be permissible if proper consent has been given (e.g., consent to obtain a blood specimen).

- **Battery.** The intentional touching of another person without consent; also, the unlawful beating of another or carrying out of threatened physical harm. Because battery always includes an assault, the two are commonly combined in the phrase *assault and battery.* The receiver of the battery does not have to be aware that a battery has been committed (e.g., a patient who is unconscious and has surgery performed on him or her without his or her approval, either expressed or implied). The law provides a remedy to the individual when consent to a touching has not been obtained or if the act goes beyond the consent given. Thus, the injured person may initiate a lawsuit against the wrongdoer for the damages suffered. Liability of hospitals, physicians, and other health care workers for acts of battery is most common in situations involving lack of or improper consent to medical procedures, such as blood collecting. For example, a small boy who refused to have his blood drawn was locked in the blood collection room by the health care worker and was forced to have his blood drawn

BOX 17–1. *(continued)*

by the health care worker. The patient's parents sued and won. As another example, a patient is feeling stressed because of pain and not knowing what medical procedures will be occurring. If a health care professional displays behavior in a threatening manner, this can lead to legal intervention. The health care worker must obviously avoid directing threatening language to a patient (e.g., "If you don't let me collect your blood, your illness will probably become critical"). If the patient feels threatened by these words, he or she can "claim intentional infliction of emotional distress." The stress of collecting blood from numerous patients in a short period can lead some health care workers to think about threatening difficult patients, but, of course, this could be detrimental to all involved.

- **Breach of duty.** An infraction, violation, or failure to perform.
- **Civil law.** Not a criminal action; the plaintiff sues for monetary damages.
- **Criminal actions.** Legal recourse for acts or offenses against the public welfare; these actions can lead to imprisonment of the offender.
- **Defendant.** The health care worker or institution against whom the action or lawsuit is filed.
- **False imprisonment.** The unjustifiable detention of a person without a legal warrant.
- **Felony.** Varies by state but generally is defined as public offenses; if the defendant is convicted, he or she will spend time in jail.
- **Invasion of privacy.** Physical intrusion upon a person; the publishing of confidential information, although true, but of such an objectionable or personal nature as to be offensive.
- **Liable.** Under legal obligation, as far as damages are concerned.
- **Litigation process.** The process of legal action to determine a decision in court. Many malpractice cases are negotiated and settled out of court.
- **Malice.** Knowing that a statement is false or making a statement with reckless disregard of the truth.
- **Malpractice.** Improper or unskillful care of a patient by a member of the health care team, or any professional misconduct, unreasonable lack of skill, or infidelity in professional or judiciary duties. Malpractice may be described as *professional negligence.*
- **Misdemeanor.** The general term for all sorts of criminal offenses not serious enough to be classified as felonies.
- **Misrepresentation.** Use of misleading information or omission of important facts.
- **Negligence.** Failure to act or to perform duties according to the standards of the profession.
- **Plaintiff.** The claimant who brings a lawsuit or an action.
- **Respondeat superior.** The concept whereby actions of one individual may be imputed to another person having control. This suggests that a technician's negligent act can be imputed to a laboratory corporation. Under this concept, supervisors and directors may be held liable for the negligent actions of their employees. This concept is also referred to as **vicarious liability.**
- **Tort.** A legal wrong in which the person who commits it is liable for damages in civil action. The tort system is a substructure of the judicial system. It is basically concerned with resolving two-party disputes over whether some harm to one party, or his or her property, was caused by the actions or inactions of another party. A tort is a harm or an injury that is civil, not criminal, in nature and does not constitute a breach of contract. Civil law does not deal with crimes. Torts and other civil wrongs must be proved by a *preponderance of the evidence.* Preponderance is taken to mean a majority; 51 percent or more implies that the defendant more likely than not committed the act.
- **Whistle-blowing.** Public disclosure of perceived wrongdoing by an employee(s) of the same organization. This usually occurs when a dedicated employee has observed something at work that may cause serious harm to one or more patients or that may be illegal. In most of these cases, the employee has reported the occurrence(s) to supervisors with no remedy to the situation. Whistle-blowers may report to governmental agencies, accreditation agencies, etc. Employees who speak out may fear reprisals that could include dismissal, blacklisting, threats of violence, and/or harassment. Numerous laws are in place, however, to protect employees who report legitimate wrongdoing.

Negligence

In the past decade, the number of legal cases in which the laboratory has been directly or indirectly involved has increased noticeably. Negligence is "a violation of a duty to exercise reasonable skill and care in performing a task."[4] Four factors, or key points, must be considered in alleged negligence cases.[4]

1. *Duty*—relates to what duties or responsibilities the hospital or health care worker had toward the patient; it also includes all the individuals who had a duty toward the patient to use the appropriate standard of care.
2. *Breach of duty*—relates to whether the duty was breached and if it was avoidable. The plaintiff must be able to show what actually happened and that the defendant acted unreasonably.
3. *Proximate causation*—relates to whether the breach of duty actually contributed to or caused injury; also concerns all the parties involved in contributing to the alleged injury. There must be a direct line from the conduct to the injury.
4. *Damages*—relates to whether the plaintiff was actually injured and when these injuries were discovered. Once negligence and causation are established, plaintiffs must be able to show that they were actually damaged by the negligent act.

Many circumstances could be considered negligence if health care workers are not extremely careful. For example, there have been legal cases in which the confusion of patient samples led to a patient's death.[5]

Patient Confidentiality

Negligence cases can also arise out of violation of the right to privacy or of **patient confidentiality.** "No one except the patient may release patient results without a clinical need to know." Patient or employee laboratory test results must be considered *strictly* confidential. Negligence can be claimed if employees' or patients' drug abuse test results are released to anyone other than the attending physician or other authorized individuals. This is particularly true regarding employee or athlete drug or alcohol abuse screening and human immunodeficiency virus (HIV) testing. Confidential materials include communications between the physician and the patient, the patient's verbal statements, and nonverbal communications, such as laboratory test results.

■ CONFIDENTIALITY AND HIV EXPOSURE

An increasing concern for health care workers collecting blood from patients who are homebound is the health care worker's rights in relation to accidental exposure to blood or body fluids, whether by a needlestick or some other means. In some states, laws allow health care workers to know the identity of a patient who has acquired immunodeficiency syndrome (AIDS) or who is HIV positive. Many states, however, do not provide for the easy acquisition of this sensitive patient information. A home health care worker who routinely collects blood specimens from homebound patients should obtain information on the state's law regarding confidentiality and HIV status.[6] It can be obtained from the health care worker's employer, from legal counsel, or from a national or state health professional organization.

It is important to use the proper blood collection techniques with safety precautions and required infection control procedures for homebound patients. If exposure to the blood occurs through a needlestick, a lancet, or another means, the home health care worker needs to be certain of obtaining the patient's HIV status to ensure that the proper immediate and long-term self-protective procedural steps can be taken. Even if the report from the HIV test is negative for the health care worker, continued negative status is not guaranteed. Just because a patient's status is HIV positive, however, the health care worker exposed to the blood may not become HIV positive.

If employed by a health care facility, the health care worker should follow the guidelines established by the facility. If he or she is self-employed, it is important to monitor his or her own HIV status. Also, counseling should be sought to obtain emotional support during this stressful time.

Clinical Alert ❗

If employed by a health care facility, the exposed health care worker must immediately file an incident report concerning the accidental exposure. If the health care worker is self-employed and working for various agencies, he or she must report the incident to these agencies. Employers are responsible for postexposure follow-up testing. The health care institutions and agencies must report accidental exposure incidents to the **Centers for Disease Control and Prevention (CDC).** The CDC maintains national surveillance of health care workers' accidental exposures. These statistics assist in developing better safeguards (e.g., new blood collection equipment) against accidental exposure.

■ MALPRACTICE

Malpractice, or professional negligence, is defined as improper or unskillful care of a patient by a member of the health care team, or any professional misconduct or unreasonable lack of skill.

The relationship between doctor and patient is, in the legal sense, a contractual one. The basic elements involved are common with those of other contracts. The elements of contracts are as follows:

- **Offer.** The physician offers to provide a service, either by opening an office or being on a hospital staff or both. Thus he or she has made him-or herself available to patients who seek care.
- **Acceptance.** The patient visits the physician for treatment of a disease or a disorder and may agree to accept medical care.
- **Consideration.** The patient accepts treatment and pays for the care provided by the physician.

By completing these steps, the physician and the patient engage in a contract that implies obligations on both their parts. The physician is obligated to provide medical care to the patient if he or she follows directions and pays for the service. There is even a question about the length of grace period in terms of payment. Also, the patient generally must refuse treatment before the physician is legally freed from his or her obligation. By agreeing to provide service, the physician is required to provide a standard of care.

If the physician is the medical director overseeing clinical laboratory testing, in most cases he or she is responsible under the law for the standard of care and the performance of all aspects of laboratory testing. Therefore, a breach of standard on the part of the health care worker collecting blood for laboratory assays could place both the physician and the health care worker at risk.

■ STANDARD OF CARE

If a patient has suffered injury due to blood collection for laboratory testing, the patient must show that the health care worker who collected the blood failed to meet the prevailing **standard of care.** All health care workers must conform to a specific standard of care to protect patients. In legal cases, the standard of care is determined by what a reasonably prudent person would do under similar circumstances. It is a measuring stick representing the conduct of the average health care worker in the community. The community has been expanded to be a national community as a result of national laboratory standards and requirements. Examples of setting the standard of care include statutes, licensing requirements, rules and regulations of regulatory or professional organizations (e.g., American Hospital Association, Joint Commission for Accreditation of Healthcare Organizations [JCAHO], Health Care Financing Administration, etc.), internal health care facility rules and regulations, and professional publications.

■ INFORMED CONSENT

Informed consent is voluntary permission by a patient to allow touching, examination, and/or treatment by health care providers. It allows patients to determine what will be performed on or to their bodies. Without informed consent, intentional touching can be considered a criminal offense. This type of consent can be obtained through word or action. Thus, the consent may be given orally, expressed by nonverbal behavior, or expressed in writing.

> The following is an example of nonverbal consent. The physician orders laboratory tests for diagnosis and the patient comes to the laboratory with a rolled-up sleeve and outstretched arm. The patient is giving consent for the health care worker to take the blood samples. Integral to consent is the patient's belief that the person to whom consent is given has the knowledge, skills, and technical ability to perform such tasks. Consequently, the patient can expect the blood collector to know the proper venipuncture, arterial puncture, and/or skin puncture technique. For the blood collection, the health care worker should briefly explain to the patient the procedure used to collect the blood specimen. It is important for the health care worker collecting the blood to stress that the physician ordered the test.

Clinical Alert !

Health care workers are becoming more cognizant of the informed consent principle because this is the largest area of litigation. Minors *must* have the consent of their parents or legal guardians for medical care, including blood collections. With the increased amount of immigration to this country, language can be a barrier to informed consent. An interpreter may be necessary so that information for consent may be given in the native tongue.

Most states have enacted legislation requiring that informed consent be obtained before most HIV testing is performed. The statutes indicate the type of information that must be given for the patient to be considered informed. These laws usually require that the patient be counseled on the following: (1) an explanation of the test, including its purpose; (2) potential uses of the HIV test; and (3) testing limitations and the meaning of its results.

■ INFORMED CONSENT FOR RESEARCH PURPOSES

Due to unethical treatment of humans in the past for research purposes, the United States passed a law in 1974, the National Research Act, which established Institutional Research Boards (IRB) at institutions (i.e., hospitals, universities) that perform research. These IRBs were established to review and approve only those research proposals that would protect the human subjects involved in the research protocol. The IRB ensures that human subjects do not bear any inappropriate risk and have properly consented to their involvement.

Frequently, in hospitals, health care facilities, and health science universities, health care workers become involved in collecting blood from research participants for research projects. The National Research Act states that any research project utilizing human subjects requires the informed consent of those subjects. In order to collect blood for a research project, the participant must understand the nature of the research study and the risks and benefits involved if they are to make an informed decision about their participation. This process requires a "consent document" that explains the nature of the research and any risks (i.e., blood collection problems) and benefits to the participant. In addition, the informed consent process must describe the level of confidentiality of the research data and the measures that the researcher will take to ensure that confidentiality is maintained. This information must be presented and signed by the participant in the research before any blood collection can occur for the research activities. In addition, working as a blood collector in the research project requires attending a course on the protection of human subjects in research projects.

■ IMPLIED CONSENT

Implied consent exists when immediate action is required to save a patient's life or to prevent permanent impairment of the patient's health. In other words, an emergency removes the need for consent. Implied consent differs legally from one state to another. Health care providers need to know the legal boundaries of implied consent because they may become involved in an emergency situation (e.g., giving cardiopulmonary resuscitation).

■ STATUTE OF LIMITATIONS

The **statute of limitations** is a law that defines how soon after an injury (e.g., malpractice) a plaintiff must file the lawsuit or be forever barred from doing so. The purpose of this law is to prevent the threat of a lawsuit from hanging over a possible defendant's (e.g., health care worker's) head forever and to force legal action before memories and records are not available and witnesses die. The statute of limitations for professional negligence in most states is 2 years. A complete and accurate medical record with laboratory testing results is the best defense in these cases because the attending physician and health care workers for the patient may have little recollection of the events in question.

■ LEGAL CLAIMS AND DEFENSE

In a malpractice lawsuit, the first pleading filed in a negligence action is the complaint. It is the first statement of a case by the plaintiff(s) against the defendant(s) and states a cause of action, notifying the defendant(s) as to the basis for suit.

Several steps follow, and if the case is not dismissed before trial, the parties to a lawsuit have the right to **discovery**—to examine the witnesses before the trial. Examination before trial is a method used to enable the plaintiff(s) and defendant(s) to learn more regarding the nature and substance of each other's case. This discovery process consists of oral testimony under oath and includes cross-examination by the lawyers. The **deposition** is the testimony of a witness that has been recorded in a written legal format. Either party in the lawsuit—plaintiff or defendant—may obtain a court order permitting examination and copying of laboratory reports, incident reports from personnel files, medical records, phlebotomy and laboratory policies and procedures, training manuals, and so forth, and other facts and information that may help in the discovery.

In addition to the deposition, the parties may undergo cross-examination at the time of the trial. They will provide testimony that will be recorded and filed with the court regarding the cause for the case.

If a health care worker receives a summons to provide a deposition before a trial and/or testimony during a trial for a lawsuit, some helpful guidelines include the following:

- Answer only the questions asked.
- Be organized in your recollection of the facts regarding the incident.
- Do not be antagonistic in answering the questions.
- Explain the laboratory and/or blood collection procedures and policies in simple terminology for the jury.
- Do not overdramatize the facts that you are presenting.
- Dress neatly and be groomed appropriately.
- Be polite, sincere, and courteous.
- Be sure to ask for clarification of questions that you did not clearly hear and questions that you did not understand.
- If you are not sure of an answer, indicate that you do not know the answer or that you are not sure.
- Above all, be truthful.

EXPERT WITNESS

Expert testimony, as well as scientific or medical data, is sometimes used to assist in establishing the standard of care required in any given situation. An **expert witness** may be used to assist a plaintiff in proving the wrongful act of a defendant or to assist a defendant in refuting such evidence. At the time of testifying, each expert's training, experience, and special qualifications will be explained during the deposition and later to the jury during the trial.

EVIDENCE

Evidence during the trial is used to prove or disprove the lawsuit. Evidence must be competent, relevant, and material. It may include such items as vacuum tube holders and tubes, needles, safety apparatuses such as biohazardous waste containers, infection control logs and reports, JCAHO standards, board certification standards for health care workers, and laboratory policies and procedures.

ADVICE TO AVOID LAWSUITS

Justice is expensive in the United States. Lawyers' fees typically range from $200 to $500 per hour, and associated costs can lead to thousands of dollars in legal fees. Also, legal proceedings are time consuming, expensive, and, most of all, emotionally devastating to both the plaintiff(s) and the defendant(s). Thus, to avoid a malpractice lawsuit, the health care provider should heed the advice in Box 17-2.

If the health care worker is involved in home health care collections, he or she needs to have the right types and amounts of insurance coverage to address liability exposures with respect to handling and transporting patients' specimens and wastes across the city.[7]

RESPONDEAT SUPERIOR

Respondeat superior (a Latin term meaning "let the master answer") is the concept whereby the actions of one individual may be imputed to another person having control. It is a legal doctrine that holds employers responsible for acts of their employees within the scope of the employment relationship. Liability predicated on respondeat superior may be imposed

---

BOX 17-2.   TIPS FOR AVOIDING MALPRACTICE LITIGATION

- Provide the patient with proper blood collection techniques comparable to national standards (e.g., National Committee for Clinical Laboratory Standards [NCCLS] guidelines, JCAHO regulations).
- Obtain consent for collection of specimens.
- Regularly participate in continuing education programs.
- Properly handle all confidential communications (e.g., HIV testing without violation).
- Maintain all required blood collection equipment on trays and/or in collection areas for proper collection, including safety apparatuses, such as gloves and disposal containers.
- Be a good listener and let the patient identify his or her anxieties.
- Report incidents immediately and document them.

on an employer only if a master–servant relationship exists between the employer and the employee and the wrongful act of the employee occurs within the scope of employment. Because the law holds negligent persons responsible for their negligent acts, employees are not released from liability when the health care institution is held liable through the application of respondeat superior. Not only may the injured party sue the employee directly, but the employer, if sued, may also seek indemnification from the employee. Indemnification is compensation for the financial loss suffered by the employee's act.

■ MEDICAL RECORDS

Medical records are vital. A health care worker cannot be expected to remember a patient from whom blood was drawn 3 to 4 years ago. The medical records must be neat, legible, and accurate. Refer to Chapter 6 for more information about medical records. They are extremely important if a medical malpractice case goes to court. Medical records have four basic purposes:

1. Allow for continuity of the patient's care plan.
2. Provide documentation of the patient's illness and treatment.
3. Document communication between the physician and the health care team.
4. Provide a legal document that can be used by patients and hospital or health care workers to protect their legal interests.

Medical records are also used for nonmedical reasons that are not directly tied to medical services, such as billing, utilization review, quality improvement, and so on.

Health care workers and their supervisors have a legal duty to keep records, documentation, and laboratory test results confidential. This duty may be waived only if a patient has given express permission for the information to be released, if the patient has sued the institution or its health care personnel, or if the health care worker is specifically obligated to release patient information (e.g., to the CDC). But even in these situations, the confidentiality of patient records and reports cannot be breached while they are communicated or in transit.

■ LEGAL CASES RELATED TO CLINICAL LABORATORY ACTIVITIES

Most phlebotomy cases are settled after a lawsuit is filed but before the court renders a judgment. It is important to remember that many cases are not cited in the literature because often health care institutions or health care workers negotiate, arbitrate, and settle out of court. The following sections discuss cases that are of interest to health care workers involved in blood collection.

Schmerber v. State of California

Nurses, technologists, and health care workers are concerned about drawing a blood sample from an unconscious patient or lacking the patient's consent when requested by police. The US Supreme Court ruled in *Schmerber v. State of California* that tests performed on a blood sample drawn by a hospital physician from a person arrested by the police were admissible in a court action. This may vary by state.

Lazernick v. General Hospital of Monroe County (PA 1977)

A patient who was pregnant for the first time had her blood typed in January 1971. The report sent to her physician indicated that her blood type was A-positive. The patient gave birth to her second child on June 1977. The child was brain damaged and paralyzed on the right side of the body as a result of hemolytic blood disease. The laboratory records in 1971 and 1977 showed that the mother's blood type was O-negative. In a malpractice suit, the parents charged that the physician's and his employees' negligence caused the child's injuries. The physician, who was chief of the laboratory when the blood test was performed, was found liable, as was the health care worker.

Walton v. Providence Hospital

A patient was admitted to Providence Hospital for treatment of pneumonia. On the second day, the patient complained of coldness and numbness in his right hand. On the fourth day, a vascular surgeon examined the hand and ordered 4000 U of heparin in hopes of restoring blood flow. The hand had to be amputated. In court, the expert witness testified that a blood pressure cuff had been left on for an extended period. The patient was awarded $40,000.

Helmann v. Sacred Heart Hospital

Failure to follow proper isolation techniques, such as proper hand washing and prevention of cross-contamination, is a major area of concern for hospitals. The patient in *Helmann v. Sacred Heart Hospital* (62 Wash. 2d 136, 381 P. 2d 605 [1963]) had multiple fractures in the area of the left hip socket. After surgery on his hip, he was returned to a semiprivate room. His roommate complained of a boil under the right arm. Eight days later, a culture was taken of the roommate's wound drainage. Three days later, the laboratory identified the wound infection as *Staphylococcus aureus*. The infected roommate was immediately placed in isolation for the wound. For the preceding 11 days, however, the hospital attendants administered care to both patients without washing their hands between patient care.

The patient with the hip injury developed a *S. aureus* infection at the site of his hip incision. The infection penetrated into the hip socket, destroying tissue and leading to additional surgery and a hip fused in a nearly immovable position. Negligence on the part of the hospital personnel was identified as the cause of the injury as a result of deviation from the accepted standard of care.

Stepp v. Review Board of the Indiana Employment Security Division

Another type of legal case involved a laboratory technician in *Stepp v. Review Board of the Indiana Employment Security Division* (521 N.E. 2d 350 [Ind. Ct. App. 1988]). Stepp was found to have been properly dismissed from her position in the laboratory because of her refusal to perform laboratory tests on patients' specimens with AIDS warnings attached.

Paros v. Hoemako Hospital

The chief X-ray technician in *Paros v. Hoemako Hospital* (681 P. 2d 918 [Ariz. Ct. App. 1984]) was found to have been properly dismissed because of a chronic hostile and argumentative attitude inconsistent with managerial supervisory responsibilities. The ruling was appealed, and the appeals court upheld the lower court's decision.

CASES RESULTING FROM IMPROPER TECHNIQUE AND NEGLIGENCE

Health care workers who collect blood by venipuncture must be thoroughly trained and skilled in proper technique, safety, and the use of collection equipment. Problems that can arise include:

- Wristband or identification error
- Hematoma
- Abscess at the puncture site
- Patient falls
- Fainting
- Nerve damage
- Emotional distress

In one case settled out of court, a health care worker had not received proper blood collection training. She performed a venipuncture by inserting the needle approximately 2 inches above the antecubital fold. The needle went through the vein, through muscle, and into the nerve, severely injuring the patient's arm, which remained permanently damaged even after three surgeries to repair the damage from the resultant hematoma and nerve injury.

Another case involved a medical technologist under pressure to collect specimens from ambulatory patients as quickly as possible. One of the patients stated prior to blood collection that she had fainted during the blood collection at a previous time. The phlebotomist, however, took no precautions to avoid syncope, collected the patient's blood, and allowed the patient to leave immediately. The patient fainted at the elevator and suffered permanent loss of smell and had a permanent "ringing sound" in her ears.

In another case, a health care worker collecting and performing bedside glucose results misread the glucometer and caused the deaths of three patients with diabetes. The errors might have been avoided with better training, supervision, and quality monitoring.

In another case, a phlebotomist collected blood at an excessive angle of needle insertion from the patient's basilic vein when the median cubital vein was clearly an option for collection. The blood collection resulted in injury to the patient's median nerve and a malpractice lawsuit. In addition, documentation errors were evident for the collection. In all, the patient was awarded thousands of dollars for the health care worker's violations regarding proper standard of care.[8]

DiMarco v. Lynch Homes–Chester County, Inc.

In *DiMarco v. Lynch Homes–Chester County, Inc.* (Pennsylvania Superior Court, April 14, 1989, 559 A. 2d 530 [PA Super 1989]), a blood collector suffered a needle puncture wound when a nursing home patient from whom she was collecting blood kicked her. The blood collector received follow-up treatment from her physician, who advised her that she may contract hepatitis up to 6 weeks after the incident. Thus, she was told, she should avoid sexual relations during this time to prevent the possibility of infecting her boyfriend. After 8 weeks, the blood collector resumed her relationship with her boyfriend. After this length of time, however, the blood collector contracted hepatitis and her boyfriend also was diagnosed with the disease. The boyfriend sued the physician and the nursing home. Through the appeals process within the state, the boyfriend won the case. The Pennsylvania Superior Court concluded that someone who renders services to another should recognize the need to protect the third party (the boyfriend) and is liable to the third party who is injured.

Booker v. Duke Medical Center

A similar case was *Booker v. Duke Medical Center* (2565.E. 2d 189 [N.C. 1979]), in which compensation was awarded to the wife of a laboratory technician who died after being exposed to viral hepatitis. The court ruled that the technician's employment exposed him to a greater risk of contracting the disease than members of the public or employees in general.

Veronica Prego v. The City of New York

In *Veronica Prego v. The City of New York* (Kings County Hospital, New York City Health and Hospital Corporation, Kings County, New York Supreme Court, Index No. 14974/88), a health care worker at Kings County Hospital pricked her finger in January 1983 on a needle used to collect blood from a patient dying of AIDS. The plaintiff tested positive for AIDS in March 1985. The health care worker stated that the hospital failed to dispose of used needles properly, claiming that needle boxes should have been provided in each room. The health care worker won the lawsuit and more than $1 million in damages.

■ HIV-RELATED ISSUES

If a health care worker becomes infected with HIV during employment at a health care facility, coverage by workers' compensation benefits are usually available. The health care worker must, however, demonstrate a causal connection between his or her HIV infection and his or her employment. This causal connection includes having a documented incident report at the health care facility involving a needlestick injury, a puncture wound, or other exposure to HIV-contaminated blood or body fluids. In addition, the health care worker's lifestyle will be investigated to determine whether the exposure occurred elsewhere. Preemployment health evaluations may prove useful later should the health care worker allege contraction of infection during the time of employment. Employers are legally responsible for monitoring postexposure follow-up.

If a health care worker resigns because of contracting AIDS, unemployment benefits may be available if the worker can show that he or she believed in good faith that continued employment would jeopardize his or her health.

In a letter to the *New England Journal of Medicine*[9], a resident physician who acquired HIV from a patient stated the following: "Workers' compensation works well to cover medical expenses and income lost because of occupational injuries that result in temporary or minor disabilities such as muscle tears or bone fractures. But these are not the accidents that a physician (health care provider) is likely to suffer at work. The main threats today are catastrophic, and workers' compensation is grossly inadequate for catastrophic illness."

■ POINT-OF-CARE HIV TESTING

Recently, the Food and Drug Administration (FDA) approved a point-of-care (POC) HIV test, the Murex Single-Use Diagnostic System (SUDS), Abbott Diagnostics, IL.[10] It provides a result in as little as 5 minutes. Other POC tests for HIV are on the horizon. Ethical and legal implications must be considered by the health care worker collecting the blood and performing this HIV test by POC methodology. Of course, prior to the HIV testing, the health care worker must counsel the patient according to the state's requirements. In addition, since this HIV procedure is 98% accurate and not 100% accurate, the potential does exist that the test result may be falsely negative or falsely positive and the patient could be given incorrect information that could be damaging. Thus, it is imperative for the health care worker performing a POC HIV test on a patient to inform the patient that the POC result must be confirmed by a Western blot analysis—the gold standard for HIV testing—in order to truly obtain the most accurate result.

■ LEGAL CASE PROTECTION

! Clinical Alert

If an incident occurs (e.g., a patient develops a hematoma), the blood collector *must* write an incident report and give it to the supervisor. The incident report can be helpful in a lawsuit to identify the real cause, the time, and other details of the incident. These reports assist the health care worker who is the defendant in the case in recalling the reason for the patient's (plaintiff's) alleged suffering. The health care worker, however, must not misrepresent or tamper with evidence in a lawsuit by writing an incident report after being sued by a patient for malpractice.

In one case in which a health care worker was sued for damaging a patient's median nerve as a result of probing with a needle to find the vein, the health care worker "after the alleged fact" wrote an incident report for the incident that occurred prior to the filed suit. Eventually, through court proceedings, it was discovered that the health care worker had not actually filed an incident report at the time of the patient's needlestick injury. The falsification of documentation with malice immensely affected the plaintiff's award for damages.

■ LAWS ON MEDICAL DEVICES AND PROTECTIVE EQUIPMENT

Blood collection involves the use of many types of equipment and supplies. Blood collectors and patients have been injured as a result of malfunctioning equipment. In 1990, the federal government issued the Safe Medical Devices Act, which states that any malfunctioning devices (e.g., in vitro diagnostics, reagent kits, clinical analyzers, blood collection equipment) must be immediately reported to the federal government with a description of the malfunctioning incident (e.g., breakage of needle in arm). After an investigation of the incident, a nationwide alert is generally provided to health care institutions regarding the failure(s) of the health care device. This law was enacted to protect health care workers and patients from injuries due to health care devices.

To avoid the possibility of malfunctioning equipment, the **Food and Drug Administration (FDA)** evaluates the safety, clinical efficacy, and medical efficacy of the equipment and supplies used in blood collection. Another federal agency, the **Environmental Protection Agency (EPA),** monitors and enforces environmental requirements for the safe disposal of chemical and biological hazards.

Another federal rule affecting health care workers who collect blood is the Occupational Safety and Health Administration (OSHA) rule for personal protective equipment (PPE) that became effective on July 5, 1994. The rule describes the following:

- PPE must be of a safe design and construction for the work to be performed.
- PPE must be provided, used, and maintained in a sanitary and workable condition.
- PPE must be selected for employees based on an assessment of the hazards of the work environment (e.g., safety shields over needle apparatus).
- Employees must be trained in the proper use of PPE.

On November 6, 2000, H.R. 5178, the Needlestick Safety and Prevention Act, was passed. This act modifies the Occupational Safety and Health Administration (OSHA) blood-borne pathogens standards to require the use of safety needles in health care facilities. In addition, the law (Public Law 106-430) mandates that employers document needlestick accidents, as well as solicit employee input on which safety devices to use.[11]

■ MALPRACTICE INSURANCE

Because hospitals are places where seriously ill patients are admitted and treated with highly sophisticated medical technology, the likelihood for problems is greater there than in other health care settings. Often, the health care staff in the hospital or clinical laboratory are part of a blanket malpractice insurance policy. If, however, the health care worker is employed by a pathologist who has a contract with an institution or owns a clinic, the staff may be protected by the pathologist's malpractice insurance policy.

Malpractice insurance rates for pathologists are generally the lowest premiums charged among physicians because of their low risk level. Laboratory personnel in administrative or technical positions in laboratories have rarely been named in malpractice suits. Part of the reason for so few cases is that under the legal concept of respondeat superior, responsibility for wrongful acts of the employee (agent–servant) rests on the employer (principal–master). Also, another reason for not being named in a suit is the *deep pocket concept.* The health care worker, with less money or no insurance, in the past has not been a target for suit. The advances in technology and increased complexity of health care have, however, increased legal exposure for allied health and nursing professionals. The health care worker that routinely deals with the public in patient–health care worker relationships is indeed liable. Therefore, each individual should examine the possibility of malpractice suits and the need for malpractice insurance from a personal standpoint.[12]

If the health care worker decides to purchase malpractice insurance, the following factors should be carefully considered[13]:

1. Does the employer carry liability insurance?
2. Is adequate dollar value coverage provided? In recent lawsuits, total damages of $1 million or more have been awarded against physicians.
3. What are the coverage limitations? How much does one have to lose if sued?
4. What are the procedures that must be followed for the policy to provide coverage? Some policies state that divulging the amount of coverage or the fact of coverage voids the policy.
5. The health care worker should not assume that the lawyers representing the hospital, laboratory, or clinic will have his or her best interests at heart. The attorney's first obligation is to serve those who have hired him or her. There have been cases in which the hospital was cleared of all charges but the health care professional was held liable for damages. For the health care worker, if an adult patient seems alert and does not object to the blood specimen collection, consent is implied. Proceeding without consent may give rise to assault and battery charges, as well as civil suits.
6. Is a job change expected soon?
7. Are specimen collecting services provided off site or in patient's homes?

With the purchase of malpractice professional liability insurance, the attorney's fee and court costs are usually covered. Some professional organizations offer professional liability insurance at a reasonable or reduced rate. With the advent of organ transplantations, renal dialysis, hyperbaric care, home care, and bedside testing, the avenues of liability are widened. A genuine concern for others and careful attention to technique are good investments of the health care worker's time. A record of continuing education courses, seminars, workshops, and academic credits should be a part of each health care worker's personal file.

■ MANAGEMENT OF RISK

CONCEPTS OF RISK

Risk can be described as "exposure to the chance of injury or loss."[14] Health care workers face many risks daily. It is important for health care workers, supervisors, and managers to reflect on their personal risk and that of their employers. Active steps should be taken to understand risk factors and to minimize areas of risk for the benefit of patients and the protection of employees and employers. Risk can be managed by using carefully planned objectives that can be categorized as preloss (to reduce or prevent losses) and postloss (how the facility can recover from a loss). **Risk management programs** reduce preventable injuries and accidents and minimize financial loss. The goals and objectives of the institution or department can guide the risk management program. A generic model of **risk management** might involve the following levels:

- *Risk identification and analysis*—analysis and measurement of identified risks.
- *Risk treatment*—use of tools (e.g., safety manuals, policies and procedures, public relations tactics) to prevent harm or losses.
- *Education*—of patients, employees, and visitors.

- *Risk transfer or postponement*—shifting risk to other parties (e.g., liability insurance, contract services, and employees).
- *Risk evaluation*—assessment of what should be done.

One way to identify risk is to review *incident* or *occurrence* reports that involve laboratory or phlebotomy services. Employees must be continually encouraged to use these tools because without an effective reporting system, proper investigations and risk assessments cannot be made. An incident or occurrence does not have to result in injury. The older term *accident report* is rarely used anymore because it implies that an error occurred, which may not always be the case. Trends of events that deviate from normal, but fortunately do not harm any patients, are most revealing and controllable.

Risk treatment has two elements: loss or risk control and risk financing.[14] Loss or risk control means that the department should attempt to reduce the frequency of errors or events that can potentially cause financial loss. Similar to quality-improvement programs, the aim would be to reduce adverse outcomes, such as excessive venipunctures on the same patient, reducing the number of hematomas, and so on. *Risk financing* refers to how to pay for losses once they occur (liability insurance or other means). If a patient faints during venipuncture and injures him- or herself, care should be taken to assist and provide free services for the person to recover. Documentation should clearly indicate the details of the incident and each step of the follow-up.

Education and communication are also vital to the risk management process. If employees do not know about new procedures, they cannot be expected to follow them.

Risk transfer through the use of liability insurance is also an important part of the risk management process. Contracting for services has also traditionally shifted some of the liability to other parties. Federal and state laws are changing, however, to include contract personnel and contract services (e.g., reference laboratories, diagnostic radiology services) under the *respondeat superior* concept. This trend suggests that health care facilities might be held liable for services performed by those with whom they have contracts.

Evaluation of all the elements of risk management just discussed may show a need for changes in procedures, employee counseling, or educational programs. Table 17–1 indicates some common sense tips for minimizing risk in a phlebotomy setting.[14–17]

Table 17–1. Lawsuit Prevention Tips for Minimizing Risks

COMMON ISSUES IN LAWSUITS AGAINST HEALTH CARE PROVIDERS	PREVENTION TIPS FOR PHLEBOTOMISTS, NURSES, AND OTHERS INVOLVED IN BLOOD COLLECTION
Documentation	Always document the time, date, and blood collector's initials on the blood collection containers.
Reporting of incidents	Document the information legibly and spell correctly. If an adverse incident occurs to the patient and/or the blood collector before, during, or after blood collection, report the incident to your immediate supervisor and complete the appropriate documentation in a legible manner.

(continued)

Table 17–1. *(continued)*

COMMON ISSUES IN LAWSUITS AGAINST HEALTH CARE PROVIDERS	PREVENTION TIPS FOR PHLEBOTOMISTS, NURSES, AND OTHERS INVOLVED IN BLOOD COLLECTION
Failure to follow health care facility's procedure	Be knowledgeable of the health care facility's and clinical laboratory's policies and procedures.
	If you must deviate from a policy or a procedure, discuss the incident with your immediate supervisor and decide on the appropriate action.
Failure to ensure patient's safety	Monitor the patient in an appropriate, timely manner during and after blood collection.
	Return bed rails to the raised position if the bed rails were raised prior to blood collection.
	Lock the patient in the blood collection chair for the duration of the blood collection procedure.
	If an outpatient says that he or she faints during blood collection, place the patient in a supine position to collect blood, and monitor the patient for at least 20 minutes after collection before allowing him or her to stand up and leave the facility.
	Remove all supplies and equipment after the procedure.
Improper treatment and performance of treatment	Use proper technique and equipment (e.g., gloves) when performing procedures.
	Follow the health care facility's and clinical laboratory's procedures when performing treatments.
	Update your collection skills and techniques through continuing education classes.
Failure to monitor and to report	Report any significant changes in a patient's condition (e.g., patient continues to bleed from puncture site after blood collection).
Equipment use	Learn how to use blood collection equipment as designed.
	Use biohazardous waste containers as indicated in procedures.
	If involved in off-site blood collections, carry biohazardous waste containers.
	If involved in off-site collections, have the correct types and amounts of insurance coverages to address liability exposures with respect to transporting biohazardous specimens.
Patients with HIV	Be conscious of actions that could result in a lawsuit: Discrimination in treatment Nosocomial transmission of the virus Breach of confidentiality
	Follow health care facility's procedures for blood collection and disposal of biohazardous waste.

CLINICAL LABORATORY IMPROVEMENT AMENDMENTS (CLIA)

In October 1988, the US Congress passed Public Law 100-578, **Clinical Laboratory Improvement Amendments (CLIA)**. This public law is administered by the **Health Care Financing Administration (HCFA)**. CLIA '88 regulations became effective on September 1, 1992, as a means to ensure the quality and accuracy of laboratory testing by creating a uniform set of provisions governing all laboratories that examine human specimens either for the diagnosis, prevention, or treatment of disease or for the impairment of, or the assessment of, the health of human beings.[16] CLIA '88 essentially applies to every clinical laboratory testing facility in the United States and requires that the facility be certified by the federal government. The certification requires an inspection by federal and/or state agencies to determine whether the laboratory testing facility uses methods to test patients' specimens that lead to accurate, reliable, and quality test results. Only laboratories or clinics that perform "waived" laboratory tests (e.g., simple tests such as dipstick urinalysis) are not required to undergo an inspection. Refer to Table 17–2. If the laboratory test is not categorized as waived by the CLIA '88 federal regulations, it falls into the category of "moderately complex" or "highly complex," depending on the difficulty of conducting the test and the risk of harm to the patient if the test is not performed correctly. For the moderately complex or highly complex testing, the inspection considers all procedural steps in laboratory testing—preanalytic, analytic, and postanalytic.

Table 17–2. Analytes on the CLIA Waived List

Amines	Metamphetamines
Amphetamines	Microalbumin
Bladder tumor associated antigen	Nicotine and/or metabolites
Cannabinoids (THC)	Opiates
Catalase, urine	Ovulation test by visual color comparison
Cholesterol, HDL	Phencyclidine (PCP)
Cholesterol, total	Prothrombin time
Cocaine metabolites	Spun microhematocrit
Creatinine	Streptococcus group A
Erythrocyte sedimentation rate	Triglyceride
Ethanol	Urine dipstick or tablet analytes, nonautomated
Fecal occult blood	Urine qualitative dipstick bilirubin
Fructosamine	Urine qualitative dipstick blood
Gastric occult blood	Urine qualitative dipstick glucose
Glucose or glucose monitoring device	Urine qualitative dipstick ketone
Glycosylated hemoglobin (HbA$_{1c}$)	Urine qualitative dipstick leukocytes
hCG, urine	Urine qualitative dipstick nitrite
Helicobacter pylori antibodies	Urine qualitative Dipstick pH
Helicobacter pylori (bacteriology)	Urine qualitative dipstick protein
Hematocrit	Urine qualitative dipstick specific gravity
Hemoglobin	Urine qualitative dipstick urobilinogen
Infectious mononucleosis antibodies	Vaginal pH
Ketones, blood	

Source: Sliva, Clara, Acting CLIA Coordinator tests waived by FDA from January 31–July 26, 2000; CDC through March 2000, downloaded 2/14/01, website: www.fda.gov/carh/clia/analyteswaived.html.

Thus, the blood collection procedures area is a major part of CLIA inspections. The HCFA states that a laboratory with moderately complex or highly complex testing must have available, and follow, written policies and procedures for the following:

- Protocols for the preparation of patients
- Specimen collection
- Specimen labeling
- Specimen preservation
- Conditions for specimen transportation

KEY TERMS

Administrative Law
Assault
Battery
Bioethics
Breach of Duty
Centers for Disease Control and
    Prevention (CDC)
Civil Law
Clinical Laboratory
    Improvement Amendments
    (CLIA)
Criminal Actions
Defendant
Deposition
Discovery
Environmental Protection
    Agency (EPA)
Ethics
Evidence
Expert Witness
False Imprisonment
Felony
Food and Drug Administration
    (FDA)
Health Care Financing
    Administration (HCFA)

Implied Consent
Informed Consent
Invasion of Privacy
Judicial Law
Law
Liable
Litigation Process
Malice
Malpractice
Medical Records
Misdemeanor
Misrepresentation
Negligence
Patient Confidentiality
Plaintiff
Preventive Law
Respondeat Superior
Risk Management
Risk Management Programs
Standard of Care
Statute of Limitations
Statutory Laws
Tort
Vicarious Liability
Whistle-blowing

STUDY QUESTIONS

For the following, choose the *one* best answer.

1. What is the legal term for improper or unskillful care of a patient by a member of the health care team, or any professional misconduct, unreasonable lack of skill, or infidelity in professional or judiciary duties?

    a. a misdemeanor
    b. malpractice
    c. litigation
    d. liability

2. What are the factors, or key points, that must be considered in alleged negligence cases?

1. duty   3. proximate causation
2. breach of duty   4. damages

Select one choice:
a. 1, 2, and 3 are correct   d. only 4 is correct
b. 1 and 3 are correct   e. all are correct
c. 2 and 4 are correct

3. One agency affecting regulations on blood collection is HCFA. It stands for which of the following?

a. Home Care Financing Administration   c. Health Care Financial Agency
b. Health Care Financing Administration d. Health Care Funding Agency

4. Which of the following legal branches writes regulations that enforce the laws?

a. administrative branch   c. US Supreme Court
b. judicial branch   d. executive branch

5. The avoidance of legal conflicts in blood collection through education and planning is considered which type of law?

a. administrative law   c. preventive law
b. executive law   d. preparatory law

6. A child who refused to have his blood drawn was locked in a room by a phlebotomist and was forced to have his blood collected. This is an example of which legal concept?

a. invasion of privacy   c. a misdemeanor
b. informed consent   d. assault and battery

7. The standard of care currently used in malpractice legal cases involving health care providers is based on the conduct of the average health care provider in which area?

a. state   c. national community
b. city   d. local community

8. Which legal concept refers to the voluntary permission by a patient to allow touching, examination, and/or treatment by health care providers?

a. implied consent   c. battery
b. assault and battery   d. informed consent

9. Which of the following evaluates the safety, clinical efficacy, and medical efficacy of the equipment and supplies used in blood collection?

a. EPA   c. CDC
b. OSHA   d. FDA

10. When should incident reports involving accidental HIV-exposures be reported?

a. at the end of the work shift   c. after 24 hours
b. immediately   d. after seeing the employee health
                                      physician

References

1. Lewis, MA, Tamparo, CD: *Medical Law, Ethics, and Bioethics for Ambulatory Care.* 4th ed. Philadelphia; F.A. Davis Company: 1998.

2. Richards, EP, Rathburn, KC: *Law and the Physician.* Boston; Little, Brown and Company: 1993.

3. Curran, WJ, Hall, MA, Kaye, DH: *Health Care Law, Forensic Science, and Public Policy.* Boston; Little, Brown and Company: 1990.

4. Rakich, JS, Longest, BB, Darr, K: *Managing Health Services Organizations.* Baltimore; Health Professions Press: 1992.

5. *Parker v. Port Huron Hospital,* 105, N.W. 2d 854 (1981).

6. Brent, NJ: Confidentiality and HIV status: The nurse's right to know, *Home Healthcare Nurse,* 1990;*8*(3):6–8.

7. Rozovsky, F, Rozovsky, L: *Home Health Care Law: Liablity and Risk Management.* Boston; Little, Brown and Company: 1996, pp. 1–13.

8. Ernst, D: Phlebotomy on trial, *MLO,* 1999, April; 46–50.

9. Aoun, H: When a house officer gets AIDS, *N. Engl J Med.,* 1989; *321*(10):695.

10. Auxter, S: Bringing rapid HIV tests to market more quickly, *Clin Lab News,* 2000; *26*(10):1, 10.

11. Needlestick Safety and Prevention Act: Public Law No. 106-430. http://thomas.loc.gov. November 6, 2000.

12. Pozgar, GD: *Legal Aspects of Health Care Administration.* Gaithersburg, MD; Aspen Publishers: 1993.

13. Markus, K: Your legal risk in giving advice or care, *Healthweek,* Oct 6, 1997; 5.

14. Troyer, GT, Salman, SL: *Handbook of Health Care Risk Management.* Rockville, MD; Aspen Publishers: 1986.

15. Bunting, RF: Risk management and prevention in the clinical laboratory, *Clin Lab Sci 5,* 1992;(Jan/Feb);1, 35–37.

16. Department of Health and Human Services (DHHS), Health Care Financing Administration (HCFA), Public Health Service: 42 CFR 405 *et seq,* 57 FR 7002–7186, Feb 28, 1992.

17. Fiesta, J: *20 Legal Pitfalls for Nurses to Avoid.* Albany, NY; Delmar Publishers: 1994.

PHLEBOTOMY CASE STUDY

■

Communication and Consent

Ms. Nancy Garcia, a 78-year-old Hispanic woman, was admitted to River Bend Hospital as a result of complications from diabetes mellitus. When the health care worker arrived at her hospital room to collect blood for laboratory tests, he introduced himself and asked her name. She did not respond and looked perplexed.

QUESTIONS

1. What should the health care worker do next?
2. What could a health care facility provide to assist in this situation?
3. Has the patient implied her consent to the venipuncture?

See Answers in Appendix.

PHLEBOTOMY CASE STUDY

■

An Ethical Dilemma

Ms. Daley was a veteran nurse on a hospital medical floor with mostly cardiac patients. The patient care assistant, Marty, had been performing phlebotomy duties on this floor for about 6 months and had developed a close friendship with Ms. Daley. They had even socialized after work on a few occasions.

One morning two individuals with similar names were admitted to this hospital unit. Their names were Frances L. Johnson and Francis T. Johnston. Ms. Daley was in charge of giving the patients their identification bracelets. Soon after admission, laboratory tests were ordered STAT on both patients so Marty went to collect the specimens. She entered the room expecting to greet Frances L. Johnson. She checked the identification bracelet and noticed that Frances L. Johnson had Francis T. Johnston's identification bracelet, even though the sign on the hospital room was correctly labeled. When Marty mentioned the mistake to Ms. Daley she said, "Oh don't worry, it's just a little mix-up and I'll fix it. Since there was no harm done, I don't see any need to report it. Thanks for letting me know."

QUESTIONS

1. What should Marty do next?
2. What corrective actions, if any, should be taken?
3. What ethical situations might arise from this situation?
4. What might the consequences have been if Marty had not noticed the error?

See Answers in Appendix.

1

APPENDIX

■

Units of Measurement and Symbols

α	alpha
Å	angstrom
amp	ampere (unit of electric current)
b.i.d.	twice per day (Latin equivalent is bis in di'e)
c	centi- (10^{-2})
°C	degrees Centigrade or Celsius (unit of temperature; convert to Fahrenheit by multiplying by 1.8 and adding 32)
cc	cubic centimeter (same as mL, $\frac{1}{1000}$ L)
cd	candela (unit of luminous intensity)
cm	centimeter
cu mm	cubic millimeter
d	deci- (10^{-1})
dL	deciliter ($\frac{1}{10}$ of a liter)
°F	degrees Fahrenheit (unit of temperature; convert to Centigrade by subtracting 32 and multiplying by 0.555)
g or gm	gram ($\frac{1}{1000}$ of a kilogram, unit of mass)
G%	grams in 100 mL
h	hecto- (10^2)
hpf	high-power field on microscope
IU	international unit
k	kilo- (10^3)
°K	degrees Kelvin (thermodynamic temperature; convert to Centigrade by subtracting 273.15)
kg	kilogram (1000 g, or 2.2 lb)
L	liter (1000 mL or 1000 cc, unit of volume)
lpf	low-power field on microscope
μ	micro- (10^{-6})
μci	microcurie ($\frac{1}{1000}$ mCi)
μg or mcg	microgram ($\frac{1}{1000}$ mg)
μm	micron

m	meter (unit of length)
m	milli- (10^{-3})
mCi	millicurie
mEq or meq	milliequivalent
mg or mgm	milligram ($\frac{1}{1000}$ g)
mg%	milligrams in 100 mL (same as dL)
min	minutes
mIU	milli-international unit ($\frac{1}{1000}$ IU)
mL	milliliter ($\frac{1}{1000}$ L, same as cc)
mm	millimeter ($\frac{1}{10}$ cm)
mm^3	cubic millimeter
mm Hg	millimeters of mercury
mmole	millimole
mol, M	mole (unit of substance)
mOsm	milliosmol
N	normality
n	nano- (10^{-9})
ng	nanogram ($\frac{1}{1000}$ mg)
p	pico- (10^{-12})
pg	picogram ($\frac{1}{1000}$ ng)
q.h. or q.2h.	every hour or every 2 hours (Latin equivalent is qua'que ho'ra or 2 ho'ra)
q.i.d.	four times per day (Latin equivalent is qua'ter in di'e)
QNS	quantity not sufficient
sec or s	second (unit of time)
SI	international system
sp *g*	specific gravity
t.i.d.	three times per day (Latin equivalent is ter in di'e)
TPN	total parenteral nutrition
TPR	temperature, pulse, respirations
U	international enzyme unit
WNL	within normal limits
WNR	within normal range
wt	weight
w/v	weight/volume
$\cong$	approximately
$\leq$	less than or equal to
$\geq$	greater than or equal to
+ or (+)	positive
− or (−)	negative
Σ	summation

APPENDIX

■

Metric Conversion Chart

LENGTH OR DISTANCE

1 inch (in.) = 2.54 centimeters (cm)
1 foot (ft) = 30.48 centimeters (cm)
39.37 inches (in.) = 1 meter (m)
1 mile (mi) = 1.61 kilometers (km)

MASS OR WEIGHT

1 ounce (oz) = 28.35 grams (g)
1 pound (lb) = 453.6 grams (g)
2.205 pounds (lb) = 1 kilogram (kg)

VOLUME

1 fluid ounce (fl oz) = 29.57 milliliters (mL)
1.057 quarts (qt) = 1 liter (liter or L)
1 gallon (gal) = 3.78 liters (liter or L)

APPENDIX

■

Formulas and Calculations

Area	square meter (sq m or m^2)
Blood volume	Total blood volume = weight (kg) × average blood volume (defined by age)
Clearance	liter/second (L/s)
Concentration and conversions	
Mass	kilogram/liter (kg/L)
Substrate	mole/liter (mol/L)

% w/v to M or vice versa:

$$M = \frac{\% \ w/v \times 10}{molecular \ wt \ (mol \ wt)}$$

% w/v to N or vice versa:

$$N = \frac{\% \ w/v \times 10}{eq \ wt}$$

mg/dL to mEq/L or vice versa:

$$mEq/L = \frac{mg/dL \times 10}{eq \ wt}$$

M to N:

$$N = M \times valence$$

N to M:

$$M = \frac{N}{valence}$$

Density	kilogram/liter (kg/L)
Dilutions	Final concentration =
	Original concentration $\times$ dilution 1 $\times$ dilution 2, etc.
Electrical potential	volt (V) = kg m^2/s^{3}A
Energy	joule (J) = kg m^2/s^2
Force	Newton (N) = kg m^2/s^2
Frequency	hertz (Hz) = 1 cycle/s
Hematology math	Mean corpuscular volume (MCV) = average volume of red blood cells (RBCs); expressed in cubic microns (μm^3) or femtoliters (fL)

$$MCV = \frac{Hct \times 10}{RBC\ count\ (in\ millions)}$$

Hct = hematocrit value

Mean corpuscular hemoglobin (MCH) = Average weight of hemoglobin in RBC; expressed in picograms (pg)

$$MCH = \frac{hgb\ (g) \times 10}{RBC\ count\ (in\ millions)}$$

hgb = hemoglobin value

Mean corpuscular hemoglobin concentration = Hemoglobin concentration of average RBC

$$MCHC = \frac{hgb\ (g)}{Hct} \times 100\%$$

RBC distribution width (RDW) = numerical expression of variation of RBC size, dispersion of RBC volumes about the mean

$$RDW = \frac{SD\ (standard\ deviation)\ of\ RBC\ size}{MCV}$$

Military Time	Military time uses a 24-hour time clock and eliminates the need for A.M. or P.M. designations. Time is expressed by up to four numbers; the first set is in hours (00 to 24) and the second set is minutes (00 to 59). Each day begins at midnight, 0000, and ends at 2359.
	The first 12 hours are equivalent in military time (3:00 A.M. is equivalent to 0300 in military time), but conversion of afternoon and evening times on a 12-hour clock to military time requires adding 12 hours (2:00 P.M. is 1400 in military time).
	Military time is usually stated in terms of hundreds (e.g., 1500 is stated as "fifteen hundred hours"; 0300 is stated as "zero three hundred").
Pressure	Pascal (Pa) = (kg/m)s^2

Quality control math:

Variance (s^2)

$$s^2 = \frac{(x - \bar{x})^2}{n - 1}$$

Standard deviation (s)

$$s = \sqrt{s^2}$$

% Coefficient of variation

$$\%CV = \frac{s}{\bar{x}} \times 100$$

Relative centrifugal force (rcf)

Measures force of centrifugation acting on blood components and allowing them to separate. Can be used to calibrate centrifuges.

$rcf = 1.118 \times 10^{-5} \times 4 \times n^2$

r = rotating radius (centimeters)

n = speed of rotation (revolutions per minute)

Solutions

Specific gravity (sp g):

$$sp\ g = \frac{wt\ of\ solid\ or\ liquid}{wt\ of\ equal\ volume\ of\ H_2O\ at\ 4°C}$$

Temperature:

Celsius or Centigrade

Kelvin

Fahrenheit

Volume

$°C = K - 273.15;\ °C = °F - 32 \times 0.555$

$°K = °C + 273.15$ or ⅚ $(°F) + 255.35$

$°F = (°C \times 1.8) + 32$

deciliter (dL)   = ⅒ of a liter

10 dL   = 1 L

centiliter (cL) = ¹⁄₁₀₀ of a liter

100 cL   = 10 dL = 1 L

milliliter (mL) = ¹⁄₁₀₀₀ of a liter

1000 mL   = 100 cL = 10 dL = 1 L

APPENDIX

■

Basic Spanish for Specimen Collection Procedures

The following translations present the health care worker with a *very basic* means of communicating with patients who speak Spanish. Before speaking with patients, the health care worker should practice using these phrases with someone who knows the correct pronunciation. Otherwise, the patient may become even more confused. Remember that in Spanish, the letter "h" is always silent. Also, if a word ends in "a" it is usually feminine gender; if it ends in "o" it is masculine. Another alternative is to have the key phrases printed on cards that the health care worker may point to or use as a reference when he or she is communicating with the patient. Also, use your hands when speaking, pantomime, point, or use facial expressions to assist in communicating.

English	Spanish
one	uno
two	dos
three	tres
four	cuatro
five	cinco
six	seis
seven	siete
eight	ocho
nine	nueve
ten	diez
twenty	veinte
thirty	treinta
forty	cuarenta
fifty	cincuenta
sixty	sesenta
seventy	setenta
eighty	ochenta
ninety	noventa

English	Spanish
one hundred	ciento/cien
Hello.	Hola.
Good day.	Buenos dias/Buendia.
Good morning.	Buenos dias.
Good afternoon.	Buenas tardes.
Good evening.	Buenas noches.
Mother	Madre/mama
Father	Padre/papa
Sister	Hermana
Brother	Hermano
Son	Hijo
Daughter	Hija
Husband	Esposo/marido
Wife	Esposa/marida
Infant/baby	Niño/niña
Grandfather	Abuelo
Grandmother	Abuela
Friend	Amigo/Amiga
Mister	Señor
Mrs.	Señora
Miss	Señorita
Doctor	Doctor/Medico
Technician	Técnico
Nurse	Enfermera
alcohol	alcohol
fasting	enayunas
gloves	guantes
needle	aguja
sterile	estéril
syringe	jeringa
tourniquet	torniquete
pathology	patología
procedure	procedimiento
hematology	hematología
complete blood count (CBC)	biometría hemática complete
blood bank	banco de sangre
coagulated	coagulado
reports	reportes
specimen	muestra
tubes	tubos
My name is . . .	Me llamo . . . /Mi nombres . . .
I work in the laboratory.	Trabajo en el laboratorio.
I speak . . .	Hablo . . .
We are going to analyze	Vamos analizar
. . . your blood.	. . . su sangre.
. . . your urine.	. . . su orina.

English	Spanish
. . . your sputum.	. . . su esputo.
Do you understand?	¿Entiende Usted (ud.)?
I do not understand.	No entiendo.
Please (pls.)	Por favor (p.f.)
Thank you.	Gracias.
You are welcome.	De nada.
Speak slower, pls.	Hable mas despacio, p.f.
Repeat, pls.	Haga me el favor de repetir, p.f.
Can you hear me?	¿Puede oírme?
Can you speak?	¿Puede hablar?
Relax.	Relajese.
What is your name?	¿Como se llama?
What is your address?	¿Que es su domicillo?
What is your birth date?	¿En que fecha nacio?
How old are you?	¿Cuantos años tiene ud.?
Have you been here before?	¿Ha estado ud. aquí antes?
Who is your doctor?	¿Quien es su doctor?
Your doctor wrote the order.	El doctor/la doctora escribio la orden.
Here is the bathroom.	Aquí esta el baño.
Here is the call light.	Aquí esta la luz de emergencia.
You may not eat/drink anything except water.	No debe de comer/beber nada solamente agua.
You may not smoke.	No puede fumar.
Have you had breakfast?	¿Ya tomo el desayuno?
We need a blood/urine/stool sample.	Necesitamos una muestra de su sangre/orina/del excremento.
Please stay in bed.	Por favor, quédese en la cama.
Please do not eat after midnight.	Por favor, no coma después de medianoche.
Please	Haga me el favor de
. . . make a fist.	. . . cerrar el puño.
. . . bend your arm.	. . . doblar el brazo.
. . . roll up your sleeve.	. . . levantarse la manga.
. . . open your hand.	. . . abrir la mano.
. . . sit down here.	. . . sientese aquí.
. . . change your position.	. . . cambiarse de posición.
. . . turn over.	. . . voltearse.
. . . change to the left.	. . . cambiarse a la izquierda.
. . . change to the right.	. . . cambiarse a la derecha.
I am going to lift your sleeve.	Voy levantar la manga.
I need to	Necesito
. . . take a blood sample.	. . . sacar una muestra de sangre.
. . . stick/prick your finger.	. . . picarle su dedo.
. . . two tubes of blood	. . . dos tubos de sangre.
Open your hand.	Abra la mano.

English	Spanish
It will hurt a little.	Le va a doler un poquito.
Please do not move.	No se mueva, por favor.
This is done quickly.	Esto se hace rapido.
The needle will stay in your arm while I am collecting the blood sample.	La aguja se quedara en su brazo/ durante el tiempo necessario para obtener la muestra.
I am finished. Thank you.	Ya termine. Gracias.
Press this gauze on your arm/finger until I can make sure that the bleeding has stopped.	Comprese esta banda en su brazo/ su dedo hasta que pare la sangre.
I am going to put a bandage on you.	Voy a ponerle una cinta adhesiva/un curita/un bandaid.
Are you lightheaded?	¿Esta usted mareado/mareada?
Do you feel as if you are going to faint?	¿Se siente como si se va a desmayar?
Do you feel all right?	¿Se siente bien?
You must lie down.	Necesita acostarse.
Collect the midstream portion of the urine in the container or bottle.	Coleccione la porción del medio de la orina en el vaso.
Void a little, then put urine in this cup.	Orine un poco, luego ponga la orina en esta taza.

Source: Joyce, EV, Villanueva, ME: *Say It in Spanish, A Guide for Health Care Professionals.* 2nd ed. Philadelphia; W.B. Saunders Co.: 2000.

APPENDIX

∎

Answers to Self Study Questions and Cases

OVERVIEW: SELF STUDY ANSWERS

CHAPTER 1
1. a, b, c, d
2. a, b, d
3. a, b, c
4. a, b, c
5. a, b, c, d
6. b, d
7. a, b, c
8. a, b, c, d
9. b, c, d

CHAPTER 2
1. a, b, c
2. c
3. b
4. a, b, c, d, e
5. a, b

6. a, b, d
7. b
8. c
9. d
10. b, c

CHAPTER 3
1. a, b, c
2. a
3. a, c
4. a
5. c, d, e
6. a, b, c, d
7. c
8. b
9. d
10. a, b, c, d

I. OVERVIEW:
CASE STUDY: ANSWERS/DISCUSSION

CASE STUDY: CHANGING ROLES IN PHLEBOTOMY PRACTICE

1. Trends in hospital management are aimed at improving the quality of health care by minimizing errors, eliminating unnecessary costs and redundancy, performing duties as a coordinated health care team rather than as individual specialists, and becoming more sensitive to patient's individual needs. Also, laboratory technology has enabled testing to be performed closer to the point-of-care or at the patient's bedside.

   Ms. Sanborn can learn more by asking administrators in her area about these changes, by reading about trends in the industry in newsletters and professional journals, by attending continuing education seminars to learn new technical skills and how to deal with change, and by networking with colleagues in other locations.

2. Ms. Sanborn already has very positive personality traits and work habits that should contribute to the team concept in a productive manner. She should remember the following skills needed for effective teams:
   - Understand the mission of the organization.
   - Know basic skills for group process and team dynamics (e.g., active listening, setting norms, etc.).
   - Understand relevance and commitment to team goals.
   - Be reliable and dependable in work assignments.
   - Be able to communicate ideas and feelings.
   - Actively participate in decision making.
   - Learn how to be flexible in decision making.
   - Constructively manage conflicts.
   - Contribute to the cohesion of the team.
   - Contribute to problem solving strategies.
   - Support and encourage other team members.

3. Ms. Sanborn has numerous positive attributes that will help her in her new role. These are efficiency in blood collection, her willingness to provide assistance, her attention to details, and her ability to communicate effectively with patients. These types of traits and work habits are universally beneficial no matter what type of health care setting she is in.

CASE STUDY: COLLECTION FROM THE DORSAL SIDE OF THE HAND

1. *Dorsal* (proximal) refers to the back of the hand in this case. The anterior hand or wrist should NOT be used for venipuncture.
2. *Supine* means lying on the back, face upward.
3. An orthopedic floor is for patients with bone and joint disorders.

CASE STUDY: COMMUNICATION AND CULTURAL SENSITIVITY: KEYS TO SUCCESS

1. The fact that Elizabeth does not speak Spanish or that Mrs. Rodriguez does not speak English well is a major barrier to effective communication between them. This barrier needs to be addressed before a successful and comfortable scenario can be achieved. In addition, having so many family members present, including the child, may also be somewhat of a distraction.

2. Mrs. Rodriguez obviously wants or needs a support group of her family members to be with her during this encounter. She may be fearful or nervous about the procedure, or she may believe that her family can help her understand what is going to happen. She may believe that if any major medical decisions need to be made, her family members can help with the decisions.

3. As mentioned in Chapter 1, communication strategies may involve the following:
   - Seek the assistance of a translator
   - Utilize written instructions in Spanish for reinforcing the messages
   - Show empathy through body language and facial expressions
   - Show respect for privacy
   - Build trust by trying to explain carefully using a model, symbols, or body language
   - Establish rapport with the patient and her family members
   - Listen actively to the patient and her family members
   - Provide as much feedback as possible

4. In this case, one or more of the family members may be able to help with the translation of various parts of the conversation. Even the child may be able to assist with some basic translations and information. They may hold her hand or comfort her as the procedure is taking place. If possible, let them participate in helping her to relax.

5. Elizabeth may want to familiarize herself with medical terms in Spanish. She could use the translations in the Appendix to practice basic requests for venipuncture and urinalysis. She could take a medical terminology course in Spanish. She could find out more about Hispanic cultures and the diversity among Hispanic cultures through their music, literature, and popular media.

II. SAFETY PROCEDURES: SELF STUDY ANSWERS

CHAPTER 4
1. d
2. b, c, d
3. b, c
4. e
5. b
6. b
7. c
8. b
9. b, c, d
10. b

CHAPTER 5
1. c, d
2. a, b, d
3. b, c, d
4. a, c, d
5. a, b, c, d
6. b
7. c
8. b
9. b

CHAPTER 6

1. a, b, c, d
2. a, b, c, d
3. a, c, d
4. a, b, c
5. a, b, c, d

6. b
7. a, b, d
8. a, b, c, d
9. a
10. c

II. SAFETY PROCEDURES:
CASE STUDY ANSWERS/DISCUSSION

CASE STUDY: ACCIDENTAL INJURY

1. Even though Sally was tired, she had a job to do. Her fatigue might have contributed to her inability to draw blood from Mr. Johnson on the first try, however, there is no way to substantiate that. She probably did the procedure correctly except she should have discarded the first needle and holder immediately after she used it. At that time she would have noticed that the biohazard container was full, and she could have notified the appropriate person for a replacement. *She should not have stuffed the other needles into the full biohazard container!!* However, she took the appropriate action by notifying her supervisor immediately of her injury.
2. Sally would have to review the exposure control plan, OSHA standards, universal precautions, and safety procedures for disposing of contaminated waste.
3. Aside from a thorough review of the procedures mentioned in Question 2, Sally would benefit from going to classes on the importance of being rested and healthy for work. In addition, it appears she needs additional practice on patients who are difficult to draw. She may benefit from observing other experienced phlebotomists while they perform difficult draws.

CASE STUDY: TRANSPORTING SPECIMENS FROM HOMEBOUND PATIENTS TO THE LABORATORY

1. Larry seemed so pleased that he successfully communicated with Mr. Gonzales that he forgot to be meticulous about checking the specimen integrity. He should have carefully placed each specimen in a *leakproof* plastic container in an upright position in the carrying container with absorbant material. He should have securely locked the container, and placed it in a safer place in his car, perhaps the floor.
2. Larry should be careful not to touch the contaminated area. He should report the spill immediately and find out the appropriate procedures for spill cleanups.

CASE STUDY: IMPROVING SPEED AND ACCURACY IN PHLEBOTOMY PRACTICE

1. Bar code technology has many benefits and applications in the clinical laboratory. The technology has been proved to be fast and accurate. Bar codes are particularly valuable in large-volume laboratories. As mentioned in Chapter 6, bar codes can be used for the following:

- Patients' names
- Patients' identification numbers
- DOB
- Test codes
- Specimen accession or log numbers
- Expiration dates for inventory of supplies and equipment
- Product codes for needles, syringes, specimen collection tubes, etc.
- Billing codes to facilitate accounting
- Sample identification numbers on laboratory analyzers

  The only drawbacks are the costs associated with starting up (equipment, software, scanners, printers, new labels) and the training time needed to teach all personnel how to operate the system.

2. Bar codes can help reduce preanalytical errors by saving transcription time and avoiding multiple entries of the same information, thereby reducing clerical errors substantially. It is faster to scan a bar code than to write down a patient's name and identification number. It is easier to scan a product bar code as it is delivered than to write down all the details of a receiving order for specimen collection supplies. Above all, identification of patients and specimens becomes more accurate and timely as each specimen works its way through the analytical phases of laboratory testing.

III. EQUIPMENT AND PROCEDURES: SELF STUDY ANSWERS

CHAPTER 7

1. a, b, c
2. d
3. a
4. b
5. c
6. b
7. a
8. a, b, c
9. c

CHAPTER 8

1. b, c
2. a, b, d
3. b
4. a, c, d
5. b, c, d
6. b, d
7. d
8. a
9. a, d, c, b
10. a, b

CHAPTER 9

1. a, b, c
2. b, d
3. c, d
4. a, b, c, d
5. b, c
6. b, d
7. b, c
8. b
9. a, b, c, d
10. c

CHAPTER 10

1. a, c, d
2. b, d
3. a, b, c, d
4. c
5. c
6. b
7. b
8. a
9. a
10. a, b, c

III. EQUIPMENT AND PROCEDURES: CASE STUDY ANSWERS/DISCUSSION

CASE STUDY: AMBULATORY HEALTH CARE COLLECTIONS

1. Under normal blood collection procedures with an evacuated tube system, the health care provider did use the proper order of draw for Mrs. Ragsdale's laboratory tests. The light blue–topped tube containing citrate should be collected prior to the red-speckled tube (gel separator tube). When using a blood collection set, however, the tubing in the assembly contains air and will *underfill* the first evacuated tube, leading to an erroneous protime result.

2. The health care provider used the proper collection procedure. A 21- or 23-gauge needle is better, however, than a 25-gauge needle because the small diameter of the 25-gauge needle may lead to hemolysis of the collected blood and erroneous laboratory tests' results.

3. The proper blood collection procedure was used for obtaining blood from Mr. Sadler. Often, hemophiliacs have sclerosed veins due to so many blood collections and transfusions. Thus, a butterfly needle assembly used on the hand or lower arm is appropriate. A "complete" assembly set, however, should be used rather than pieces from different manufacturers. Mismatched medical equipment has led to 50 percent of mucocutaneous blood-borne pathogen exposures* of health care workers to HIV-positive and/or HCV infected patients.

CASE STUDY: VENIPUNCTURE SITE SELECTION

1. The preferred site would be the dorsal side of the left wrist, below the IV site. The preferred phlebotomy method would be to use a winged infusion set in combination with evacuated tubes that could handle a short draw in case of difficulty.

2. The right arm of Mrs. McDonald should never be used for venipuncture because of her partial mastectomy. This type of surgical procedure often results in removal of lymph nodes resulting in edematous areas. Since she is a diabetic, foot veins should be eliminated because of an increased likelihood of infectious complications. Since the left arm had an IV located below the anticubital area, this location could not be used for venipuncture due to contamination with IV fluid. The area below the IV site is acceptable for tourniquet application and venipuncture. The winged infusion system is most effective for the smaller veins of the wrist. It is also less painful for the patient.

3. It would be helpful to the clinical laboratory and other members of the health care team to document that the blood sample was drawn from below the IV site since the patient was diabetic, had a mastectomy on the right side, and had an IV located in the left arm.

4. Site selection can be facilitated by the following: proper positioning, use of a pillow or towel under the wrist, rotation of the patient's arm, palpation, warming the site, and dangling the arm for a short while to increase blood flow to the area.

*Ippolito, G, Puro, V, Petrosillo, N, et al.: *Prevention, Management & Chemoprophylaxis of Occupational Exposure to HIV.* Virginia; Advances in Exposure Prevention Publisher: 1997.

CASE STUDY: FINDING THE RIGHT SITE

1. The phlebotomist should clarify on which side the mastectomy was performed and draw from a vein in the other arm.
2. and 3. Often when a mastectomy is performed, lymph nodes are also removed from the area adjacent to the malignant site. Once they have been removed they never grow back. Since lymph nodes function to move lymph fluid throughout the body, the absence of lymph nodes causes fluid build-up in that region of the body. While the swelling probably is not significant after 5 years, even a minor fluid build-up might have a dilution effect on the specimen if it is collected from that side of the body.

IV. SPECIAL PROCEDURES AND POINT-OF-CARE TESTING: SELF STUDY ANSWERS

CHAPTER 11

1. a, b
2. b, d
3. a, b, d
4. c
5. a, d
6. d
7. b
8. a, b
9. a, b, d
10. c
11. b, c
12. b, c, d

CHAPTER 12

1. c
2. c
3. d
4. a
5. d
6. c
7. a
8. b
9. a
10. b

CHAPTER 13

1. c
2. d
3. b
4. c

5. d
6. b
7. b
8. a
9. a
10. c

CHAPTER 14

1. b
2. b
3. c
4. c
5. c
6. b
7. b
8. c
9. b
10. b

CHAPTER 15

1. b
2. a, b, c, d
3. a, b
4. b
5. b
6. a, c
7. a, b, c, d
8. a, b, c, d
9. b, d
10. a, b, c

IV. SPECIAL PROCEDURES AND POINT-OF-CARE TESTING: CASE STUDY ANSWERS/DISCUSSION

CASE STUDY: HOME CARE COLLECTIONS

1.

Laboratory Assay	*Color of Blood Collection Tube Top*
Calcium, ionized	green
APTT	light blue
CBC count	purple
Protime	light blue
Chemistry screen	red or red-speckled
Digoxin	red or red-speckled
Plasma potassium	green

2. The order of draw was incorrect for blood vacuum tube collections. The correct order should have been red, light blue, green, and purple. The correct order prevents contamination of nonadditive tubes by additive tubes, and minimizes cross-contamination between the different anticoagulants.
3. The order of draw should have been the same as for vacuum tubes; therefore, the order of draw for this specimen was correct. Care should have been taken to mix the purple-topped tube immediately after filling it.

CASE STUDY: BEDSIDE GLUCOSE TESTING

1. The problem in this bedside glucose testing case is that the patient's meter was reading outside the control confidence limits. Thus, the glucose results are out of control and not considered accurate or reliable.
2. The phlebotomist, the nurse, and other health care providers involved in the bedside glucose testing for this patient should troubleshoot for:
   a. Correct timing of the analytic procedure.
   b. Reagents and controls stored at correct temperature and within appropriate expiration dates.
   c. Instrument blotting or wiping technique performed according to manufacturer's directions.

In this case, the control solution had expired March 2, 1998.

CASE STUDY: NEWBORN NURSERY COLLECTIONS

1. Blood collected from a baby for a bilirubin determination should be collected in an amber microcollection tube or a tube covered with foil so that the microcollection tube is not exposed to light. Light breaks down bilirubin.
2. Because bilirubin breaks down in the presence of light, the longer a blood specimen is exposed to light, the more bilirubin is broken down. Thus, the bilirubin value will be falsely decreased.
3. Probably, the phlebotomist who collected Baby McPherson's blood on Sunday morning collected the blood in a clear microcollection tube and allowed it to remain in direct light for an extended period prior to delivering it to the clinical laboratory.

CASE STUDY: COLLECTING BLOOD FROM AN INFANT

1. For this microcollection, Ms. Wiggins needed to have the following equipment:
   a. Sterile automatic disposable pediatric safety lancet devices
   b. 70% isopropyl alcohol swabs in sterile packages
   c. Sterile cotton balls or gauze sponges
   d. Plastic microcollection containers
   e. Puncture-resistant sharps container
   f. Disposable sterile gloves (nonlatex if infant is allergic)
   g. Compress (towel or washcloth) to warm heel if necessary
   h. Marking pen
   i. Laboratory request slips or labels

   For the procedure, after Ms. Wiggins washes her hands outside of the nursery and then dons the gown, gloves, and mask, she picks up her blood collection tray with two clean paper towels and enters the nursery area. The tray is then placed on a diaper on the small metal cart next to the infant. Then, the infant must be identified properly. The phlebotomist then collects the blood after ensuring that the infant's heel is adequately warm for the collection.

2. For Infant Jim Jenkins, the microcollection tube with EDTA was used first to collect blood for the hemoglobin procedure, then the microcollection tube with lithium heparin was used next to collect blood for the potassium test, and finally a microcollection tube without additives was used to collect blood for the thyroxine test.

V. QUALITY MANAGEMENT AND LEGAL ISSUES: SELF STUDY ANSWERS

CHAPTER 16

1. a, b, c, d
2. a, b, c, d
3. a, b, c
4. a, b, c, d
5. a, c, d

CHAPTER 17

1. b
2. e
3. b
4. d
5. c
6. d
7. c
8. d
9. d
10. b

V. QUALITY MANAGEMENT AND LEGAL ISSUES: CASE STUDY ANSWERS/DISCUSSION

CASE STUDY: COMMUNICATION AND CONSENT

1. The phlebotomist should check with the floor nurse to determine whether Ms. Garcia speaks English and/or whether she has a hearing disability. If the patient speaks only Spanish, an interpreter or a written description of the phlebotomy procedure should be available in Spanish to assist in this situation. If the patient has a hearing disability, efforts should be made to write down instructions for the patient.

2. If a patient has a hearing disability, writing tools should be kept at the bedside of the patient. If a large segment of the patient population speaks another language, the hospital should provide interpreters who know the basic use of that language. Also, instruction sheets on phlebotomy steps should be made available in other languages for patients who do not speak English.

3. The patient has not consented to the venipuncture, nor did she appear to understand the verbal communication. The efforts mentioned in the above answers will facilitate seeking consent and minimize the risk of legal or financial loss to the hospital. Above all, these efforts will provide a cooperative, professional interaction for the patient and health care worker.

CASE STUDY: AN ETHICAL DILEMMA

1. and 2. Marty took the correct action by informing the nurse in charge. However, in this case, it is important to share the incident with another supervisor because of possible legal ramifications later. More importantly, it is impossible to tell from the scenario how long the identification was incorrect and there could have been other procedures, treatments, or care plans that were performed with the patients incorrectly identified. Thus, someone else may be able to trace all possible errors associated with the mix-up and remedy the situation before any harsh outcomes for either of the patients has occurred. Marty should make sure the corrections have been made and then continue with her careful evaluation of the patient and venipuncture procedure.

3. There are several ethical issues associated with this case. The first involves the relationship between the two employees. It appears that Ms. Daley was using her friendship with Marty to cover up her own mistake and not report it. These actions were unethical. Secondly, Marty had to make a decision about whether or not to report Ms. Daley's mistake to another supervisor or third party, thereby directly violating Ms. Daley's request. The ethical and professional decision would be for Marty to report it to another supervisor and document the incident, even though she would jeopardize her friendship.

4. There are many legal, ethical, and most importantly, clinical consequences that can be extremely damaging to both of the patients, both employees, and the health care organization itself. The clinical consequences of misidentifying a patient can result in severe injury, including death. Legal consequences might include malpractice, negligence, and large financial penalties to all parties involved. Ethical consequences involve violations of institutional policy, negative feelings toward both employees and their families, and negative afterthoughts for many years.

Glossary

ABO Blood Group System a method by which red blood cell antigens are classified (e.g., individual's blood cells with type A antigens have type A blood); those with B antigens have type B blood, etc.

Acid-Citrate-Dextrose (ACD) an additive commonly used in specimen collection for blood donations to prevent clotting. It ensures that the RBCs maintain their oxygen-carrying capacity.

Acidosis a pathologic condition existing when the blood pH decreases to less than 7.35.

Active Listening a set of skills that enables one to become a more effective listener. The skills include concentrating on the speaker, getting ready to listen by clearing one's mind of distracting thoughts, use of silent pauses when appropriate, providing reassuring feedback, verifying the conversation that took place, keeping personal judgments to oneself, paying attention to body language of the person speaking, and maintaining eye contact.

Acute Care health care delivered in a hospital setting that is usually associated with a hospital stay of less than 30 days.

Administrative Law a type of law that is initiated by the executive branch of government. Federal agencies write regulations that enforce laws created through the legislative body.

Adrenals glands that produce hormones as a result of emotional changes like fright or anger. Hormone production causes an increase in blood pressure, widened pupils, and heart stimulation.

Adulteration means of tampering with a specimen, usually urine, to make the specimen test negatively for drugs. Water is the most common substance added to the specimen or ingested to dilute the urine so that drug concentrations are below the detection limit.

Age-Specific Care Considerations providing services that are age appropriate and considerate (e.g., special considerations are needed for different ages of children (toddler vs. teen) and also for geriatric patients). Factors typically relate to age-related fears/concerns, communication styles, procedures for comforting the patient, and safety.

Alkalosis a pathologic condition that results when the blood pH increases to more than 7.45. In serious cases, it can lead to coma.

Allen Test a procedure used prior to drawing specimens (for ABGs) from the radial artery. It assures that the ulnar and radial arteries are providing collateral circulation to the hand area. Basically, it entails compressing the arteries to the hand and emptying the hand of arterial blood, then releasing the compression to see if the circulation is immediately restored. A negative test would indicate that collateral circulation is not sufficient and an alternative artery (brachial or femoral) should be used for ABG collections.

Alveolar Sacs grape-like structures in the lungs that allow for diffusion between air and blood.

Ambulatory Care health care services that are delivered in an out-patient, or non-hospital, setting. It implies that the patients are able to ambulate, or walk, to the clinic to receive their services.

American Hospital Association (AHA)   nonprofit group or alliance of member hospitals and health care organizations that promote the interests of hospitals. Annual state and national conferences are held each year to discuss important legislation, financial considerations, regulations, and accreditation issues that affect hospitals. AHA is an advocacy group for health care organizations, particularly hospitals.

American Nurses Association (ANA)   professional organization for nurses.

American Society for Clinical Laboratory Scientists (ASCLS)   professional organization for laboratory personnel that provides continuing education, conference activities, and certification examinations for specified groups.

American Society of Clinical Pathologists (ASCP)   professional organization that certifies many types of laboratory personnel based on passing a certification examination. ASCP offers clinical and research conferences, many types of continuing education activities, and ongoing certification programs.

Amniotic Fluid   fluid from the amniotic sac (i.e., the membranes that hold a developing embryo and fetus).

Anabolism   a body function whereby cells use energy to make complex compounds from simpler ones. It allows the synthesis of body fluids (e.g., sweat, tears, saliva, etc.).

Analytic Phase   refers to the phase in laboratory testing whereby the specimen is actually assessed or evaluated, and results are confirmed and reported.

Anatomic Pathology   major area of laboratory services whereby autopsies are performed, and cytology procedures and surgical biopsy tissues are analyzed.

Anatomy   study of the structural components of the body.

Anterior   surface region of the body characterized by the front (or ventral) area and including the thoracic, abdominal, and pelvic cavities.

Anticoagulant(s)   substance introduced into the blood or a blood specimen to keep it from clotting.

Antiseptics   chemicals used to clean human skin by inhibiting the growth of microorganisms (e.g., 70 percent isopropyl alcohol, iodine).

Aorta   the largest artery in the body.

Arterial Blood Gases (ABGs)   analytical test that measures oxygen and carbon dioxide in the blood. Provides useful information about respiratory status and the acid-base balance of patients with pulmonary disorders.

Arteries   highly oxygenated blood vessels that carry blood away from the heart.

Arterioles   smaller branches of arteries.

Assault   a legal term referring to the unjustifiable attempt to touch another person or the threat to do so in circumstances that cause the other person to believe that it will be carried out, or to cause fear. An assault may be permissible if proper consent has been given (e.g., consent to obtain a blood specimen).

Assessments   used as a quality improvement measurement term to refer to both the analytic (quantitative) and non-analytic (qualitative) components of health care. In the clinical laboratory, assessments are used to ensure test sensitivity, specificity, precision and accuracy, and/or effective communication styles, timeliness, etc.

Atria   two of the four chambers of the heart.

Autologous Transfusion   a patient donates his or her own blood or blood components for use later; this is the safest type of transfusion (i.e., using one's own blood). It prevents transfusion-transmitted infectious diseases and eliminates the formation of antibodies from other donors.

Bacteremia   presence of bacteria in the blood; an infection of the blood.

Bar Codes   series of light and dark bands of varying widths that relate to alphanumeric symbols. They can correspond to the patient's name and/or identification numbers.

Basal State   for phlebotomy procedures, this refers to the patient's condition in the early morning, approximately 12 hours after the last ingestion of food. In hospitals, most laboratory tests are analyzed on basal state specimens.

Basilic Vein   vessel of the forearm that is acceptable for venipuncture.

Battery   a complex legal term referring to the intentional touching of another person without consent and/or beating or carrying out threatened physical harm. "Battery" always includes an assault, and is therefore commonly used with the term "assault and battery."

Bioethics   moral issues, dilemmas, or problems that are the result of modern medical practices, health care services, clinical research, and/or technology (i.e., often the bioethical issues involve "life-and-death" situations). *Bio* refers to "life" and *ethics* refers to a branch of philosophy dealing with the distinction between right and wrong.

Bleeding-Time Test   test useful for assessing platelet plug formation in the capillaries. It is generally done along with other coagulation tests and often used as a preoperative (presurgical) screening test. Basically it utilizes an automated, sterile incision-making instrument to puncture the skin and then the blood clotting process is timed. Phlebotomists must be specially trained to perform this procedure accurately.

Blood   circulating fluid and cells in the cardiovascular system.

Blood Cultures   tests that aid in identifying the specific bacterial organism causing infections in the blood. In the case of a patient that is experiencing fever spikes, it is recommended that the blood culture specimens be collected before and after the fever spike, when bacteria are most likely present in the peripheral circulation. Care must be taken by the phlebotomist not to contaminate the specimen, so special preparation of the collection site is required.

Blood-Drawing Chair   chair specifically designed to hold a patient comfortably and safely in a proper position during and after a blood collection procedure. The design typically includes a moveable armrest on both sides of the chair.

Blood Gas Analysis   refer to "arterial blood gas."

Blood Pressure   assessment of the functioning of the cardiovascular system using an instrument called a sphygmomanometer or blood pressure cuff. It is measured as systolic pressure, when the heart receives blood, and diastolic pressure, when the heart's ventricles relax.

Blood Urea Nitrogen (BUN)   analytic testing procedure to determine the amount of urea in the blood.

Blood Vessels   key component of the circulatory system, these vessels transport blood throughout the body.

Blood Volume   the total amount of blood in an individual's body. This is particularly important in pediatric phlebotomies because withdrawing blood can cause a significant decrease in the total blood volume of a small infant, thus resulting in anemia. Blood volume is based on weight and can be calculated for any size person.

Body Planes   imaginary dividing lines of the body that serve as reference points for describing distance from or proximity to the body. Body planes include the sagittal, frontal, transverse, and medial planes.

Brachial Artery   an artery located in the cubital fossa of the arm and used as an alternative site for ABG collections. Phlebotomists must be specially trained to perform collections from this site.

Breach of Duty   a legal term referring to an infraction, violation, or failure to perform.

Buffy Coat   in blood specimens that contain anticoagulants, the WBCs and platelets form a thin white layer above the RBCs called the buffy coat.

Butterfly System   also called a winged-infusion or scalp needle set, the system can be used for difficult venipunctures due to small or fragile veins. The needle is typically smaller, and has a thin tubing with a luer adapter at the end so that it can be used on a syringe or an evacuated tube system during venipuncture.

Calcaneus   heel bone.

Cannula   a tube that can be inserted into a cavity or blood vessel and used as a channel for transporting fluids. The term is most commonly used in dialysis for patients with kidney disease. The cannula is used to gain access to venous blood for dialysis or for blood collections. Specialized training and experience are required to draw blood from a cannula.

Capillaries   microscopic blood vessels that carry blood and link arterioles to venules.

Capillary Action   a term used when referring to microcollection procedures that indicates the free flowing movement of blood into the capillary tube without the use of suction.

Capillary Blood Gas Analysis   using microcollection methods on infants (usually the heel site) to collect specimens for blood gas analyses; these analytical tests measure oxygen and carbon dioxide in the blood. Provides useful information about respiratory status and the acid-base balance of patients with pulmonary disorders.

Capillary Tubes   disposable narrow-bore pipettes that are used for pediatric blood collections and/or microhematocrit measures. The tubes may be coated with anticoagulant such as heparin and for safety reasons are usually made of plastic.

Cardiac (Striated Involuntary) Muscles   muscles that make up the wall of the heart.

Cardiopulmonary Resuscitation (CPR)   the method used to revive the heart and/or breathing of a patient whose heart or respiration has stopped. It is advisable for health care workers to be appropriately trained in the use of CPR.

Cardiovascular System   body system that provides for rapid transport of water, nutrients, electrolytes, hormones, enzymes, antibodies, cells, and gases to all cells of the body.

Cartilage   substance similar to bone except that cells are surrounded by a gelatinous material that allows for flexibility.

Catabolism   chemical reactions in the body that break down complex substances into simpler ones while simultaneously releasing energy. The process provides energy for all body functions.

Cause-and-Effect Diagrams (Ishikawa)   a quality improvement tool that uses diagrams to identify interactions between equipment, methods, people, supplies, and reagents.

Centers for Disease Control and Prevention (CDC)   federal agency responsible for monitoring morbidity (disease) and mortality (death) throughout the country.

Central Intravenous Line   a commonly used VAD. Refer to "vascular access device."

Centriole   a cellular structure that plays a role in cellular division.

Cephalic Vein   vein of the forearm that is acceptable for venipuncture.

Cerebrospinal Fluid (CSF)   fluid that surrounds the brain and meninges within the spinal column.

Chain-of-Custody   process for maintaining control and accountability of a specimen from the point of collection to its final disposition. The process documents the identity of each individual that handles the specimen and each time a specimen is transferred.

Chain of Infection   the process by which infections are transmitted; components include the source of the infection (non-sterile items, contaminated equipment/supplies, etc.), the mode of transmission (direct contact, airborne, medical instruments, etc.), and the susceptible host (patient).

Circulatory System   body system referring to the heart, blood vessels, and blood; responsible for transporting oxygen and nutrients to cells and transports carbon dioxide and wastes until they are eliminated, transports hormones, regulates body temperature, and helps defend against diseases.

Citrate-Phosphate-Dextrose (CPD)   anticoagulant typically used for blood donations.

Citrates   type of anticoagulant additive for blood collection tubes; prevents the blood clotting sequence by removing calcium and forming calcium salts.

Civil Law   different from criminal law; in civil law, the plaintiff sues for monetary damages.

Clean-Catch Midstream   a urine specimen that is used for detecting bacteria and/or for microscopic analysis. Normally, the specimen should be free of contamination because the patient should be instructed to clean and decontaminate themselves prior to urination. The urine specimen should actually be collected in a sterile container. Urine should be voided and the specimen should be collected during the mid portion of urination.

Clinical Laboratory Improvement Amendments (CLIA)   federal guidelines that regulate all clinical laboratories across the United States. Regulations apply to any site that tests human specimens, including small POL's, or screening tests done at the patient's bedside.

Clinical Pathology   major area of laboratory services where blood and other types of body fluids and tissues are analyzed.

Coagulation   a phase in the blood clotting sequence in which many factors are released and interact to form a fibrin meshwork or blood clot.

Competency Statement   performance expectations that include entry-level skills, tasks, and roles performed by the designated health care worker.

Confidentiality   the protected right and duty of health care workers not to disclose any information acquired about a patient to those who are not directly involved with the care of the patient.

Continuous Quality Improvement (CQI)   a theoretical framework and management strategy to improve health care structures, processes, outcomes, and customer satisfaction. It is ongoing and involves all levels of the administrative structure of an organization.

Creatinine Clearance Test   analytic procedure to determine whether or not the kidneys are able to remove creatinine from the blood.

Criminal Actions   legal recourse for acts against the public welfare; these actions can lead to imprisonment of the offender.

Critical Value   a laboratory result that indicates a pathophysiologic state at such variance with normal as to be life-threatening; these values should be defined and reported to the patient's physician as soon as possible.

Cross–Match Testing   laboratory analyses that involves exposure of a donor's blood to a patient's blood to see if they are compatible or incompatible.

Culture   a system of values (individualism, importance of education and financial security), beliefs (spiritual, family bonding), and practices (food, music, traditions) that stem from one's concept of reality. Culture influences decisions and behaviors in many aspects of life.

Culture and Sensitivity (C&S)   microbiologic test to determine the growth of infectious microorganisms in bodily specimens (e.g., urine), and to determine which antibiotics are most effective on the microorganism.

Custody and Control Form (CCF)   part of the "chain-of-custody" process that requires specific documentation related to donor identification procedures, specimen collection steps, security for the collector, the donor, and the specimen, and tampering with the specimen.

Cyanotic   bluish in color due to oxygen deficiency.

Cytoplasm   contained within a cellular membrane, it contains mostly water with dissolved nutrients and contains other structures or organelles of the cell.

Decontaminated   prior to venipuncture, cleaning with a sterile swab or sponge to prevent microbiological contamination of either the patient or the specimen. This is usually accomplished with a sterile swab containing 70 percent isopropyl alcohol (or isopropanol).

Defendant   individual (e.g., a health care worker), against whom a legal action (civil or criminal) or lawsuit is filed.

Deoxyribonucleic Acid (DNA)   molecule containing thousands of genes that make up an individual's genetic code. Often referred to as a *double-helix,* DNA is inherited from parents and carries the code for an individual's characteristics such as eye or hair color, height, etc.

Department of Health and Human Services (HHS)   federal agency involved in many aspects of health delivery, regulation, and monitoring. One responsibility is the establishment of scientific and technical guidelines for federal drug testing programs and standards for certification of laboratories engaged in urine drug testing for federal agencies.

Department of Transportation (DOT)   federal agency responsible for the transportation industry in the United States. They develop drug testing guidelines for specified types of transportation personnel and standards for testing specified categories of drugs.

Deposition   a legal term referring to the testimony of a witness that is recorded in a written legal format.

Diabetes Mellitus   metabolic disease in which carbohydrate utilization is reduced due to a deficiency in insulin and characterized by hyperglycemia, glycosuria, water and electrolyte loss, ketoacidosis, and in serious conditions, coma. In milder forms of non-insulin dependent diabetes mellitus, dietary regulation may keep the disorder under control.

Diastolic Pressure   the second measure reported in a blood pressure measurement.

Differentials   a laboratory test that categorizes blood cells and any abnormalities present.

Digestive System   body system referring to organs in the gastrointestinal (GI) tract that break down food chemically and physically into nutrients that can be absorbed by the body's cells and allow the elimination of waste products of digestion.

Discovery   a legal term referring to the right to examine the witness(es) before a trial; it consists of oral testimony under oath and includes cross-examination by lawyers.

Disinfectants   chemical compounds used to remove or kill pathogenic microorganisms; typically used on medical instruments or countertops.

Disposable Sterile Lancet   sterile sharp device, preferably retractable, used in skin puncture collections to penetrate the skin at specified depths (e.g., no more than 2.0 mm for infant heelsticks).

Diurnal Rhythms   opposite of nocturnal (nighttime), "diurnal" rhythms are variations in the body's functions or fluids that occur during daylight hours or every 24 hours (e.g., some hormone levels decrease in the afternoon). Also referred to as circadian rhythms.

Dorsal   surface region of the body characterized by the back (or posterior) area and including the cranial and spinal cavities.

Double Bagging   practice of using two trash bags for disposing of waste from patient's rooms, particularly those in isolation.

E-mail   electronic mail often used in health care facilities. Guidelines for using e-mail, including a patient's consent to use e-mail, are now required of health care facilities.

Endocrine Glands   ductless glands that release their secretions (hormones) directly into the bloodstream.

Endoplasmic Reticulum   cell structure that acts as a transport channel between the cell membrane and the nuclear membrane.

Environmental Protection Agency (EPA)   federal agency that, among other responsibilities, regulates the disposal of hazardous substances, and monitors and regulates disinfectant products.

Erythropoiesis   production of erythrocytes or red blood cells.

Erythropoietin (EPO)   hormone produced in the kidney that initiates the production of red blood cells.

Ethics   a branch of philosophy that deals with distinguishing right from wrong and with moral consequences of human actions.

Ethylenediamine Tetra-acetic Acid (EDTA)   anticoagulant additive used to prevent the blood clotting sequence by removing calcium and forming calcium salts. EDTA prevents platelet aggregation and is useful for platelet counts and platelet function tests. Fresh EDTA samples are also useful for making blood films or microscopic slides because there is minimal distortion of platelets and WBCs.

Eutectic Mixture of Local Anesthetics (EMLA)   a topical anesthetic (pain reliever) that is an emulsion of lidocaine and prilocaine and can be applied to intact skin.

Evacuated Tube System   method of blood collection using double-sided needles whereby the needle is attached to a holder/adapter and allows for multiple specimen tube fills and changes without blood leakage.

Evidence   a legal term referring to materials (e.g., tubes, needles, safety devices, waste containers, log books, lab reports, etc.), submitted during a legal case to prove or disprove a lawsuit.

Exocrine Glands   glands that secrete fluids through channels or ducts (e.g., sweat, saliva, mucus, digestive juices).

Expert Witness   a legal term referring to a witness who is specially qualified or has expertise in certain areas pertaining to the case.

Exposure Control Plan   a required document in health facilities that details the process for medical treatment, prophylaxis, and/or follow-up after an employee has been exposed to potentially harmful or infectious substances (e.g., in the case of a needlestick injury).

Extrinsic Factors   substances involved in the clotting process that are stimulated when tissue damage occurs.

False Imprisonment   a legal term referring to the unjustifiable detention of an individual without a legal warrant for his or her arrest.

Fasting Blood Tests   tests performed on blood taken from a patient who has abstained from eating and drinking (except water) for a particular period of time.

Fax Machines   facsimiles are often used to transmit health care information. Guidelines for their use and confidentiality of patient information are required.

Feathered Edge   a term used to describe blood smears on microscopic slides; it is a visible curved edge that thins out smoothly and resembles the tip of a bird's feather.

Felony   a legal term referring to a public offense that may require a jail sentence.

Femoral Artery   located in the groin area of the leg and lateral to the femur bone, it is the largest artery used as an alternative site for ABG collections. Phlebotomists must be specially trained to perform collections from this site.

Fevers of Unknown Origin (FUO)   indicates the patient has an undiagnosed infection which usually results in ordering blood cultures.

Fibrin   substance that forms a blood clot.

Fibrinolysis   the final phase of the hemostatic process whereby repair and regeneration of the injured blood vessel occurs and the clot slowly begins to dissolve or break up (lysis).

Fistula   an artificial shunt or passage, commonly used in the arm of a patient undergoing kidney dialysis; the vein and artery are fused through a surgical procedure. Only specially trained personnel can collect blood from a fistula.

"5 Q" Framework   used as a quality improvement term to refer to The Westgard and associates model for quality. The "5 Qs" are quality planning, quality laboratory practices, quality control of processes, quality assessment to monitor performance, and quality improvement when problems occur.

Flowcharts   a quality improvement tool used to break a process into its component parts so that people can understand how it works.

Fomites   inanimate objects that can harbor infectious agents and transmit infections (e.g., toilets, sinks, linens, door knobs, glasses, phlebotomy supplies, etc.).

Food and Drug Administration (FDA)   federal agency responsible for safety, clinical efficacy, and medical efficacy of the country's food and drug supply. This includes equipment and supplies used in blood collection.

Forensic Specimens   specimens that are involved in civil or criminal legal cases, including specimens for analysis of drugs of abuse.

Frontal Plane   imaginary line running lengthwise on the body from side to side, dividing the body into anterior and posterior sections.

Gastric Analysis   gastric fluid analysis to determine gastric function. Involves passing a tube through the patient's nose and into the stomach. It requires specialized training.

"Gateway Drugs"   drugs such as tobacco and alcohol.

Gauge Number   refers to the size (diameter) of the internal bore of a needle. The larger the number, the smaller the bore size and vice versa.

Genes   located on a chromosome, it is a unit of heredity capable of reproducing itself exactly during cell division; it is made of segments of DNA.

Glucose Tolerance Test   diagnostic test for detecting diabetes. The test is performed by obtaining blood and urine specimens at timed intervals after fasting, then after ingesting glucose. Each specimen is analyzed for its glucose content to determine if the glucose level returns to normal within 2 hours after ingestion. Diabetic patients' glucose is metabolized differently and may need to be analyzed up to 4 or 5 hours after ingestion. Special instructions are needed for the patient and special training for the phlebotomist should occur if they will be collecting such specimens.

Golgi Apparatus   cell structure that stores proteins.

Granulocytes (Basophils, Neutrophils, Eosinophils)   mature leukocytes (WBCs) in the circulating blood; when stained and viewed microscopically, granules are present.

Health Care Financing Administration (HCFA)   federal agency responsible for oversight of health care financing and regulation in the health care industry. Among other responsibilities, HCFA develops, administers, and regulates the CLIA Amendments.

Health Insurance Portability and Accountability Act (HIPAA)   federal law (1996) expanded in 2000 to protect security and confidentiality of electronic health information, including e-mail and faxes.

Heart   a key component of the cardiovascular system, it is the pump that forces blood throughout the body.

Heel Stick   pediatric phlebotomy procedure that requires puncturing specified areas of an infant's heel.

Hematocrit   a commonly ordered laboratory test to assess the circulatory system; it describes the concentration of RBCs and therefore provides an indirect measure of the oxygen-carrying capacity of the blood.

Hematoma   a localized leakage of blood into the tissues or into an organ. In phlebotomy, it can occur as a result of blood leakage during the vein puncture, thereby causing a bruise.

Hematopoiesis   the process of blood cell formation that occurs in the bone marrow.

Hemoconcentration   increased localized blood concentration of large molecules such as proteins, cells, and coagulation factors. This can be caused by excessive application of a tourniquet.

Hemoglobin   the molecules that carry oxygen and carbon dioxide in the RBCs.

Hemolysis   rupture or lysis of the blood cells.

Hemostasis   maintenance of circulating blood in the liquid state and retention of blood in the vascular system by prevention of blood loss.

Heparin   an anticoagulant that prevents blood clotting by inactivating thrombin and thromboplastin, the blood clotting chemicals in the body.

Heparin or Saline Lock   part of a vascular access device, a heparin or saline lock is put in place to be used for medication administration or blood collection. It must be "flushed" routinely to prevent clot formation in the line. If a heparin lock is used, blood from this site should not be used for coagulation studies due to possible contamination of the specimen with residual heparin.

Histograms   bar graphs often used as quality improvement tools.

Holder (Adapter)   plastic apparatus needed in specimen collections using the evacuated tube method. The adapter/holder secures the double-pointed needle: one end of the needle goes in the patient's vein, and the other end of the needle is placed an evacuated tube.

Hollander Test   involves gastric fluid to determine gastric function in terms of stomach acid production. It uses insulin to stimulate gastric secretions. Special training is required prior to assisting with this procedure.

Home Health Care Services   provision of health care services in a patient's home under the direction of a physician.

Homeostasis   literally means *remaining the same;* also referred to as a *steady state condition,* it is a normal state that allows the body to stay in a healthy balance by continually compensating with necessary changes.

Hormones   body substances secreted from glands that play a role in growth and development, fluid and electrolyte balance, energy balance, and acid-base balance.

Human Immunodeficiency Virus (HIV)   a virus spread by sexual contact or exposure to infected blood.

Hyperventilation   a condition whereby chemoreceptors in the brain cause a faster and deeper rate of respiration in order to blow off excess carbon dioxide.

Hypobilirubinemia   abnormally low levels of bilirubin in the blood.

Hypothyroidism   when referring to infantile hypothyroidism, it is a disorder that may be congenital and results in defective development of an embryo.

Hypoxia   a condition in which body tissues are not receiving enough oxygen.

Illicit Drugs   illegal drugs including opiates, cocaine, amphetamines, etc.

Implanted Port   type of vascular access device (VAD) surgically implanted beneath the skin; it is a small chamber attached to an indwelling line. Access to these ports must be by specially trained personnel and specially designed noncoring needles.

Implied Consent   a complex legal term that varies from state to state in its interpretation. Basically it entails conditions when immediate action is required to save a patient's life or to prevent impairment of a patient's health (i.e., medical emergency care operates with the notion of implied consent in many cases).

Infection Control Programs   guidelines designed to address surveillance, reporting, isolation procedures, education, and management of community acquired and health care associated infections.

Inferior Vena Cava   one of the two large veins that brings oxygen-poor blood to the heart from the lower trunk of the body (e.g., legs).

Informed Consent   a complex legal term; basically, it refers to voluntary permission by a patient to allow touching, examination, and/or treatment by health care workers after they have been given information about the procedures and potential risks and consequences. It allows patients to decide what may be performed on or to their bodies.

Inpatients   hospitalized patients.

Insulin   a chemical produced by the pancreas that is released into the bloodstream to facilitate glucose absorption from the blood into the tissues where it is used for energy. When insulin is not produced (as in diabetes mellitus), blood glucose levels increase because it cannot be absorbed into the tissues.

Integumentary System   body system referring to skin, hair, sweat and oil glands, teeth, and fingernails; involved in protective and regulatory functions.

Intravenous (IV) Catheter   vascular access device inserted into a blood vessel for administration of medications, nutrients, and blood collection.

Intrinsic System   part of the coagulation process that involves the clotting factors contained in the blood.

Invasion of Privacy   a legal term referring to objectionable or personal intrusion upon an individual such that it is offensive (e.g., the publishing of confidential information).

Isolation Procedures   methods used to protect individuals (health care workers) from patients with infectious diseases. Formally divided into two types (category-specific and disease-specific), newer guidelines combine isolation practices for moist and potentially infectious body substances to be used for all patients. The new categories of isolation are based on the mode of transmission and include airborne, droplet, and contact precautions.

JCAHO 10-step Process   strategy for quality assessment of health care performance.

Judicial Law   legal processes designed to resolve disputes.

Lactose Tolerance Test   a test to determine lactose intolerance. Some individuals have difficulty digesting lactose, a milk sugar. This test is similar to the glucose tolerance test (which is usually performed one day before) and requires timed testing for lactose after fasting, then after ingestion of lactose at 1, 2, and 3-hour intervals.

Lateral   directional term meaning toward the sides of the body.

Latex Allergy   reaction to certain proteins in latex rubber, a natural ingredient in some varieties of gloves. Allergic reactions range from skin redness, rash, hives, or itching to respiratory symptoms and, in rare instances, shock.

Law societal rules or regulations designed to protect society and resolve conflicts; laws are rules that must be observed.

Liable a legal term that refers to a legal obligation when damages are concerned.

Light Sensitive refers to laboratory specimens; some chemical constituents (bilirubin, vitamin B_{12}, carotene, and folate, urine porphyrins) decompose if exposed to light and therefore should be protected/covered during transportation and handling.

Lipemic when referring to serum, it is a cloudy or milky appearance, usually due to a temporarily elevated lipid level after the ingestion of fatty foods.

Lithium Iodoacetate antiglycolytic agent and anticoagulant; *not* to be used for hematology testing or enzymatic determinations.

Litigation Process a legal action to determine a decision in court. Many malpractice cases are negotiated and settled out of court.

Long-term Care health care services that are provided for more than 30 days. Usually it is related to chronic conditions (i.e., rehabilitation or services for the elderly in nursing homes).

Lymphatic System body system responsible for maintaining fluid balance, providing a defense against disease, and absorption of fats and other substances from the blood stream.

Lymphocytes type of white blood cell that is non-granular in appearance; plays a role in immunity and in the production of antibodies.

Lymphostasis obstruction and/or lack of flow of the lymph fluid.

Lysosomes cell structures that release digestive enzymes into vacuoles, or small pouches, for digestion of food particles.

Malice a legal term referring to a reckless disregard for the truth (e.g., knowing that a statement is false).

Malpractice a legal term referring to improper or unskillful care of a patient by a member of the health care team or any professional misconduct, unreasonable lack of skill, or infidelity in professional or judiciary duties; often described as "professional negligence."

Mastectomy removal of a breast.

Material Safety Data Sheets (MSDSs) required information about any chemical used in the workplace; MSDS generally lists information about the chemical, precautionary measures, and emergency information about accidental exposures to the chemical.

Meconium the first intestinal discharges of the newborn infant, greenish in color; consists of epithelial cells, mucus, and bile.

Medial directional term meaning toward the midline of the body.

Median Cubital Vein forearm vein that is most commonly used for venipuncture.

Medicaid federal program designed to provide health insurance for the elderly and members of special groups.

Medical Records definitive documents (paper or electronic) that contain a chronological log of a patient's care. It must include any information that is clinically significant or relevant to the patient's care.

Medicare a shared federal and state funded program designed to provide health insurance for the poor.

Megakaryocytes large cells located in the bone off of which platelets are formed.

Melanin pigment in the skin that provides color and protects underlying tissues from absorbing ultraviolet rays.

Memorandum for Record (MFR)   a document used to officially add information, correct omissions of information, or clarify incorrect notations in specimen collection procedures for drug testing purposes.

Meninges   protective membranes that cover the brain and spinal cord.

Metabolic Acidosis   a pathologic condition that occurs when the kidneys cannot eliminate acidic substances (i.e., diabetes mellitus). It can result in kidney (renal) failure and death.

Metabolic Alkalosis   a pathologic condition that results from excessive vomiting or an abnormal secretion of certain hormones that cause excess elimination of hydrogen ions (from CO_2).

Metabolism   an important bodily function that allows the formation or breakdown of substances (e.g., proteins) for the purpose of using energy.

Microcontainers   specialized collection devices designed for small quantities of blood; some containing anticoagulants. These devices are typically used for pediatric, geriatric patients with fragile or inaccessible veins, and/or fingersticks.

Misdemeanor   a legal term referring to many types of criminal offenses that are not serious enough to be classified as felonies.

Mitochondria   cell structure that produces energy for the cell.

Mode of Transmission   refers to the method by which pathogenic agents are transmitted (e.g., direct contact, air, medical instruments, other objects, and other vectors).

Monocytes   type of white blood cells that is non-granular and also plays a role in defense.

Multiple-Sample Needles   used with the evacuated tube method of blood collection, these needles are attached to a holder/adapter and allow for multiple specimen tube fills and changes without blood leakage.

Muscular System   body system referring to all muscles of the body.

National Committee for Clinical Laboratory Standards (NCCLS)   nonprofit organization that recommends quality standards and guidelines for clinical laboratory procedures.

National Phlebotomy Association (NPA)   professional organization for phlebotomists that offers continuing educational activities and a certification examination for phlebotomists.

Negligence   a legal term referring to the failure to act or perform duties according to the standards of the profession.

Neonatal Screening   typically refers to mandatory (required by law) laboratory testing of infants for specified disorders such as PKU and hypothroidism. There is wide variability in what tests are required by each state.

Neonates   a newborn infant; term used during the first 28 days after birth.

Nervous System   body system referring to organs that provide communication in the body, sensations, thoughts, emotions, and memories.

Neurons   specialized nerve cells that transmit nerve impulses.

Nosocomial Infections   infections acquired after admission into a health facility.

Nucleolus   cell structure located inside the nucleus, aids in cellular metabolism and cellular reproduction.

Nucleus   cell structure that is the control center; it governs the functions of each individual cell (e.g., growth, repair, reproduction, and metabolism).

Occluded Veins   closed or constricted veins.

Occult Blood   analysis that detects hidden (occult) blood in the stool.

Occupational Safety and Health Administration (OSHA)   an agency of the U.S. Department of Labor, requiring employers to provide a safe work environment, including measures to protect workers exposed to biological and occupational hazards. OSHA is also responsible for responding to complaints, monitoring employer practices, and imposing sanctions (fines or closure) on employers who are non-compliant.

Osteochondritis   inflammation of the bone and its cartilage.

Osteomyelitis   inflammation of the bone due to bacterial infection.

Outcomes   used as a quality improvement term to refer to what is accomplished for the patient (i.e., healing, return to wellness, or return to normal functions). Poor patient outcomes have been described as the "5 Ds: death, disease, disability, discomfort, dissatisfaction."

Ova and Parasites (O&P)   laboratory analysis performed on stool specimens that determines the presence of parasitic microorganisms or eggs of parasitic organisms.

Oxalates   anticoagulants that prevent blood clotting sequence by removing calcium and forming calcium salts.

"Panic Value"   also referred to as a "critical value." Refer to "critical value" for definition.

Parental Involvement   when referring to pediatric phlebotomy procedures, a parents' support and presence during the procedure is often helpful in reducing stress/anxiety for the patient. On the other hand, some parents are reluctant to be involved so the phlebotomist must assess each situation to determine the level of parental involvement that would optimize the phlebotomy encounter.

Pareto Charts   quality improvement tool incorporating bar charts that show the frequency of problematic events.

Parkinson's Disease   a neurological disease characterized by muscular tremors and rigidity of movement.

Pathogenic Agents   disease-causing bacteria, fungi, viruses, or parasites that are transmitted by direct contact, air, medical instruments, other objects, or vectors.

Pathology   the study of all aspects of disease and abnormal conditions of the body.

Patient Confidentiality   refer to "confidentiality."

Patient-Focused Testing   laboratory testing designed with the patient as a top priority; that it is usually performed at the patient's bedside with a rapid turn around time.

Patient's Bill of Rights   a statement originally developed in 1973 by the AHA to affirm the rights of patients. Key elements involve the right to respectful and considerate care; accurate information about diagnoses, treatment and prognoses; informed consent; refusal of treatment; privacy; confidentiality; advance directives; review records about own treatment; identity and role of personnel involved in care; information about research procedures; billing information; and business relationships of those providing care.

"Peak"   a term used for therapeutic drug monitoring to describe the blood sample that is taken when the drug is at its highest concentration in the patient's serum (e.g., the "peak" level).

Pediatric Phlebotomies   procedures performed on infants and children that require specialized training and management. Often done by skin puncture, pediatric phlebotomies also entail matching the procedure with the specimen requirements for testing, the patient's age and emotional condition, and possible parental involvement.

Pericardial Fluid   fluid from the heart cavity.

Peripherally Inserted Central Catheter (PICC)   type of vascular access device (VAD) inserted into the peripheral venous system with a lead into the central venous system. A PICC is usually placed in the arm in the basilic or cephalic vein. A PICC should not be used for blood collections because it may collapse during aspiration of the blood.

Peristalsis   part of the digestive process whereby food is moved in wavelike contractions through the intestines.

Peritoneal Fluid   fluid from the abdominal cavity.

Personal Protective Equipment (PPE)   equipment designed to protect the health care worker from hazards in the workplace (e.g., goggles, gloves, gowns, etc.).

Petechiae   minute, pinpoint hemorrhagic spots in the skin that may be indicative of a coagulation abnormality. For phlebotomists, it should be a warning sign that the patient may bleed excessively.

Phenylketonuria (PKU)   a congenital disorder, usually diagnosed at birth, that can cause brain damage resulting in severe retardation, often with seizures, and other neurologic abnormalities.

Phlebotomist   individual who practices phlebotomy (i.e., a blood collector); *phlebo* is related to the word "vein" and *tomy* relates to "cutting."

Physician's Office Laboratories (POLs)   non-hospital laboratories usually based in a physician's office/clinic at the private practice.

Physiology   study of the functional components of the body.

Pituitary Gland   also referred to as the *master gland*, stimulates other glands to produce hormones as needed. It controls and regulates hormone production through chemical feedback.

Plaintiff   a legal term referring to the person who initiates a lawsuit or legal action.

Plasma   liquid portion of the blood in which blood cells are suspended.

Platelets (Thrombocytes)   blood cells that aid in blood clot formation.

Pleural Fluid   fluid from the lung cavity.

Pneumatic Tube Systems   transportation system used in many health care facilities for specimens and paper-based documentation. Considerations for use of these systems involves evaluation of speed, distance, control mechanisms, shock absorbency, sizes of carriers, and breakage/spillage rates.

Point-of-Care   refers to tests and procedures that are actually performed at the patient's bedside or at the "point-of-care." The tests are not sent to a laboratory in a remote location; rather, they are rapid methods designed to produce quick results.

Posterior   surface region of the body characterized by the back (or dorsal) area and including the cranial and spinal cavities.

Postprandial Glucose Test   a glucose test performed after ingestion of a meal; useful for screening patients for diabetes because glucose levels in serum specimens drawn 2 hours after a meal are rarely elevated in normal patients. In contrast, diabetic patients have elevated glucose values 2 hours after a meal.

Preanalytical Phase   refers to the laboratory testing phases in which tests are ordered, and specimens are collected and prepared for testing. Preanalytical variables include patient variables (fasting vs. nonfasting, stress, availability, etc.), transportation variables (specimen leakage, tube breakage, excessive shaking, etc.), specimen processing variables (centrifugation, delays, contamination of the specimen, exposure to heat or light), and specimen variables (hemolysis, inadequate volume, inadequate mixing of the tube, etc.).

Premature Infant   an infant born before it is "full term," (i.e., 37 weeks or 8½ months after conception).

Preventive Law   a legal term referring to the use of education and planning to avoid legal conflicts.

Primary Care   health care services that are provided to maintain and monitor normal health and provide preventive services.

Privacy   the patient's right to respectful consideration of the confidential nature of his or her health information.

Process   used as a quality improvement term to refer to what is actually done to the patient in a health care encounter. Process assessments are common throughout the specimen collection process to see if proper procedures and standards were followed.

Proficiency Testing (PT)   testing that is part of the quality management of laboratory services and involves subscribing to an outside source to provide "unknown" or "blind" specimens to see how one laboratory's results compare with other laboratories' results. Performance reviews on proficiency tests are part of the accrediting process for most laboratories.

Protective (Reverse) Isolation   precautionary measures and procedures designed to protect patients who are particularly susceptible or at increased risk of acquiring infections (e.g., patients with low WBC counts (neutropenic or leukopenic), patients with burns, and/or immunosuppressed patients).

Pulmonary Circuit   when blood leaves the heart and enters the right and left pulmonary arteries, they carry *deoxygenated* blood.

Pulse Rate   rate used to assess normal functioning of the cardiovascular system; it is measured off of the pulse located in an artery. Normal pulse rate is about 75 beats per minute.

Quality Control Material   daily controls that are used in analytic testing to determine acceptable ranges of test results (i.e., tolerance limits).

Radial Artery   located on the thumb side of the wrist, this artery is most commonly used to collect blood specimens for arterial blood gases. Phlebotomists must be specially trained to perform collections from this site.

Random Urine Sample   urine sample taken at random time(s).

Red Blood Cells (RBCs or Erythrocytes)   blood cells that function to transport oxygen and carbon dioxide in the body.

Reference Ranges   when referring to laboratory values, these are laboratory test values that are considered within "normal" limits.

Reproductive System   body system referring to organs involved in sperm production, secretion of hormones (e.g., testosterone, estrogens, and progesterone), ovulation, fertilization, menstruation, pregnancy, labor, and lactation.

Requisition Form   paper-based method for requesting laboratory tests.

Respiratory Acidosis   a pathologic condition that results when the respiratory system is unable to eliminate adequate amounts of CO_2 (i.e., a collapsed lung or blocked respiratory passages).

Respiratory Alkalosis   a pathologic condition that results from hyperventilation or the loss of too much CO_2 from the lungs.

Respiratory System   body system referring to parts that assist in respiration or breathing (e.g., nose, pharynx, larynx, trachea, bronchi, and lungs).

Respondeat Superior   a legal term referring to the concept by which the actions of an individual are attributed to the supervisors or employers in control. In these cases, the supervisor may be liable for the negligent actions of their employee. It is also referred to as "vicarious liability."

Rh Factor   a method to categorize blood according to the presence or absence of the Rh antigen.

Ribosomes   cell structure that assembles amino acids into proteins.

Risk Management   management programs to reduce risks associated with health care delivery. Risk management programs reduce preventable injuries, accidents, and minimize financial loss to the organization.

RUMBA Model   a quality improvement model used to check for the feasibility of monitoring a particular procedure or process. "RUMBA" stands for relevant, understandable, measurable, behavioral, achievable.

Sagittal Plane   imaginary line running lengthwise on the body from front to back, dividing the body into right and left halves.

Sclerosed Veins   veins that have become hardened.

Secondary Care   specialized health care services usually provided by a physician who is an expert on a particular group of diseases, organ systems, or an organ (e.g., an ophthalmologist diagnoses and treats disorders of the eyes).

Septicemia   formally called "blood poisoning," the term now means the presence of toxins or multiplying bacteria in the blood.

Serum   when blood is allowed to clot, sera results plus blood cells meshed in a fibrin clot. Serum contains the same constituents as plasma except that the clotting factors are contained within the clot.

Sexually Transmitted Diseases (STDs)   pathogenic diseases that are transmitted via sexual contact (e.g., gonorrhea, genital herpes, syphilis, and human immunodeficiency virus).

Single-Sample Needle   used for collecting a blood sample from a syringe.

Single-Specimen Collection   term commonly used for urine drug testing to refer to a single-specimen requirement.

Skeletal (Striated Voluntary) Muscles   muscles that are attached to bones.

Skeletal System   body system referring to all bones and joints.

Skin Test   test that determines whether a patient has had contact with a particular antigen and therefore has produced antibodies to that antigen. A wide range of disease states stimulate antibody responses in individuals. Examples of skin tests include tuberculosis, fungal, ragweed, milk allergies, etc.

Sodium Fluoride   an additive (antiglycolytic agent) present in specific blood collection tubes that is used for glycolytic inhibition tests.

Sodium Polyanethole Sulfonate (SPS)   an additive typically used in blood culture bottles to prevent clotting.

Source   the origin of an infection (e.g., human hands, lab coats or other clothing, contaminated medical instruments, etc.).

Specimen Collection Manual   electronic or paper-based document required by accrediting agencies that includes instructions for patient preparation, type of collection containers, amounts of specimen required for specified tests, timing requirements, preservatives or anticoagulants needed, special handling instructions, proper labeling requirements, and other test-specific or situation-specific requirements for specimens.

Split-Specimen Collection   term commonly used for urine drug testing to refer to the specimen requirement for two specimens. The donor should not be allowed to "split" his or her own specimen; the specimen should be split by the "collector" using one original specimen and depending on the volume and integrity of the original specimen.

Sputum   fluid from the lungs that often contains pus.

Stakeholders   individuals, groups, organizations, and/or communities that have an interest in or are influenced by health care services. Stakeholders can be internal to the organization, or external (i.e., outside the organization).

Standard of Care   the practices or guidelines that a reasonably prudent person would follow in any particular circumstance. Many agencies, licensing boards, certifying boards, and accrediting organizations write standards of care or standards of practice to guide health care workers in their duties.

Standard Precautions   a set of safeguards designed to reduce the risk of transmission of microorganisms; guidelines apply to all patients and all body fluids, non-intact skin, and mucous membranes and include use of barrier protection (protective equipment such as gloves, gowns, etc.), hand washing, and proper use and disposal of needles and other sharps.

Stat   an emergency situation that requires immediate action; in the case of blood collection and analysis, tests that are ordered "stat" should be given the highest priority for collection, delivery to the laboratory, analysis, and reporting.

Statute of Limitations   a legal term referring to the time limit after an injury that a plaintiff must file a lawsuit or be forever barred from doing so. The statute of limitations for professional negligence in most states is 2 years.

Statutory Laws   statutes and ordinances that are legally binding but in certain instances may require the courts (judicial law) to step in.

Steady State   also referred to as *homeostasis,* it is a condition that allows the normal body to stay in balance by continually compensating with necessary changes, thereby remaining in a healthy condition.

Sterile Gauze Pads   typically used in blood collection procedures either during the decontamination process and/or after the blood collection to aid in stopping the bleeding; it is a sterile cotton mesh pad that is packaged in individual units.

Sterile Technique   use of procedures that produce an aseptic condition (i.e., free from all living microorganisms and their spores).

Structure   used as a quality improvement term to refer to the physical or organizational properties of the setting where health care is provided.

Sucrose Nipple or Pacifier   a sucking device for infants and toddlers that is used to pacify or comfort the child.

Superior Vena Cava   one of the two large veins that brings oxygen-poor blood to the heart from the head, neck, arms, and chest region.

Supine   reclining position.

Surveillance   monitoring and data collection on specific populations that are at risk for infections, have previously acquired infections, have been accidentally exposed to a communicable disease, contaminated equipment or hazardous reagents, and patients in specified areas of the facility.

Susceptible Host   a component in the "chain of infection;" the degree to which an individual is at risk for acquiring an infection. Factors affecting susceptibility are age, drug use, degree and nature of the patient's illness, and status of the patient's immune system.

Sweat Chloride Test   used in the diagnosis of cystic fibrosis.

Syncope   loss of consciousness caused by diminished blood flow to the brain (e.g., fainting).

Synovial Fluid   joint fluid.

Syringe Method   method of venipuncture whereby a syringe is used to collect blood that is then transferred to collection tubes.

Systemic Circuit   part of the cardiovascular system that carries blood to the tissues of the body.

Systolic Pressure   the first measure reported for a blood pressure measurement.

Tertiary Care   health care that is highly specialized and oriented toward unusual and complex diagnoses and therapies. Sophisticated instrumentation and technology or invasive procedures are used in an acute care facility.

Therapeutic Drug Monitoring (TDM)   testing procedures to evaluate drug levels in a patient's blood. This is valuable for drug dosage and to monitor the patient for a variety of other factors (clinical effectiveness, toxicity, etc.).

Therapeutic Phlebotomy   removal of blood for therapeutic reasons (i.e., in conditions where there is an excessive production of blood cells).

Thrombi   blood clot(s) formed somewhere within the cardiovascular system; it may occlude a vessel or attach to the wall of a vessel.

Tissue (Interstitial) Fluid   term describing the fluids found in between and around tissues that are not blood.

Tort   a legal wrong in which the person who commits it is liable for damages in civil, not criminal, court. The tort system is part of the judicial system concerned with resolving 2-party disputes over whether some harm has been committed to one party or his/her property.

Tourniquet   a soft rubber strip typically about 1 inch wide and 15 to 18 inches long used on the arm to help find a site for venipuncture. The ends are stretched around a patient's arm about 3 inches above the venipuncture area. The tightening of the tourniquet causes venous filling in the veins and enables better visualization and feel of the prominent veins in the area.

Toxicology   scientific study of poisons (including drugs), how they are detected, their actions in the human body and treatment of the conditions they produce.

Trace Evidence   evidence found at the scene of a crime or on a person involved in a crime (e.g., fingerprints, hairs, fibers, glass fragments, drugs, firearms, etc.).

Trace Metals   elements such as aluminum or lead that may be present in the blood. Specially prepared blood collection tubes are required during phlebotomy so they are free of metals that may cause interference with the testing process.

Transverse Plane   imaginary line running crosswise or horizontally on the body, dividing the body into upper and lower sections.

Troponin T   a protein released and detected after a myocardial infarction (MI); it is elevated only when heart damage has occurred; thus, it is valuable in the early diagnosis of MI and in monitoring the effectiveness of therapy after an MI.

"Trough"   a term used for therapeutic drug monitoring to describe the blood sample that is taken just prior to the next dose or when the drug is at a low concentration in the patient's serum (e.g., the "trough" level).

Turbid   cloudy or milky in appearance.

Universal Precautions   a term now replaced by "standard precautions," and sometimes referred to as "standard universal precautions." Refer to "standard precautions" for current definition.

Urinary System   body system referring to processes enabling the production and elimination of urine. Consists of kidneys, ureters, bladder, and urethra.

Vacuum (Evacuated) Tube   color-coded specimen-collection tube that contains a vacuum so as to aspirate blood when a needle enters a patient's vein. The tubes are part of a blood collection method that also requires a double-pointed needle and a special plastic holder (adapter). One end of the double-pointed needle enters the vein, the other pierces the top of the tube and the vacuum aspirates the blood into the tube. Tubes may contain anticoagulants.

Vascular Access Devices (VADs)   a variety of specially-designed devices to allow entrance into a vein or artery. One of the most commonly used VADs is a central venous catheter (CVC) which is usually inserted into the subclavian vein (in the chest area below the clavical), the jugular vein, or the superior vena cava.

Vasoconstriction   rapid constriction of the blood vessels to decrease blood flow to the area.

Veins   blood vessels that carry blood toward the heart after oxygen has been delivered to the tissues.

Venae Cavae   largest veins of the body.

Ventral   surface region of the body characterized by the front (or anterior) area and including the thoracic, abdominal, and pelvic cavities.

Ventricles   two of the four chambers of the heart.

Venules   minute veins that flow into larger veins.

Vicarious Liability   a legal term whereby actions of one individual may be imputed to another person having control (i.e., the actions of an employee may be blamed on the supervisor in charge). The term is synonymous with *"respondeat superior."*

Visceral (Nonstriated, Smooth, Involuntary) Muscles   muscles that line the walls of internal structures (e.g., veins and arteries).

Whistle-blowing   disclosure of a legal wrongdoing by an employee of the same organization (i.e., an illegal action is reported by an employee to appropriate authorities such as a governmental agency, accreditation agency, etc.). Employees who speak out to reveal illegal actions may fear reprisals that could jeopardize their safety or their job. Thus, numerous laws are in place to protect employees who report legitimate wrongdoings.

White Blood Cells (WBCs or Leukocytes)   blood cells that provide for defense against infectious agents.

Winged Infusion System   also called a butterfly set or scalp needle set, the system can be used for difficult venipunctures due to small or fragile veins. The needle is typically smaller, it has a thin tubing with a luer adapter at the end so that it can be used on a syringe or an evacuated tube system during venipuncture.

Zone of Comfort   area of space surrounding a person/patient that is considered "private or personal;" if a stranger (or phlebotomist) gets too close to the individual (i.e., beyond the zone of comfort), the person/patient may begin to feel uncomfortable.

Index